Veterinary Infection: Prevention and Control

Veterinary Infection: Prevention and Control

Editor: Ryan Jaxon

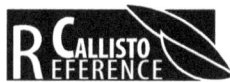

R CALLISTO REFERENCE

www.callistoreference.com

Callisto Reference,
118-35 Queens Blvd., Suite 400,
Forest Hills, NY 11375, USA

Visit us on the World Wide Web at:
www.callistoreference.com

ISBN: 978-1-64116-279-1 (Hardback)

Cataloging-in-Publication Data

Veterinary infection : prevention and control / edited by Ryan Jaxon.
    p. cm.
Includes bibliographical references and index.
ISBN 978-1-64116-279-1
1. Communicable diseases in animals. 2. Communicable diseases in animals--Prevention.
3. Veterinary medicine. 4. Animals--Diseases. I. Jaxon, Ryan.
SF781 .V48 2020
636.089 69--dc23

Table of Contents

Permissions

List of Contributors

Index

Preface

Infectious diseases of animals are a substantial hazard to animal health and welfare, with implications for agronomic health, food supply and economy. Changes in agricultural practices and global climate conditions are conducive to the spread of infectious diseases. Arthropod-borne diseases and zoonotic infections are on the rise. Zoonotic or phonetic infections pose not only a threat to animal health, but can adversely affect humans. Foot rot, anthrax, rabies, swine vesicular disease, glanders, etc. are veterinary infections. Certain diseases are specific to one type of stock, such as scrapie and classical swine fever, while others can affect all animals with a specific trait, such as foot and mouth disease which affects all cloven-hoofed animals. Infection prevention and control typically involves decreasing host exposure to pathogens, decreasing host susceptibility and increasing resistance to infectious pathogens. Immunization, proper feeding and nutrition, judicious use of antimicrobials and other drugs, management of underlying disease, adequate pain control, etc. are certain measures that can be adopted to prevent such infections. This book unravels the recent studies in the field of veterinary infections. Also included herein is a detailed explanation of the various strategies for the prevention and control of veterinary infectious diseases. The extensive content of this book provides the readers with a thorough understanding of the subject.

This book is the end result of constructive efforts and intensive research done by experts in this field. The aim of this book is to enlighten the readers with recent information in this area of research. The information provided in this profound book would serve as a valuable reference to students and researchers in this field.

At the end, I would like to thank all the authors for devoting their precious time and providing their valuable contribution to this book. I would also like to express my gratitude to my fellow colleagues who encouraged me throughout the process.

Editor

Sequencing and comparative analysis of flagellin genes *fli*A and *fli*B in bovine *Clostridium chauvoei* isolates

Jabbari, A.R.[1*], Azizian, Kh.[1], Esmaelizad, M.[2]

[1]*Department of Anaerobic Bacterial Vaccines Research and Production, Razi vaccine and Serum Research Institute, Agricultural Research Education and Extension Organization (AREEO), Karaj, Iran*

[2]*Department of Biotechnology, Razi Vaccine and Serum Research Institute, Agricultural Research Education and Extension Organization (AREEO), Karaj, Iran*

Key words:

Clostridium chauvoei, flagellin, polymorphism

Correspondence

Jabbari, A.R.
Department of Anaerobic Bacterial Vaccines Research and Production, Razi vaccine and Serum Research Institute, Karaj, Iran

Email: a.jabbari@rvsri.ac.ir

Abstract:

BACKGROUND: *Clostridium chauvoei* is the etiological agent of blackleg as an endogenous infection in cattle. Flagella have been known to play a critical role in the protective immunity of animals to clostridial infections. *C.chauvoei* has two copies of *fli*C gene, namely *fli*A and *fli*B. **OBJECTIVES:** The aim of this study was the determination and nucleotide sequence analysis of both copies of *fli*C genes in vaccinal strain and Iranian *C. chauvoei* isolates. **METHODS:** Six specific primers for amplification of *fli*A, *fli*B, and flagellin (*fli*C) genes were designed by Oligo software. Polymerase chain reaction was performed to amplify a fragment of 700 bp for both copies of flagellin (*fli*A and *fli*B) genes. The nucleotide percentage identity and divergence among isolates were deduced using BlAST and MegAlign softwares. **RESULTS:** It was found that divergence in *fli*B was more than *fli*A by sequence alignment analysis. Six highly conserve regions, thirty-one SNPs and 13 amino acid polymorphisms were found in *fli*C gene (between *fli*A and *fli*B sequences) of Iranian *C. chauvoei* isolates. In comparative analysis, genomic similarity of the *fli*A and *fli*B genes between the vaccinal strain and examined field isolates was proved to be as high as 97.3 % and 98.2%, respectively. **CONCLUSIONS:** The *fli*C copies were identified as excellent biomarkers to study the molecular epidemiology and strain diversity among *C. chauvoei* isolates. The existence of genetic variation between two alleles of *fli*C gene in *C. chauvoei* is reported for the first time in Iran. In spite of some genetic variations, the immunologic cross protection test showed a high protection power of the local vaccine (produced by Razi Institute) against homologous and heterologous challenge.

Introduction

Blackleg in cattle has been recognized in Iran since 1938 (Ardehali et al., 1984). The disease is distributed in most cultivated areas, especially in plain rice fields, low hills, and sandy spots. The disease is generally known to affect cattle, but sheep, goats, swine, camels, deer, and mink are also susceptible (Ardehali and Darakhshan, 1975). Blackleg is a fatal disease for young animals between 10 months and two years of age (Blood et al., 1983; Miyashiro et al., 2007; Uzal et al., 2003).

Clostridium chauvoei is a gram positive and spore forming anaerobic bacterium. *C. chauvoei* is the causative agent of blackleg with high mortality rate (Bagge et al., 2009). Death can occur due to septicemia (Kojima et al., 2001). Many Symptoms observed in blackleg are also created by *C. septicum*, *C. novyi*, and *C. perfirgens* (Kojima et al., 2001; Miyashiro et al., 2007). Distinguishing *C. chauvoei* from *C. septicum* based on physiologic and toxigenic characteristic is very difficult. Similarity, in 16s rRNA sequence between *C. chauvoei* and *C. septicum* is 99.3% that indicates similarity at phenotypic levels (Miyashiro et al., 2007).

Flagella are well controlled organelle and essential for microbial motility in many bacterial genera. While the genetics, regulation, assembly, and physical structure of the Gram negative bacterial flagellin has been extensively investigated, less is known about the flagella of Gram positive bacteria, and, in particular, clostridial flagella (Dauga et al., 1998; Ji et al., 2001). Different studies suggest that flagella are important factors in pathogenesis of bacteria (Attridge and Rowley, 1983; Morooka et al., 1985). Flagellin in *C. chauvoei* is important to induce protective immunity in host, but in contrast, in other clostridia, toxoid is very important for immunization (Tamura and Tanaka, 1984).

Flagellum is composed of four parts: (1) basal body consists of MS rings (*FliF*) and rod (Gram negative bacteria have L ring (FlgH) and P ring (FlgI) in addition to MS rings); (2) hook and associated hook-filament junction (FlgK and FlgL); (3) filament cap (*FliD*); and (4) Flagellar filament (*FliC*) which is composed from repeating the flagellin protein subunit, encoded by *fli*C gene (Macnab, 2004; Wilson and Miles, 1975). Comparison of the amino acid sequence of the flagella of many bacterial species has revealed a distinctive domain structure of the protein. The N- and C- terminal parts of the molecule, which are responsible for secretion and polymerization, are conserved among species, whereas the central regions, which produce the surface-exposed antigenic part of the flagellar filament, are highly variable (Reid et al., 1999).

The number of *fli*C gene copies in clostridia genera are different. The *C. chauvoei* has two copies of *fli*C gene in genomic DNA, which are named *fliA* and *fliB*. The *C. septicum* has three copies and *C. difficile* has only one copy of *fli*C gene (Sasaki et al., 2002). The particular structure of the flagellin gene with terminal conserved regions allow gene amplification and sequence analysis to study the variations in the central region.

The aim of this study was to identify molecular identification of two copies of *fli*C gene, *fliA* and *fliB*, in bovine *C. chauvoei* isolates.

Materials and Methods

Bacterial strains and culture: The *C. chauvoei* (Vaccine strain and three field isolates), which is used in this study, was collected from Anaerobic Bacterial Department of Razi Vaccine and Serum Research Institute of Iran (Table 1). All of the strains tested for biochemical identification fermented glucose, maltose, lactose, and sucrose. They did not ferment salicin, inulin, glycerol, and manitol.

PCR amplifications (DNA extraction): The bacterial isolates were cultured on Thio-glycolate consisted of liver broth, incubated at 37 °C for 48 hours in anaerobic condition. Bacterial cells were pelleted at 4000 rpm for 30 minutes and washed two times by sterile phosphate buffer saline. The pellets were re-suspended in 200 ul of HPLC-grade water. After boiling for 20 minutes and centrifugation, approximately 5 ul of supernatant was used as template for PCR assay.

Amplification of *fli*C gene: Two specific primers (CFC 5′-cat tgc tac agc agg taa ta<c> 3′ and CRC 5́-gaa cag cac cta act ttg at<c>3́) were designed to amplify a fragment of 1000 bp of *fli*C gene. This PCR was tested for differentiation of *C. chauvoei* from other pathogenic clostridia, including *C. septicum*, *C. tetani*, *C. novyi*, and *C. perfrigens*.

Amplification of *fli*C Gene Copies (*fliA* and *fliB*):

Two specific reverse primers for *fliA* (CRA, 5′-cca ctc tta act gtt aat act gca <t>-3') and *fliB* (CRB 5′-cca cct tta aca gtt aaa aca gca <c>-3′) were designed by Oligo software. The forward primer CFC was used commonly with both CRA and CRB reverse primers. Polymerase chain reactions were performed to amplify a fragment of 700 bp for both *fliA* and *fliB* genes.

PCR reactions were consisted of 1.5mM MgCl2; 0.5 unit Taq DNA Polymerase; 0.25 mM dNTPs; DNA template 100 ng/reaction; and 10 pmol of each primers in 50 µl total volume. The PCR program was run with initial denaturation at 95 °C for 5 min and 35 cycles of denaturation at 94 °C for 1 min; annealing temperature, 52 °C for 1 min; extension, 1 min at 72 °C; and a final extension at 72 °C for 10 min. Five microliters of the PCR products were separated by electrophoresis on a 1% agarose gel, stained with ethidium bromide (0.25 µg/ ml) and documented with a gel documentation system.

Nucleotide sequencing and analysis: PCR products were purified (purification kit, Roche, Cat No. 11732668001) and were sequenced in two directions (Macrogen Co. South Korea). The nucleotide sequences of *fliA* and *fliB* genes were analyzed by Megalign software. The alignments of Iranian isolates were compared to each other and the *fli*C gene sequences of reference strains in the GenBank.

Results

*Fli*C-PCR: A fragment of 1000 bp length was amplified from *C. chauvoei* by *fli*C specific (CFC and CRC) primers. Two copies of *fli*C (*fliA* and *fliB*) gene were amplified from PCR product of the previous step with a 700 bp size.

Two specific primers (CFC and CRC) could differentiate *C. chauvoei* from *C. septicum*, *C. novyi* type A, *C. tetani*, and *C. perfringens*.

Nucleotide sequence analysis: The dendrogram based on nucleotide sequences of *fli*C gene copies (*fliA* and *fliB*) of *C. chuvoei* is shown in Figure 1. All *fliA* and *fliB* sequences were located in two separated branches. Multiple alignment of *fliA* and *fliB* sequences recognized thirty-one single nucleotide polymorphisms: one SNP in nucleotide position 150, three SNPs in nucleotide positions (187-189), five SNPs in nucleotide position (484-495), two SNPs in position (515-516), three SNPs in positions (530-535), four SNPs in position (552-561), eight SNPs in positions (571-585), and five SNPs in nucleotide positions (592-604) were identified between *fliA* and *fliB* in all *C. chauvoei*. Six highly conserved regions between *fliA* and *fliB* at nucleotide positions (134-149), (153-186), (190-238), (271-483), (496-514), and (517-529) were observed. Nucleotide sequence alignment showed that the divergence in *fliB*s is more than *fliA*s (Table 2). Insilico translation of nucleotide sequences observed 13 single amino acid polymorphisms (SAPs) between *fliA* and *fliB* protein sequences.

Discussion

Flagellin, as a main virulence factor of *C. chauvoei*, is known as the cause of blackleg in animals (Alm and Guerry, 1993). Tamura et al (1984) demonstrated that the *fli*C protein has immunogenicity and protective roles (Kojima et al., 2000; Tamura and Tanaka, 1984; Tanaka et al., 1987). Sequence of N-terminal of flagellin protein has been used to obtain relations between several bacteria (Sasaki et al., 2002). Flagellin in flagellar structure has hairpin model in which the N-C terminal folds to inner flagellum and the central domain is exposed to environment. Diversity in internal domains causes antigenic diversity in Entero-

Table 1. Explanation of *Clostridium* species which were used in this study.

Isolate code	Clostridum sp	Source	Organ/tissue	District
CH 721	*C. chauvoei*	cattle	Muscle Muscle	Saveh
CH 740	*C. chauvoei*	cattle	Muscle	Semnan
CH 743	*C. chauvoei*	cattle	Muscle	Ilam
CH 701	*C. chauvoei*	vaccine	Muscle	Haydarabad
SEP 907	*C. septicum*	sheep	Abomasum	Haydarabad
CPA105	*C. perfringens*	Cattle	Intestine	Tehran
TT502	*C. tetani*	soil	-	NA
NA814	*C. novyi*	sheep	Liver	Isfahan

Table 2. The percent of identity and the sequence distances among the *C. chauvoei* isolates which was designed by MegAlign software.

					Percent of Identity							
	1	2	3	4	5	6	7	8	9	10		
1	■	97.9	93.5	93.3	93.9	93.4	90.2	89.5	91.8	88.7	1	Ab058932
2	0.2	■	92.6	93.3	91.7	91.1	88.6	87.9	91.0	86.7	2	Ch 743 *fliB*
3	0.0	0.0	■	90.7	98.2	88.4	85.6	85.0	86.6	92.5	3	Ch 721 *fliB*
4	4.1	4.3	4.3	■	92.7	87.1	85.6	84.9	87.1	86.9	4	Ch 740 *fliB*
5	0.2	0.3	0.0	4.2	■	87.7	84.1	83.5	85.2	91.5	5	Ch vac *fliB*
6	7.4	7.4	7.3	11.1	8.1	■	96.8	95.9	97.3	93.2	6	Ab 058931
7	8.0	8.2	8.3	11.9	9.1	2.8	■	97.0	99.0	89.0	7	Ch 721 *fliA*
8	8.7	9.7	8.6	13.0	9.3	3.9	1.4	■	93.8	88.1	8	Ch 740 *fliA*
9	6.8	7.1	6.5	11.1	7.3	1.9	1.9	4.0	■	90.1	9	Ch vac *fliA*
10	6.8	7.0	5.6	11.0	6.7	2.0	3.0	3.6	1.3	■	10	Ch 743 *fliA*
	1	2	3	4	5	6	7	8	9	10		

Divergence (row label on left side)

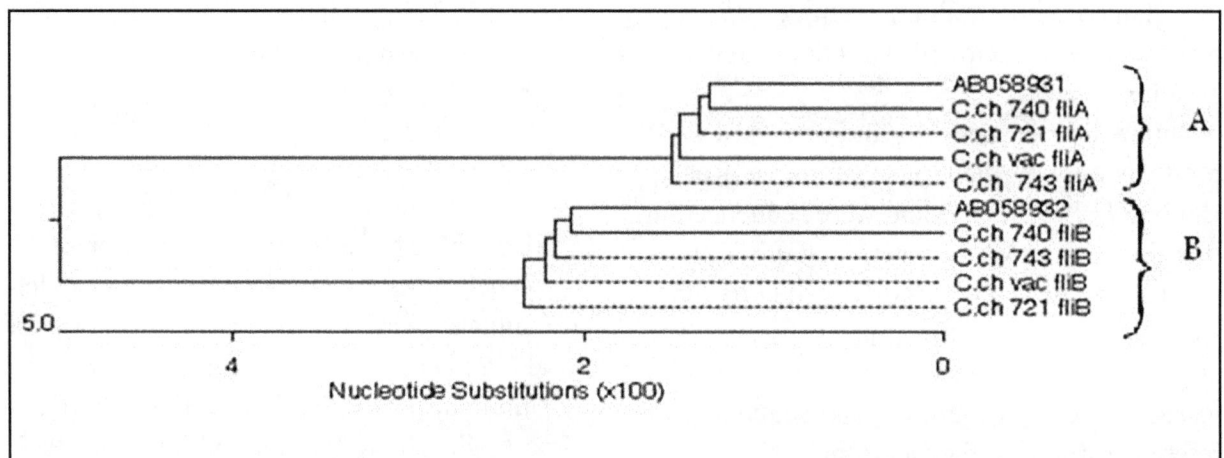

Figure 1. Dendrogram was designed by MegAlign software, based on nucleotide sequences of *fliA* and *fliB* of *C. chuvoei*.

bacteriaceae (Joys, 1988; Kostrzynska et al., 1991; Tino, 1977). In Some species of bacteria, such as *Escherichia coli* and *Salmonella*, only one of the flagella subunits is involved in the organization of flagellum, but in many of the bacteria, flagellar filament is organized from multi-flagella subunits, such as campylobacter and some of the clostridia.

Terponema pallidum has periplasmic flagella, this flagella is composed of several flagellin subunits (Alm and Guerry, 1993). Sasaki et al. (2002) demonstrated that one or more tandem copies of *fliC* in different clostridia belonged to cluster I are available, as *C. chauvoei* and *C. novyi* type A, have two copies of *fliC* gene and *C. septicum* has three copies of *fliC* gene. Kojima (2000) sequenced only one copy of *fliC* gene in *C. chauvoei*. In this study two copies of *fliC* gene in four Iranian vaccine and field isolates of *C. chauvoei* were sequenced. Phylogenic analysis showed more than five percent divergence between *fliA* and *fliB* sequences placed in two branches A and B (Fig. 1).

Comparing Iranian isolates to Japanese strain (AB058931-2) showed high similarity (93-97%) in both *fliA* and *fliB* copies of *fliC* gene (Table 2). Six highly conserved regions were detected in different copies of *fliC* gene. On the other hand, thirty-one single nucleotide polymorphisms including thirty specific nucleotide patterns were observed between *fliA* and *fliB* of *C. chauvoei*. Nucleotide sequence alignment showed more divergence in *fliB* (> 2%) than *fliA* sequences (Table 2).

In this study, a set of primers (CFC and CRC) are promising primers to differentiate *C. chauvoei* from *C. septicum*, *C. novyi* type A, *C. tetani* and *C. perfringens*. On the other hand, conserved regions, single nucleotide polymorphisms, and specific nucleotide patterns of *fliC* gene, which were identified in this study, might help us to better understand the *fliC* gene structure and design better specific primers and probes for diagnostic techniques such as real time PCR.

Although physiological traits, biochemical tests, and toxins are still used to characterize *C. chauvoei*, this information does not possess the discrimination required for source attribution and epidemiological investigations (Ji et al., 2001).The existence of genetic variation between two copies of *fliC* in *C. chauvoei* is reported for the first time in Iranian isolates. This finding can be considered as a scientific base for molecular identification and discrimination among the field isolates. It will be helpful to find out the genetic diversity of the *C.* *chauvoei* isolates according to their different origin, host, and geographical areas.

Acknowledgments

The authors wish to thank the Razi Vaccine and Serum Research Institute for Grant supporting this project.

References

1. Alm, R.A., Guerry, P. (1993) Distribution and polymorphism of the flagellin genes from isolates of *Campylobacter coli* and *Campylobacter jejuni*. J Bacteriol. 175: 3051-3057.

2. Ardehali, M., Darakhshan, H. (1975) Isolation and characterization of *Clostridium chauvoei* strains isolated from cases of blackleg in cattle in Iran. Arch Razi Inst. 27: 37-41.

3. Ardehali, M., Darakhshan, H., Moosawi M. (1984) The existence and present situation of clostridial diseases of domestic animals in Iran. Arch Razi Inst. 34: 27-32.

4. Attridge, S., Rowley, D. (1983) The role of the flagellum in the adherence of *Vibrio cholerae*. J Infect Dis. 147: 864.

5. Bagge, E., Lewerin, S.S., Johansson, K. (2009) Detection and identification by PCR of *Clostridium chauvoei* in clinical isolates, bovine faeces and substrates from biogas plant. Acta Vet Scand. 51: 8.

6. Blood, D.C., Radostitis, O.M., Henderson, J.A. (1983) Veterinary Medicine: A Textbook of the Diseases of Cattle, Sheep, Goats and Horses. (6th ed.) Bailliere Tindall, oxford, London, Uk.

7. Dauga, C., Zabrovskaia, A., Grimont, P.A.D. (1998) Restriction fragment length polymorphism analysis of some flageelin genes of *Salmonella enterica*. J Clin Microbiol. 36: 2835-2843.

8. Ji, W.S., Hu., J.L., Qiu, J.W., Peng, D.R., Shi, B.L., Zhou, S.J., Wu, K.C., Fan, D.M. (2001) Polymorphism of flagellin A gene in *Helicobacter pylori*. World J Gastroentrol. 7: 783-787.

9. Joys, T.M. (1988) The flagellar filament protein. Can J Microbiol 34: 452-458.

10. Kojima, A., Uchida, I., Sekizaki,T., Sasaki, Y., Ogikubo, Y., Kijima, M. (2000) Cloning and expression of a gene encoding the flagellin of *Clostridium chauvoei*. Vet Microbiol. 76: 359-372.

11. Kojima, A., Uchida, I., Sekizaki, T., Sasaki, Y., Ogikubo, Y., Tamura, Y. (2001) Rapid detection and identification of *Clostridium chauvoei* by PCR based on flagellin gene sequence. Vet Microbiol. 78: 363-371.

12. Kostrzynska, M., Betts, J.D., Austin, J., Trust, T.J. (1991) Identification, characterization, and spatial localization of two flagellin species in *Helicobacter pylori* flagella. J Bacteriol. 173: 937-946.

13. Macnab, R.M. (2004) Type III flagellar protein export and flagellar assembly. Biochim Biophys Acta. 1694: 207-217.

14. Miyashiro, S., Nassar, A., Souza, M., Carvalho, J., Adegas, J. (2007) Identification of *Clostridium chauvoei* in clinical samples cultures from blackleg cases by means of PCR. Braz J Microbiol 38: 491-493.

15. Morooka, T., Umeda, A., Amako, K. (1985) Motility as an intestinal colonization factor for *Campylobacter jejuni*. J Gen Microbiol. 131: 1973-1980.

16. Reid, S.D., Selander, R.K., Whittam, T.S. (1999) Sequence diversity of flagellin (*fliC*) alleles in pathogenic *Escherichia coli*. J Bacteriol. 181: 153-160.

17. Sasaki, Y., Kojima, A., Aoki, H., Ogikubo, Y., Takikawa, N., Tamura, Y. (2002) Phylogenetic analysis and PCR detection of *Clostridium chauvoei*, *Clostridium haemolyticum*, *Clostridium novyi* types A and B, and Clostridium septicum based on the flagellin gene. Vet Microbiol. 86: 257-267.

18. Tamura, Y., Tanaka, S. (1984) Effect of antiflagellar serum in the protection of mice against *Clostridium chauvoei*. Infect Immun. 43: 612-616.

19. Tanaka, M., Hirayama, N., Tamura, Y. (1987) Production, characterization, and protective effect of monoclonal antibodies to *Clostridium chauvoei* flagella. Infect Immun. 55: 1779-1783.

20. Tino, T. (1977) Genetics of structure and function of bacterial flagella. Annu Rev Genet. 11: 161-182.

21. Uzal, F.A., Paramidani, M., Assis, R., Morrris, W., Mivakawa, M.F. (2003) Outbreak of *Clostridial myocarditis* in calves. Vet Rec. 152: 134-136.

22. Wilson, G.S., Miles, A.A. (1975) Topley and Wilson's Principles of Bacteriology, Virology and Immunology. (6th ed.). The Williams and Wilkins Co, Baltimore, Maryland, USA.

Antimicrobial activity of Zatacin against bacterial diarrheal pathogens

Mahboubi, M.[1*], Falsafi, T.[2], Torabi Goodarzi, M.[3]

[1]*Department of Microbiology, Biology Center, Medicinal Plant Center of Barij, Kashan, Iran*

[2]*Department of Biology, Faculty of Basic Sciences, Alzahra University, Vanak, Tehran, Iran*

[3]*Razi Vaccine & Serum Research Institute (Central Area branch), Arak, Iran*

Key words:

calf, diarrhea, *Zataria multiflora*, zatacin, antibacterial

Correspondence

Mahboubi, M.
Department of Microbiology,
Biology Center, Medicinal Plant
Center of Barij, Kashan, Iran

Email: mahboubi1357@yahoo.com

Abstract:

BACKGROUND: Calf diarrhea is an important disease that is caused by different pathogens including bacteria, virus and parasites and is associated with economic losses. OBJECTIVES: In this study, we evaluated the antibacterial activities of Zatacin (*Z. multiflora* aerial part ethanol extract), colistin, co-Trimoxazole and enrofloxacin against clinical isolates of *Salmonella* sp, *E. coli* and *Campylobacter* sp isolated from diarrheic calves. METHODS: Disc diffusion method and microbroth dilution assay were used for antimicrobial evaluation. RESULTS: In disc diffusion method, the antibacterial activity of Zatacin increased dose dependently. The sensitivity of different isolates of *E. coli*, *Salmonella* sp and *Campylobacter* sp to Zatacin was almost the same. The antibacterial activity of Zatacin was lower than that of enrofloxacin but it was higher than co-Trimoxazole and colistin. The means of MIC values of Zatacin for *E.coli* were higher than that of *Campylobacter* sp and *Salmonella* sp but its means of MBC values for *E. coli* were lower than that of two other bacteria. CONCLUSIONS: Zatacin can be used as an antimicrobial agent in treatment of infectious causes of calf scours instead of antibiotics with undesired adverse effects on animal and humans.

Introduction

Salmonella sp, *Campylobacter* sp and *Escherichia coli* are the specific bacterial agents of dairy and beef calf diarrhea. Diarrhea in dairy and beef cattle is the leading cause of mortality and morbidity in cattle industries. Diarrhea is the result of increase in bacterial colonization 5 to 10000-fold in duodenum, jejunum and ileum of cattle (Isaacson et al., 1978). Increase in colonization of small intestine has been associated with impaired glucose, xylose and fat absorption (Youanes and Herdt, 1978). Diarrhea is caused in all species of domestic animals including young animals, pregnant and lactating animals and bacteremia, acute septicemia, abortion, arthritis and respiratory diseases may occur.

The main therapies in calf diarrhea are fluid therapies, antibiotics and nursing care. The use of antibiotics in treatment of the disease carries the risk of bacterial flora and developing drug resistance to important anti-bacterial agents such as colistin, enrofloxacin and co-trimoxazole.

Zatacin is a natural herbal product made from ethanol extract of *Zataria multiflora* Boiss aerial part for treatment of calf diarrhea. *Z. multiflora* is an aromatic plant belonging to Labiatae family and has been traditionally used for treatment of infectious diseases. There are many researches on their pharmacological activity as its traditional uses include antinociceptive effects (Hosseinzadeh et al., 2000; Jaffary et al., 2004; Ramezani et al., 2004), anti-inflammatory effects (Hosseinzadeh et al., 2000, AshtaralNakhai et al., 2007), immune stimulation (Shokri et al., 2006), antioxidant activity (Sharififar et al.,2007; Babaie et al., 2007), and their antimicrobial activities (Misaghi and AkhondzadehBasti, 2007; Sharififar et al., 2007; Fazeli et al.,2007; Moosavy et al., 2008; Khosravi et al., 2008; Mahboubi and Ghazian Bidgoli, 2010). The aim of this investigation was to evaluate the in vitro antimicrobial activities of Zatacin against clinical isolates of *Escherichia coli*, *Salmonella* sp. and *Campylobacter* sp from diarrhea in calves.

Materials and Methods

Disc antibiotics: Co-Trimoxazole (Sulpha/Trimethoprim) COT 25 mcg (23.75/1.25 mcg); Enrofloxacin EX 10 mcg, Colistin (Methane Sulphonate) Cl 10 mcg; Co-Trimoxazole Ezy MIC Strips (COT 0.016-256 mcg ml⁻¹), Enrofloxacin powder, Colistin Ezy MIC Strip (Cl 0.016-256 mcgml⁻¹) were provided by HiMedia Laboratories Pvt. Ltd.

Bacterial strains: *Salmonella* sp (12 clinical isolates), *Campylobacter* sp (12 clinical isolates) and *Escherichia coli* (12 clinical isolates) were isolated from clinical cases of diarrhea in newborn calves. The bacterial isolates were confirmed by biochemical

tests. All strains were cultured on nutrient agar and incubated in suitable condition at 37 °C overnight. 1-2 colonies of each strain were dissolved in normal saline and turbidity was adjusted to 0.5 McFarland spectrophotometrically (Optical density 600 was 0.6).

Disc diffusion assay: The antibacterial activities of Zatacin and antibiotic discs (co-trimoxazole, enrofloxacin, colistin) were evaluated by disc diffusion assay. The above bacterial suspensions were cultured on Muller Hinton Agar by sterile swab and blank discs or antibiotic discs were put on cultured plates. The different dilutions of Zatacin were put on blank discs (5, 10, 15 and 20 µl). The plates were incubated at 37 °C overnight and then the diameters of inhibition zone in millimeter (in triplicate) were measured. Inhibition zone diameters were expressed as millimeter ±standard deviation (mm±SD) (Mahboubi et al., 2015).

Antibacterial activity of Zatacin by microbroth dilution assay and E-test: One milliliter of Zatacin contained 0.63 mg phenolic compounds (thymol and carvacrol). A serial concentration of Zatacin was prepared in purified water (15-0.015 mg ml⁻¹). 100 µl of each serial dilution was added to each well of 96 micro plates. Bacterial suspension was diluted in broth medium (Muller Hinton Broth or *Brucella* broth) to reach the 1×10^6 CFUml⁻¹. 100 µl of diluted bacterial suspension was added to each well. The plates were shaken for 30 min and then incubated at 37 °C overnight. Then, the first well with no growth was determined as MIC value, and the well that showed no growth on solid media as MBC value. 100 µl of tetrazolium chloride (0.02%) was added to each well to confirm the results. All experiments were done in triplicate. The

Table 1. The inhibition zone diameters (mm) of Zatacin against calf diarrheal pathogens by disc diffusion assay. * = µl/disc,** based on the observed means at level 0.05, there were seven subsets, a was the most sensitive compound followed by b,c,.....

	E. coli		Salmonella		Campylobacter		total
	Means±SE	Min-Max	Means±SE	Min-Max	Means±SE	Min-Max	Means**
Zatacin* (5)	7.57±0.25	6.1-10.4	6.8±0.14	6.1-8.6	6.2±0.05	6.1-8.1	6.74[g]
Zatacin* (10)	10.5±0.43	6.45-14.8	10.9±0.39	7.1-18.8	9.2±0.16	6.1-17.6	10.2[f]
Zatacin* (15)	14.02±0.6	0.1-20.15	16.2±0.34	12.1-20.9	14.6±0.47	8.1.19.90	14.9[d]
Zatacin* (20)	17.9±0.67	11.5-22.1	20.6±0.39	16.7-25.4	19.9±0.3	15.4-24.8	19.6[b]
Colistin	16.5±0.19	14.8-19.1	16.1±0.45	12.6-21.8	16.9±0.36	11.7-21.4	16.6[c]
co-Trimoxazole	15.1±0.06	6.1-30.7	15.7±2.01	6.1-30.6	9.53±1.09	6.1-33.9	13.02[e]
Enrofloxacin	28.5±1.2	12.3-35.2	29.2±0.58	23.1-34	28.2±0.78	13.2-32.9	28.6[a]

Table 2. The antimicrobial activity of antimicrobial agentsagainst clinical isolates of calf diarrhea by micro-broth dilution assay and E-test. The reported MIC and MBC values have been expressed as the means±SE of MIC or MBC against clinical isolates.

	Zatacin (mg/ml)		Co-Trimoxazole(µg/ml)		Enrofloxacin(µg/ml)		Colistin(µg/ml)	
	MIC	MBC	MIC	MBC	MIC	MBC	MIC	MBC
E. coli	0.60±0.1	1.1±0.05	1.48±1.26	1.48±1.26	1.25±0.45	2.3±0.9	0.85±0.06	0.85±0.06
Salmonella	0.445±0.0	5.2±0.5	4.2±3.9	8.4±4	0.29±0.05	0.5±0.12	1.2±0.12	1.2±0.12
Campylobacter	0.445±0.0	2.2±0.4	192±63	192±63	0.88±0.4	1.7±0.9	1±0.17	1±0.17

results were analyzed by SPSS 17.0 (SPSS for Windows; SPSS Inc, Chicago, IL) and expressed as means±SE (Mahboubi et al., 2015). The MIC values of enrofloxacin were determined by micro broth dilution while the MIC values of colistin and co-trimoxazole were determined by disc diffusion method with their E- Strips.

Results

The antibacterial evaluation of Zatacin (5, 10, 15 and 20 µl/disc) against 36 clinical isolates of E. coli, Salmonella sp and Campylobacter sp. in comparison with colistin, co-trimoxazole and enrofloxacin by disc diffusion method showed that the measured inhibition zone diameters for higher concentration of Zatacin against all strains were larger than the lower concentrations. On the other hand, the antibacterial activity of Zatacin increased dose dependently. The sensitivity of different isolates of E. coli, Salmonella sp and Campylobacter sp. to Zatacin was almost the same but higher concentrations of Zatacin had larger inhibition zone diameters against clinical isolates of Salmonella sp. The inhibition zone diameters of enrofloxacin on clinical isolates of E. coli, Salmonella sp and Campylobacter sp. were larger than the inhibition zone diameters of Zatacin even in concentration of 20 µl/disc, while the inhibition zone diameters of co-trimoxazole on clinical isolates of E. coli and Salmonella sp were equal to the inhibition zone diameters of Zatacin (15 µl/disc). The inhibition zone diameters of co-trimoxazole on clinical isolates of Campylobacter sp were comparable to 10 µl/disc Zatacin. The inhibition zone diameters of colistin on 36 clinical isolates of E. coli, Salmonella sp. and Campylobacter sp. were comparable to 15 µl per disc Zatacin (Table 1).

Antimicrobial activity evaluation of Zatacin against the clinical diarrheal bacteria by micro broth dilution assay revealed that the mean of MIC values for different clinical isolates of E. coli were higher than this amount for Salmonella sp. and Campy-

lobacter sp. The mean of MBC for clinical isolates of *Salmonella* sp were two-fold toward *Campylobacter* sp (2.15 versus 5.2 mg/ml), while the mean of MBC value for clinical isolates of *E. coli* was 1.13 mg/ml. In other words, with respect to MIC and MBC values of Zatacin against different clinical isolates of bacteria, Zatacin had a higher bactericidal effect against clinical isolates of *E. coli*, followed by *Salmonella* sp and *Campylobacter* sp (Table 2).

Discussion

Calf diarrhea is the most important cause of death in dairy and beef calves. *E. coli* is the single most important cause of bacterial diarrhea in most newborn calves and is transmitted from environment. *Salmonella* sp infects the calves at six days of age or older. Antibiotic treatment of infected calves with *salmonella* sp damages the *Salmonella* organism and releases a toxin that will poison the animal, resulting in endotoxic shock. The administration of electrolyte solutions and antimicrobial agents plays an important role in treatment of calf diarrhea. Regardless of the appearance of the antimicrobial resistant bacteria among calves, the use of some antibiotics has been prohibited in food producing animals due to the occurrence of non-dose related anemia and concerns regarding the mutagenicity or carcinogenicity of related product in humans (Constable, 2004). The aim of this study was to evaluate the in vitro efficacy of herbal preparation with the commercial name of Zatacin (BarijEssence Pharmaceutical Co. Kashan, Iran) against bacterial diarrhea infection. Zatacin is made from the ethanol extract of *Z. multiflora* flowering aerial part. Some studies have evaluated the antimicrobial effects of

Z. multiflora ethanol extract against different kinds of microorganisms (Owlia et al., 2006; Fazeli et al., 2007). It has been reported, *Z. multiflora* aerial parts ethanol extract (80%) with 21% extract yield exhibited the antibacterial activity against *Bacillus cereus*, *Staphylococcus aureus*, *Escherichia coli*, *Proteus vulgaris* and *Shigella flexeneri* with MIC values 0.4% (v/v), while *S. typhi* was less sensitive than others with MIC value 0.8% (Fazeli et al., 2007).

The antimicrobial activity of *Z. multiflora* ethanol extract against *S. aureus* ATCC 25923 was %25 (Owlia et al., 2006). Therefore, hydro alcoholic extract of *Z. multiflora* aerial parts exhibited the antibacterial activity against Gram positive and Gram negative bacteria.

Furthermore, *Z. multiflora* aerial part ethanol extract with LD_{50} 3.47 g/kg has shown the anti-inflammatory effect against acute and chronic inflammation (Hossein zadeh et al., 2000).

In this investigation we evaluated the antibacterial activity of *Z. multiflora* aerial part ethanol extract (Zatacin) against clinical isolates of *E. coli*, *Salmonella* sp. and *Campylobacter* sp from calf diarrheal infection. In disc diffusion method, the inhibition zone diameters of Zatacin were lower than that of enrofloxacin, while Zatacin (20 μl/disc) had higher inhibition zone diameters than that of colistin and co-Trimoxazole. *Campylobacter* sp and *Salmonella* sp had higher inhibition zone diameters for Zatacin than that of *E. coli*. Also, in micro broth dilution assay, with respect to the means of MIC values, clinical isolates of *E. coli* had less sensitivity to Zatacin than *Campylobacter* sp and *Salmonella* sp (0.601 versus 0.445 mg/ml), but in evaluating the MBC values, *E. coli* exhibited more sensitivity to

Zatacin than *Campylobacter*, and *Salmonella* sp.

Z. multiflora contains alkanes, fatty acids, phytosterols, hydroxycinnamic acid, flavonoids, tannins, resins and saponins (Sajed et al., 2013). Furthermore, Zatacin has been standardized by thymol and carvacrol. Thymol and carvacrol as terpenoid compounds of *Z. multiflora* essential oil have high antimicrobial activity (Mahboubi and Ghazian Bidgoli, 2010). The higher antibacterial activity of thymol than carvacrol was reported against *E. coli* (Bassolé et al., 2010). Thymol disrupts the outer and inner membranes and interacts with membrane proteins and intracellular targets (Xu et al., 2008), periplasmic enzymes (Juven et al., 1994). The synergistic activity of thymol and carvacrol has been reported (Zhou et al., 2007). Therefore, the antimicrobial activity of Zatacin against bacterial infections involved in calf diarrheal diseases may be related to the components that are found in *Z. multiflora* aerial parts ethanol extract and especially to thymol and carvacrol or synergistic effects of compounds. Regardless of its antimicrobial activity, Zatacin may have antinociceptive (Hosseinzadeh et al., 2000; Jaffary et al., 2004; Ramezani et al., 2004), anti-inflammatory (Hosseinzadeh et al., 2000, Ashtaral Nakhai et al., 2007), and immune modulating effects (Shokri et al., 2006).

Conclusion: Therefore, Zatacin may be used as a natural antibacterial agent in treatment of calf diarrheal diseases that are caused by Gram negative bacteria such as *E. coli*, *Salmonella* sp or *Campylobacter* sp instead of chemical antibiotics with no reported side effects for human and calves. Furthermore, it is essential to demonstrate its efficacy in farms.

Acknowledgements

This study was supported by Barij Essence Research Center. The authors are thankful to Mrs Laleh Hejazi for her considerable help.

References

1. Ashtaral Nakhai, L., Mohammadirad, A., Yasa, N., Minaie, B., Nikfar, S.H., Ghazanfari, G.H., Zamani, M.J., Dehghan, G.H., Jamshidi, H.R., Shetab Boushehri, V., Khorasani, R., Abdollahi, M. (2007) Benefits of *Zataria multiflora* Boiss in experimental model of mouse inflammatory bowel disease. J Evid Based Complementary Altern Med. 4: 43-50.

2. Babaie, M., Yasa, N., Mohammadirad, A., Khorasani, R., Abdollahi, M. (2007) Antioxidative stress potential of *Zataria multiflora* Boiss (Avishan shirazi) in rats. Int J Pharmacol. 3: 510-514.

3. Bassolé, I.H.N., Lamien-Meda, A., Bay-ala, B., Tirogo,S., Franz, C., Novak, J., Nebié, R.C., Dicko, M.H. (2010) Composition and antimicrobial activities of *Lippia multiflora* Moldenke, *Menthax piperita* L. and *Ocimum basilicum* L. essential oils and their major monoterpene alcohols alone and in combination. Molecules. 15: 7825-7839.

4. Constable, P.D. (2004) Antimicrobial use in the treatment of Calf diarrhea. J Vet Intern Med. 18: 8-17.

5. Fazeli, M.R., Amin, G.H., Ahmadian Attari, M.M., Ashtiani, H., Jamalifar, H., Samadi, N. (2007) Antimicrobial activities of Iranian sumac and avishan-e-shirazi (*Zataria multiflora*) against some food-borne bacteria. Food Control. 18: 646-649.

6. Hosseinzadeh, H., Ramezani, M., Salmani, G.H.A. (2000) Antinociceptive, anti-inflam-

matory and acute toxicity effects of *Zataria multiflora* Boiss extracts in mice and rats. J Ethnopharmacol. 73: 379-385.

7. Isaacson, R.E., Moon, H.W., Schneider, R.A. (1978) Distribution and virulence of *Escherichia coli* in the small intestines of calves with andwithout diarrhea. Am J Vet Res. 39: 1750-1755.

8. Jaffary, F., Ghannadi, A., Siahpoush, A. (2004) Antinociceptive effects of hydroalcoholic extract and essential oil of *Zataria multiflora*. Fitoterapia. 75: 217-220.

9. Juven, B.J., Kanner, J., Schved, F., Weisslowicz, H. (1994) Factors that interact with the antibacterial action of thyme essential oil and its active constituents. J Appl Bacteriol. 76: 626-631.

10. Khosravi, A.R., Eslami, A.R., Shokri, H., Kashanian, M. (2008) *Zataria multiflora* cream for the treatment of acute vaginal candidiasis. Int J Gynaecol Obstet. 101: 201-202.

11. Mahboubi, M., Valian, M.M., Kazempour, N. (2015) Chemical composition, antioxidant and antimicrobial activity of *Artemisia sieberi* oils from different parts of Iran and France. J Essent Oil Res. 27: 140-7.

12. Mahboubi, M., Ghazian Bidgoli, F. (2010) Anti staphylococcal activity of essential oil from *Zataria multiflora* and its synergy with vancomycin. Phytomedicine. 17: 548-550.

13. Misaghi, A., Akhondzadeh Basti, A. (2007) Effects of *Zataria multiflora* Boiss. essential oil and nisin on *Bacillus cereus* ATCC 11778. Food Control. 18: 1043-1049.

14. Moosavy, M.H., Akhondzadeh Basti, A., Misaghi, A., Zahraei Salehi, T., Abbasifar, R., Ebrahimzadeh Mousavi, H.A., Alipour, M., Emami Razavi, N., Gandomi, H., Noori, N. (2008) Effect of *Zataria multiflora* Boiss. essential oil and nisin on *Salmonella typhimurium* and *Staphylococcus aureus* in a food model system and on the bacterial cell membranes. Food Res Int. 41: 1050-1057.

15. Owlia, P., Saderi, H., Matloob, F.N., Rezaee, M.B. (2006) Antimicrobial Effect of *Zataria multiflora* Boiss extract and oxacillin against *Staphylococcus aureus*. Iranian Journal of Medical and Aromatic Plants. 22: 22-26.

16. Ramezani, M., Hosseinzadeh, H., Samizadeh, S.H. (2004) Antinociceptive effects of *Zataria multiflora* Boiss fractions in mice. J Ethnopharmacol. 91: 167-170.

17. Sajed, H., Sahebkar, A.H., Iranshahi, M. (2013) *Zataria multiflora* Boiss. (Shirazi thyme)-An ancient condiment with modern pharmaceuticaluses. J Ethnopharmacol. 145: 686-98.

18. Sharififar, F., Moshafi, M.H., Mansouri, S.H., Khodashenas, M., Khoshnoodi, M. (2007) In vitro evaluation of antibacterial and antioxidant activities of the essential oil and methanol extract of endemic *Zataria multiflora* Boiss. Food Control. 18: 800-805.

19. Shokri, H., Asadi, F., Bahonar,A.R., Khosravi, A.R. (2006) The role of *Zataria Multiflora* essence (Iranian herb) on innate immunity of animal model. Iran J Immunol. 3: 164-168.

20. Xu, J., Zhou, F., Ji, B.P., Pei, R.S., Xu,N. (2008) The antibacterial mechanism of carvacrol and thymol against *Escherichia coli*. Lett Appl Microbiol. 47: 174-179.

21. Youanes, Y.D., Herdt, T.H. (1978) Changes in small intestinal morphologyand flora associated with decreased energy digestibility in calves with naturally occurring diarrhea. Am J Vet Res. 48: 719-725.

22. Zhou, F., Ji, B., Zhang, H., Jiang, H., Yang, Z., Li, J., Li, J., Ren, Y.,Yan, W. (2007) Synergistic effect of thymol and carvacrol combined with chelators and organic acids against *Salmonella typhimurium*. J Food Prot. 70: 1704-1709.

3

Frequency of selected virulence-associated genes in intestinal and extra-intestinal *Escherichia coli* isolates from chicken

Eftekharian, S.[1], Ghorbanpoor, M.[1*], Seyfi Abad Shapouri, M.R.[1], Ghanbarpour, R.[2], Jafari, R.[3], Amani, A.[4]

[1]*Department of Pathobiology, Faculty of Veterinary Medicine, Shahid Chamran University of Ahvaz, Ahvaz, Iran*

[2]*Molecular Microbiology Research Group, Faculty of Veterinary Medicine, Shahid Bahonar University, Kerman, Iran*

[3]*Department of Clinical Sciences, Faculty of Veterinary Medicine, Shahid Chamran University of Ahvaz, Ahvaz, Iran*

[4]*DVSc (Poultry Diseases) Graduate, Faculty of Veterinary Medicine, Shahid Chamran University of Ahvaz, Ahvaz, Iran*

Key words:

aerobactin, chicken, *Escherichia coli*, fimbriae type 1, temperature sensitive hemagglutinin (tsh)

Correspondence

Ghorbanpoor, M.
Department of Pathobiology,
Faculty of Veterinary Medicine,
Shahid Chamran University of
Ahvaz, Ahvaz, Iran

Email: m.ghorbanpoor@scu.ac.ir

Abstract:

BACKGROUND: Although *Escherichia coli* (*E. coli*) is a part of intestinal normal microflora of warm-blooded animals, including poultry, outbreaks occur in poultry raised below standard sanitation and during the course of respiratory or immunosuppressive diseases. Avian pathogenic *E. coli* (APEC) harbors several genes associated with virulence and pathogenicity. APEC strains are responsible for some diseases in poultry including colibacillosis, swollen head syndrome, yolk sac infection, omphalitis and coli granuloma. **OBJECTIVES:** The aim of this study was examination of the presence and frequency of three important virulence genes in intestinal and extra-intestinal (liver) *E. coli* isolates from chicken of Khuzestan province in the southwest of Iran. **METHODS:** Totally 120 (60 intestinal and 60 liver) *E. coli* isolates were examined by polymerase chain reaction (PCR) for the presence of aerobactin (iutA), temperature sensitive hemagglutinin (tsh) and fimbriae type 1 (fimH) genes. **RESULTS:** The results showed that tsh, iutA and fimH are respectively present in 78.3%, 70% and 61.7% of liver isolates while in intestinal ones the frequency of these genes was 21.7%, 41.7% and 41.7% respectively. The most prevalent genotypes in extra intestinal and intestinal isolates were tsh+fimH+iutA+ and tsh-fimH-iutA-respectively. **CONCLUSIONS:** It seems that these sets of virulence genes are significantly more prevalent (P<0.05) in extra intestinal isolates and probably these genes play an important role in the pathogenesis of APEC isolates in the southwest of Iran. Although these virulence genes were not present in all APEC isolates their frequencies were high and using the products of these genes in vaccines may be effective in protecting against infections caused by this bacterium.

Introduction

Escherichia coli (*E. coli*) strains are a part of intestinal normal microflora of warm-blooded animals, including humans and poultry (Brzuszkiewicz et al., 2011; Salehi 2014). Although *E. coli* is a normal inhabitant of the intestine of poultry, outbreaks occur in poultry raised below standard sanitation and during the course of respiratory or immunosuppressive diseases (Kheirandish et al., 2012). The pathogenic *E. coli* strains, known as avian pathogenic *E. coli* (APEC), can cause localized or systemic infections in poultry, such as acute fatal septicemia or subacute pericarditis and airsacculitis (Cavicchio et al., 2015). APEC has a broad range of virulence factors similar to other extra-intestinal pathogenic *E. coli* (ExPEC) strains include adhesins (F1, P, stg fimbriae, curli and EA/I), iron acquisition system (aerobactin, iroprotein, yersinibactin), autotransporters (tsh, vat, AatA), the phosphate transport system, sugar metabolism and the Ibex protein (Wang et al., 2015; Schouler et al. 2007).

APEC strains infect poultry by initial respiratory tract colonization followed by systemic spread (Wang et al., 2014). An important aspect of pathogenesis in several diseases starts with bacterial adhesion to host cells that can result in internalization by bacterial-induced endocytosis (Ramirez et al., 2009). *E. coli* colonization in host tissue is mediated by fimbrial adhesions. Type 1 fimbriae, expressed by APEC, have the ability to bind to D-mannose and thus to many kinds of eukaryotic cells such as lung, intestinal, bladder and kidney epithelial tissues (La Ragion et al. 2002), and so is associated with *E. coli* colonization in extra intestinal tissues (Mcpeak et al. 2005). APEC strains can survive in environments with low iron availability such as inside the host by expression of iron acquisition system. This system includes production of sidrophores such as aerobactin which acts as iron chelates in the host (Naka-

zato et al. 2009). Temperature sensitive hemagglutinin (tsh) has a hemagglutinin activity in APEC at 26-30ºC and is repressed at 42ºC (La Ragion et al. 2002). This protein is encoded by the tsh gene that is located in high molecular weight plasmids (Dizois et al. 2003). The tsh is a serine protease auto transporter protein and to date, its role in avian coli septicemia is still to be elucidated (Nakazato et al. 2009).

The purposes of the study were to determine the presence and frequency of three important virulence genes (tsh, iutA and fimH) in fecal and extra-intestinal infection *E. coli* isolates from chicken of Khuzestan province in the southwest of Iran.

Materials and Methods

Bacterial isolates: Totally 120 *E. coli* were isolated from either the liver of chickens with clinical signs of colibacillosis (60 isolates), or from feces of apparently healthy chickens (60 isolates) from different poultry farms of Khuzestan province in the southwest of Iran. The isolates were cultured on sheep blood agar and their pure cultures were identified morphologically and biochemically (Markey et al, 2013). All isolates were stored at −60ºC in skimmed milk broth to which 15% glycerol was added after growth.

The reference *E. coli* strains J96 and Mg1655 were used as positive and negative controls for all probes, respectively.

Polymerase chain reaction (PCR): *E. coli* isolates were examined by PCR for the presence of aerobactin (iutA), temperature sensitive hemagglutinin (tsh) and fimbriae type 1 (fimH) genes. The specific sequence of these genes was downloaded from GenBank and analyzed for specific primers of the genes using primer 3 software. Description, primer sequences and sizes of amplified fragments for the characteristics studied have been summarized in Table 1.

Template DNA of all isolates was prepared

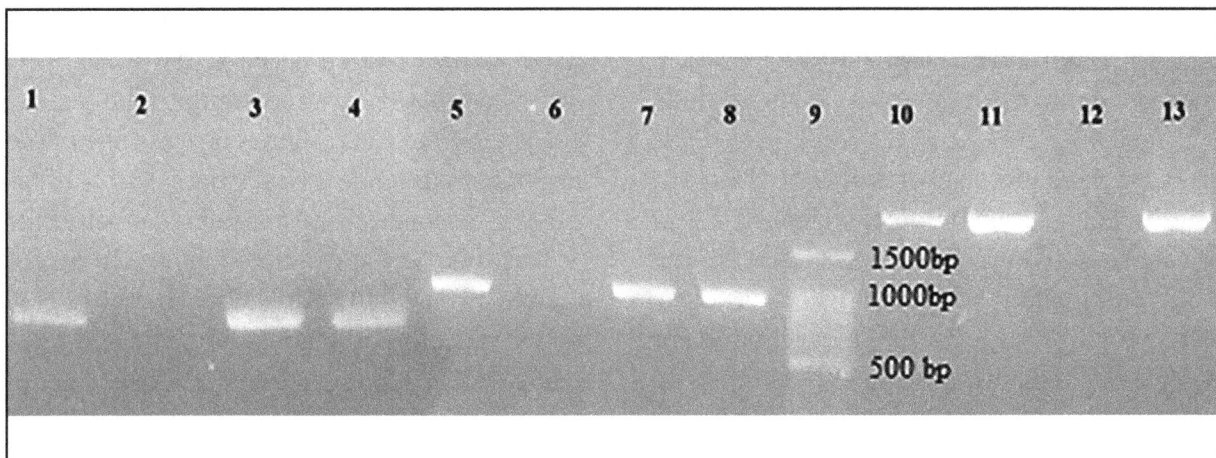

Figure 1. Agarose gel electrophoresis of the PCR products obtained from tsh, fimH and iutA genes of *E. coli* (Lane 1-4: 750bp PCR product of tsh gene; Lane 5-8: 902bp PCR product of fimh gene; Lane9: 100 bp ladder and Lane 10-13: 2272bp PCR product of iutA gene. Lane 2, 6 and 12 are negative controls).

Table.1. Sequence of oligonucleotide primers for amplification of three virulence genes of avian isolates of *E. coli*.

Primer	Target gene	Sequence	Product length (bp)
FimHf & FimHr	Fimbriae type 1 (fimH)	Forward: 5′-ATGAAACGAGTTATTACCCTGT-3′ Reverse: 5′-TTATTGATAAACAAAAGTCACGCCA-3′	902
IutAf & IutAr	Aerobactin (iutA)	Forward: 5′-CAGAGTTTTGTTTCTGACGGTCC -3′ Reverse: 5′-ACGTGCAACCTGGTAACCA-3′	2272
Tshf & Tshr	Temperature Sensitive Hem-agglutinin (tsh)	Forward: 5′-ATGATGATAAGCAAAAAGTATACGC -3′ Reverse: 5′-TCAGAACAGCACAGAGTAGTTCAG -3′	750

Table 2. The frequency of different genotypes of three virulence genes in 60 intestinal and 60 extra intestinal *E. coli* isolates from chicken.

Genotype	No of positive fecal isolates	No of positive liver isolates	Total
tsh+iutA+fimH+	5/60	21/60	26/120
tsh+iutA+fimH-	4/60	12/60	16/120
tsh+iutA-fimH+	1/60	8/60	9/120
tsh-iutA+fimH+	9/60	7/60	16/120
tsh+iutA-fimH-	3/60	6/60	9/120
tsh-iutA+fimH-	7/60	2/60	9/120
tsh-iutA-fimH+	10/60	1/60	11/120
tsh-iutA-fimH-	21/60	3/60	24/120

by boiling (Delicato et al. 2003) and the DNA was stored at −60°C until used. Presence of the iutA, fimH and tsh genes was verified by simplex PCR analysis. PCR was performed with a thermal cycler (Mastecycler Gradient, Eppendorf, Germany) in a 25 µl reaction containing 12.5 µl master mix (Ampelicon, Denmark), 5.5 µl PCR water, 1 µl (10 Pico mole) of each primer (Bioneer, South Korea) and 5 µl of template DNA. DNA polymerization was performed using thermal cycler and J96 strain of *E. coli* as positive and Mg 1655 strain as negative controls. Amplification of fimH was obtained with an initial denaturation step at 95°C for 5 minutes followed by 35 cycles involving denaturation at 95 °C for 30 seconds, annealing at 55°C for 30 seconds, and synthesis at 72 °C for 1 min. The final extension was down for 5 min at 72°C. For amplification of iutA gene the conditions were the same as fimH with the exception that annealing step was at 60°C for 1 min and extension at 72 for 2.5 min. Amplification of tsh gene was done as fimH but annealing was at 60°C for 1 min. PCR products were electrophoresed on 1.5% (w/v) agarose gels. Each 60 ml gel contained 1.7 μl of safe stain (Cinnagene, Iran). Gels were run for approximately 60 min at 100 v. Products were visualized using a UV trans-illuminator (UVtech, England) and size determination was achieved using a 100 base pair (bp) ladder (Cinnagene, Iran).

Statistical analysis: Statistical analysis was performed using SPSS software (version 22) and Chi square test. Significance was accepted when the p-value was < 0.05.

Results

The monoplex PCR results obtained for some APEC and non-APEC strains are shown in Figure 1. Frequency, patterns and combinations of three virulence-associated genes for all 120 isolates of *E. coli* are summarized in Table 2. The iutA gene was present in 42 (70%) liver and 25 (41.7%) fecal isolates and this difference was statistically significant (p=0.002). Frequency of fimH gene in liver isolates was 61.7% (37 isolates out of 60) while this gene was present in 41.7% (25 isolates out of 60) of fecal isolates and this difference was also significant (p=0.022). Our data also indicated that tsh was present in 47 (78.3%) liver and in 13 (21.7%) intestinal isolates. Statistical analysis revealed that tsh is also more frequent in liver isolates (p<0.001). The fimH+iutA+tsh+ genotype was most prevalent (35%) among all liver isolates, while the fimH-iutA-tsh-genotype was the greatest (35%) genotype among fecal isolates.

Discussion

In this study the 120 including 60 fecal and 60 liver *E. coli* isolates from chicken were investigated for the presence of three virulence-associated genes (iutA, tsh and fimH) described for APEC. According to the results, at least 95% of liver isolates possess one of the examined virulence genes, whereas 65% of fecal *E. coli* isolates were considered positive for at least one of the examined genes. In agreement with our results Kafshdouzan et al. (2013) by examination of avian pathogenic and fecal *E. coli* isolates for 6 virulence associated genes also reported that 85% of APEC and 66% of isolates from apparently healthy birds possess at least one of the examined genes. McPeake et al. (2005) showed that APEC virulence associated genes may be present in *E. coli* isolates from apparently healthy birds.

In this study 70% of APEC isolates were identified positive for iutA while 41.7% of fecal isolates were positive for this gene. Similar to our study, Kafshdouzan et al. (2013) found that IutA, is detectable in 67.4% of APEC isolates. Rodriguez-siek et al. (2005) also reported 81.2% of *E. coli* isolates from poultry colibacillosis are positive for iutA gene. Delicato et al. (2002) identified only 12% of fecal isolates positive for iutA, compared to 63% of isolated *E. coli* from cases of colibacillosis.

In our study the tsh gene was found in 78.3% of liver and 21.7% of fecal isolates, so the importance of tsh in APEC pathogenesis is confirmed. In contrast to our results for this gene, McPeake et al. (2005) demonstrated that occurrence of tsh gene in *E. coli* isolates from healthy birds is 93.3%; But, Delicato et al. (2002) identified only 4% of fecal isolates positive for tsh compared to 39.5% of isolated *E. coli* from cases of colisepticaemia. Same as in our study, Maurer et al. (1998) detected tsh in 46% of clinical isolates and showed the absence of this gene in all commensal *E. coli*. Furthermore, Campos et al. (2005) reported that tsh gene was found in 50% of APEC strain.

In the present study frequency of fimH genes in liver and fecal *E. coli* isolates from chickens were 61.7% and 41.7% respectively.

The fimH genes that encode type 1 fimbriae, were detected in almost 50% of examined isolates, in contrast with previous data (Delicato et al., 2003; Maurer et al., 1998; Roussan et al., 2014) showing their ubiquity among commensal and clinical isolates. Ghanbarpour et al., (2011) also reported 96.4% of fecal isolates positive for fimH compared to 95% of isolated *E. coli* from cases of colibacillosis. This difference may be due to discrepancy in time and different place of studies. Such differences may also be due to the different primers used in different investigations.

In the present study the fimH+iutA+tsh+ genotype was significantly more prevalent in liver (35%) than fecal (8.3%) isolates. McPeake et al. reported that APEC plasmids possess several virulence associated genes, though some of these have been reported in *E. coli* strains isolated from apparently healthy birds (McPeake et al., 2005).

In conclusion, cases of avian colisepticaemia within Khuzestan province in the southwest of Iran could not be linked to any individual genotype of causative agent. However, these results suggest fimH+iutA+tsh+genotype may play a significant role in colisepticaemia in this area and although these virulence genes were not present in all APEC isolates their frequency is high and using the products of these genes in vaccines may be effective in protecting against infections caused by this bacterium.

Acknowledgements

This work was supported by a grant from the Research Council of Shahid Chamran University of Ahvaz.

References

1. Brzuszkiewicz, E., Thürmer, A., Schuldes, J., Leimbach, A., Liesegang, H., Meyer, F.D., Boelter, J., Petersen, H., Gottschalk, G., Daniel, R. (2011) Genome sequence analyses of two isolates from the recent *Escherichia coli* outbreak in Germany reveal the emergence of a new pathotype: entero-aggregative-haemorrhagic *Escherichia coli* (EAHEC). Arch Microbiol. 193: 883-91.

2. Campos, T.A., Stehling, E.G., Ferreira, A., Castro A.F.P., Brocchi, M., Silveria, W.D. (2005) Adhesion properties, fimberial expression and PCR detection of adhesion related genes of avian *Escherichia coli* strains. Vet Microbiol. 106: 275-285.

3. Cavicchio, L., Dotto, G., Giacomelli, M., Giovanardi, D., Grilli G., Franciosini, M.P., Trocino, A., Piccirillo, A. (2015) Class 1 and class 2 integrons in avian pathogenic *Escherichia coli* from poultry in Italy. Poult Sci. 3: 1–7.

4. Delicato, E.R., Guimaraes de Brito, B., Gaziri, L.C.J., Vidotto, M.C. (2003) Virulence associated genes in *Escherichia coli* isolates from poultry with colibacillosis. Vet Microbiol. 94: 97-103.

5. Dizois, C.M., Daigle, F., Curtiss, R. (2003) Identification of pathogen specific and conserved genes expressed invivo by an avian pathogenic *Escherichia coli* strain. Proc Nati Acad Sci USA. 100: 247-252.

6. Ghanbarpour, R., Sami, M., Salehi, M., Ouromiei, M. (2011) Phylogenetic background and virulence genes of *Escherichia coli* isolates from colisepticemic and healthy broiler chickens in Iran. Trop Anim Health Prod. 43:153-7.

7. Kafshdouzan, K.H., Zahraei Salehi, T., Nayeri Fasaei, B., Madadgar, O., Yamasaki, S.H., Inenoya, A., Yasuda, N. (2013) Distribution of virulence associated genes in isolated *Escherichia coli* from avian colibacillosis. Iran J Vet Med. 7: 1-6.

8. Kheirandish, R., Salehi, M., Ghanbarpour, R., Alidadi, S., Askari, N. (2012) Coligranuloma in a pigeon. Eurasian J Vet Sci. 28: 237-239.

9. La Ragion, R.M., Woodward, M.J. (2002) Virulence factor of *Escherichia coli* serotypes associated with avian colisepticaemia. Res Vet Sci. 73: 27-35.

10. Markey, B.K., Leonard, F.C., Archambault,

M., Cullinane, A., Maguire, D. (2013) Clinical Veterinary Microbiology. (2ⁿᵈ ed.) Mosby.

11. China.Maurer, J.J., Brown, T.P., Steffens, W.L., Thayer, S.G. (1998) The occurrence of ambient temperature-regulated adhesins, curli, and the temperature-sensitive hemagglutinin Tsh among avian Escherichia coli. Avian Dis. 42: 106–118.

12. McPeake, S.J., Smyth, J.A., Ball, H.J. (2005) Characterization of avian pathogenic *Escherichia coli* (APEC) associated with colisepticaemia compared to faecal isolates from healthy birds. Vet Microbiol. 110: 245-253.

13. Nakazato, G., Campos, T.A., Stehling, E.G., Brocchi, M., Silveria, W. (2009) Virulence factor of avian pathogenic *Escherichia coli* (APEC). Pesq Vet Bras. 29: 479-486.

14. Ramirez, R.M., Almanza, Y., Garcia, S., Heredia, N. (2009) Adherence and invasion of avian pathogenic *Escherichia coli* to avian tracheal epithelial cells. World J Microbiol Biotechnol. 25: 1019-1023.

15. Rodriguez-siek, K.E., Giddings, C.W., Doetkott, C., Johnson, T.J., Nolan, L.K. (2005) Characterizing the APEC pathotype. Vet Res. 36: 241-256.

16. Roussan, D.A., Zakaria, H., Khawaldeh, G., Shaheen, I. (2014) Differentiation of avian pathogenic *Escherichia coli* strains from broiler chickens by multiplex polymerase chain reaction (PCR) and random amplified polymorphic (RAPD) DNA. Open J Vet Med. 4: 211-219.

17. Salehi, M. (2014) Determination of intimin and Shiga toxin genes in *Escherichia coli* isolates from gastrointestinal contents of healthy broiler chickens in Kerman City, Iran. Comp Clin Pathol. 23: 125-129.

18. Schouler, M., Reperant, M., Laurent, S., Bree, A., Grasteau, S.M., Germon, P., Rasschaert, D., Schouler, C. (2007) Experimental pathogenic *Escherichia coli* strains of avian and human origin: link between phylogenetic relationships and common virulence patterns. J Clin Microbiol. 45: 3366-3376.

19. Wang, S., Bao, Y., Meng, Q., Xia, Y., Zhao, Y., Wang, Y., Tang, F., ZhuGe, X., Yu, S., Han, X., Dai, J., Lu, C. (2015) IbeR facilitates stress-resistance, invasion and pathogenicity of avian pathogenic *Escherichia coli*. PLoS One. doi: 10.1371.

20. Wang, S., Dai, J., Meng, Q., Han, X., Han, Y., Zhao, Y., Yang, D., Ding, C., Yu, S. (2014) DotU expression is highly induced during in vivo infection and responsible for virulence and Hcp1 secretion in avian pathogenic Escherichia coli. Front Microbiol. doi: 10.3389.

4

An outbreak of a mixed infection due to fungal (*Trichophyton mentagrophytes* var. *mentagrophytes*) and parasitic (*Geckobiella donnae*) agents on green iguanas

Sharifzadeh, A.[1], Khosravi, A.R.[1], Shokri, H.[2*], Balal, A.[1], Arabkhazaeli, F.[3]

[1]*Mycology Research Center, Faculty of Veterinary Medicine, University of Tehran, Tehran, Iran*

[2]*Department of Pathobiology, Faculty of Veterinary Medicine, Amol University of Special Modern Technologies, Amol, Iran*

[3]*Department of Parasitology, Faculty of Veterinary Medicine, University of Tehran, Tehran, Iran*

Key words:

dermal co-infection, *Geckobiella donnae*, green iguana, *Trichophyton mentagrophytes* var. *mentagrophytes*

Correspondence

Shokri, H.
Department of Pathobiology,
Faculty of Veterinary Medicine,
Amol University of Special
Modern Technologies, Amol,
Iran

Email: hshokri@ausmt.ac.ir

Abstract:

BACKGROUND: Green iguana (*Iguana iguana*) is one of the newly imported exotic pets which has been observed with increasing regularity in veterinary clinics in Iran. Despite their popularity, information about their diseases is scarce. **OBJECTIVES:** The aim of this study was to assess the pathogenic agents in green iguanas with skin disorders. **METHODS:** The animals were brought to Small Animal Hospital, Faculty of Veterinary Medicine, Tehran, Iran, with chronic pruritic dermatitis, scabs, loss of spines and deep ulcerative dermatitis located over the body. During physical exam, deposits of dry seborrhea were taken and processed for diagnosis. The clinical specimens were cultured on sabouraud dextrose agar containing chloramphenicol and cycloheximide and mycosel agar. **RESULTS:** Microscopic examination revealed fungal elements as *Trichophyton mentagrophytes* var. *mentagrophytes* and psoroptid mites as *Geckobiella donnae*. **CONCLUSIONS:** This was the first report of the presence of fungal and parasitic agents as the etiological agents of dermatological disorders in green iguanas.

Introduction

Many different mycotic diseases have been reported in captive reptiles. Etiological agents of cutaneous and systemic infections in reptiles are attributed to a wide variety of filamentous fungi and yeasts, although they have often been inadequately identified (Pare et al., 2006). As a rule, fungal infection of reptiles has been regarded as opportunistic, caused by normally saprophytic organisms that invade living tissue strictly under favorable circumstances for the pathogen. Predisposing factors such as suboptimal cage temperatures and inappropriate environmental conditions are often involved (Kostka et al., 1997, Schumacher, 2003).

Dermatophytosis is caused by fungi in the genera *Microsporum*, *Trichophyton* and *Epidermophyton*. There are three ecological groups of dermatophytes: anthropophilic (mostly associated with humans), zoophilic (associated with animals) and geophilic (found in the soil) (Nweze, 2010). Dermatophytes are also reportedly cited among the most frequent cause of dermatological problems in domestic animals (Cabañes, 2000). Human beings are usually infected from animals mostly through direct contact or via fungus-bearing hair and scales from infected animals. In the last few years, the interest in having animals as pets has increased dramatically in many countries with an increasing number of such pets co-habiting and feeding with their owners and members of their households in the majority of cases (Nweze, 2011).

Parasites, especially mites, are well-known causes of dermatological problems in reptiles. Parasitic mites are chiefly ectoparasites of the skin, mucous membranes, or feathers, but a few are endoparasites. Mites are distributed worldwide on both plants and animals and cause direct injury as well as the spread of disease (Scott et al., 2001). Mite families of importance to lizards include: Trombiculidae, Macronyssidae and Pterygosomatidae (Peterson, 2006).

Skin diseases represent one of the most important reasons for veterinary intervention in reptile medicine. Whereas most skin diseases in commonly kept reptile species are primarily caused by inappropriate husbandry and feeding, few of the infectious agents that primarily cause dermatitis are known. Green iguana (*Iguana iguana*) are probably the most popular lizards kept as pets. Readily available, they are also fairly inexpensive, especially when acquired at a small size (50-100 grams). In recent years, although increasing attention has been paid to keeping green iguanas as pet animals in Iran and allowing a close relationship with humans in indoor areas, little is known about the zoonotic hazards of this animal. In this manuscript, we will focus on fungal (*Trichophyton mentagrophytes* var. *mentagrophytes*) and parasitic (*Geckobiella donnae*) agents involved in severe and persistent dermatological problems in a green iguanas.

Materials and Methods

Green iguanas (9 months) were presented with a history of skin darkness lesions, thickening, scaling and crusting on the neck, tail and distal aspects of the legs (Fig. 1). Due to the scaling nature of the lesions, it was suspected to have dermatophyte invasion. Clinical specimens were taken from involved cutaneous surface by scraping epidermal scales with sterile surgical blade. Direct microscopic examination was done using 10% potassium hydroxide (KOH) /dimethylsulfoxide (DMSO). The clinical specimens were cultured on sabouraud dextrose agar (Merck Co., Darmastdt, Germany) containing chloramphenicol (0.005%) and cyclohexamide (0.04%), mycosel agar and on dermatophyt test media (Merck Co., Darmastdt, Germany). The cultures were incubated at 30°C for 3 weeks.

Results

Direct microscopy showed hyphae and hyaline-septated arthroconidia (Fig. 2a) with lots of red mites in epidermal scales, suggesting mixed dermatophyte-mite co-infection. After 8 days, the colonies of *T. mentagrophytes* var. *mentagrophytes* had changed to white to cream in color, granular surface and with central folding or downy areas (Fig. 2b). Reverse pigmentation was usually a yellow to brown color. Microconidia were hyaline, single-celled, and smooth-walled and were predominantly spherical to subspherical in shape. Varying numbers of coil and spiral hyphae along with smooth, thin-walled, clavate shaped, multicelled macroconidia were also observed in lactophenol cotton blue staining. The identification of this dermatophyte was confirmed by studying the macroscopic and microscopic characteristics as well as positive hydrolysis of urea within five days and in vitro hair perforation test within 12 days and development of granular appearance on the 1% peptone agar (Merck Co., Darmstadt, Germany).

Mite identified as *Geckobiella donnae* had oligotrichous idiosoma. Dorsal idiosomal setae c3 was present. The prodorsal shield resembled an inverted pentagon with anterior sides almost parallel. There were two pairs of

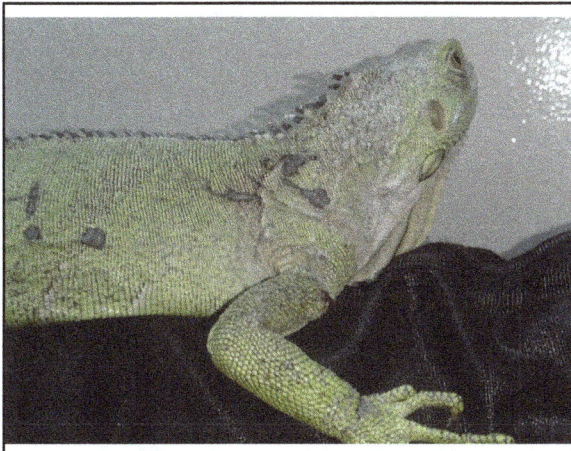

Figure 1. Green iguana with thickening of dark discoloration of the skin surrounding necrosis on the right ventral abdominal region.

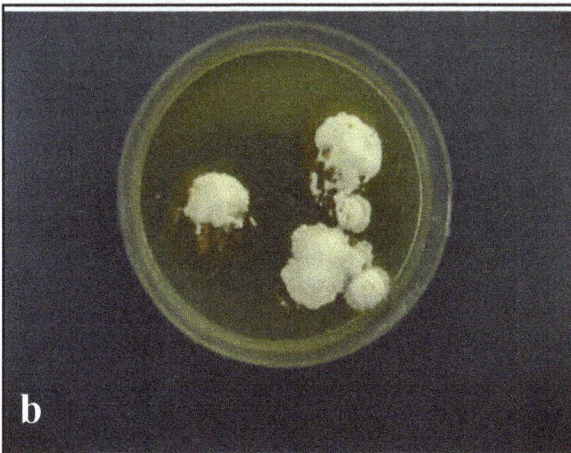

Figure 2. (a) Microscopic appearance of the isolate showing hyphae bearing arthroconidia (b) Culture of scales on Sabouraud at 30 °C.

short setae on the shield (Fig. 3a). Coxal group III-IV were considerably apart from the coxal group I-II and stout tarsi I-IV had blunt endings. Base of the capitulum was simple and one pair of ventral, slender and smooth setae was visible behind the palps. Palps were slender and about two times longer than the length of base of gnathosoma (Fig. 3b). Seta d on femur I was branched.

Discussion

Dermatophytosis is a well-recognised zoonotic infection of keratinized structures such as nails, hair shafts, claws and stratum corneum by dermatophytes. Zoophilic dermatophytes, in particular *Trichophyton mentagrophytes* var. *mentagrophytes*, are the prominent aetiological agents (Mancianti et al., 2002). The identification of dermatophyte species is essential for appropriate diagnosis and treatment in veterinary dermatology. Routine identification of dermatophytes relies on the use of appropriate culture growth media and the examination of gross colony and microscopic morphology. Results of this study describe the first report of the occurrence of a mixed infection with *Trichophyton mentagrophytes* var. *mentagrophytes* and *Geckobiella donnae* in green iguanas in Tehran, Iran. To our knowledge this is the first report of *Trichophyton mentagrophytes* var. *mentagrophytes* being implicated in a disseminated cutaneous infection in iguanas. The isolation of the fungi in pure culture confirmed this fungus as the etiologic agent of the infections in this reptile species. In a previous study by Khosravi et al. (2012), all green iguanas were suffering from *T. mentagrophytes* var. *interdigitale* infection. Chung et al. (2014) reported a 1-year-old female green iguana presented with a nodular, darkly discolored skin lesion surrounded by necrosis in the right ventral abdominal region suffering from *Microsporum canis*. Totally, cutaneous fungal infections in iguanas are attributed to a wide variety of filamentous fungi and yeasts, which often have been inadequately identified (Pare et al., 2006). Although rodents and soil were known to harbour different *T. mentagrophytes* varieties, it was possible that husbandry was

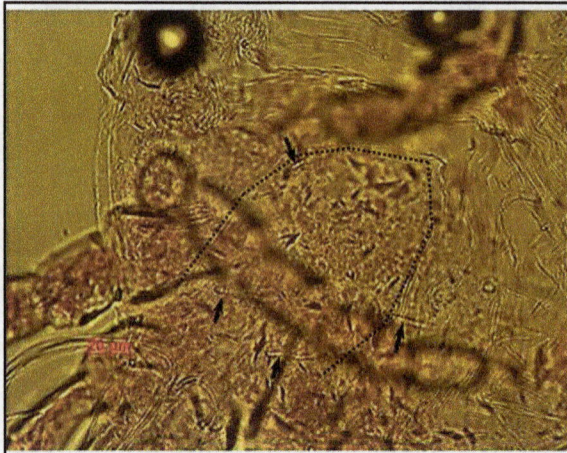

Figure 3a. Dorsal shield of *Geckobiella donnae* shaped as an inverted pentagon with anterior sides almost parallel (outlined) and 2 pairs of short setae (arrows) (x400).

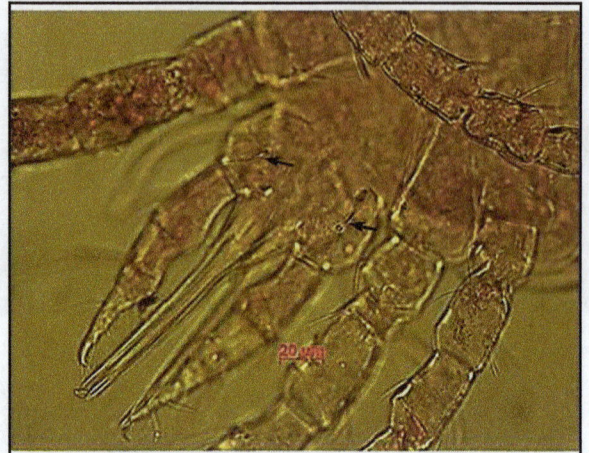

Figure 3b. Gnathosoma of *Geckobiella donnae*. Note the slender and long with a pair of smooth setae visible behind them (arrows) (x400).

suboptimal, and this would be a predisposing factor contributing to the onset of infection.

Pterygosomatidae, the only family in the superfamily Pterygosomatoidea, comprises various species of bright red mites found primarily on lizards, tortoises, and arthropods all over the world. The described genera includes Cyclurobia, Geckobia, Geckobiella, Hirstiella, Ixodiderma, Pterygosoma, Scaphothrix, Teqttisistlana and Zonurobia, which are mostly external parasites of lizards. They attach under scales, between the toes, or in areas known as mite pockets and often are confused with chiggers. They feed on body fluids of their host and cause benign to severe pathological disorders such as anemia and intense skin irritation. Apparently, some species are vectors of protozoan diseases of lizards (Krantz and Walter, 2009). *Geckobiella* spp. (as well as other Pterygosomatids) is scansorial and not usually found in mite-pockets. These mites live under the imbricate scales of their hosts (Delfino et al., 2011). All instars of this genus are parasitic on the Iguanidae (Paredes-León et al., 2012). Parasitism by *Geckobiella* may cause problems during the molting process of their hosts and some species are potential vectors of *Plasmodium* and *Haemogregarina* (Murgas et al., 2013). The mites tend to localize around the eyes, under the chin, in the dewlap, axillary and inguinal areas, on limbs in folds of skin associated with joints, and on the tail. They can cause irritation to the lizards, resulting in a pruritic response (Hoppmann and Barron, 2007). Previous studies in Turkey (Gazyacsi et al., 2011) and Greece (Farmaki et al., 2013) reported a number of red mites, erythema, darkness, and itching on the skin of green iguanas and *Hirstiella* spp. was diagnosed after microscopic examination. In the iguanas in the present case, mites were generally picked up from periocular, dorsal and tail sites and skin examination showed erythema, darkness, and pruritis. This was the first report of *Geckobiella donnae* on a green iguanas in Iran and the source of the infestation in the present iguana case was not known. In summary, this case suggests that fungal and parasitic co-infection with multiple organ involvement should be included as a possible etiology in the differential diagnosis of cutaneous infections in reptiles. Moreover, it also demonstrates diagnostic techniques available to aid in identification of fungal and parasitic agents in reptiles.

Acknowledgments

This study was funded by Research Council of Faculty of Veterinary Medicine, University of Tehran, Tehran, Iran.

References

1. Cabanes, F.J. (2000) Animal dermatophytosis. Recent advances. Rev Ibero Micol. 17: S8-12.

2. Chung, T.H., Kim, E.J., Choi, U.S.D. (2014) Multiorgan fungal infection caused by *Microsporum canis* in a green iguana (*Iguana iguana*). J Zoo Wildl Med. 45: 393-396.

3. Delfino, M.M.S., Ribeiro, S.C., Furtado, I.P., Anjos, L.A., Almeida, W.O. (2011) Pterygosomatidae and Trombiculidae mites infesting *Tropidurus hispidus* (Spix, 1825) (Tropiduridae) lizards in northeastern Brazil. Braz J Biol. 71: 549-555.

4. Farmaki, R., Simou, C., Papadopoulos, E., Koutinas, A.F., Saridomichelakis, M.N. (2013) Effectiveness of a single application of 0.25% fipronil solution for the treatment of hirstiellosis in captive green iguanas (*Iguana iguana*): an open-label study. Parasitology. 140: 1144-1148.

5. Gazyagci, R., Aktas, M.S., Sari, B. (2011) Theefirst record of the mite (*Hirstiella* sp.) on a green iguana from Turkey and its therapy with fipronil-a case report. Vet Arh. 81: 793-797.

6. Hoppmann, E., Barron, H.W. (2007) Dermatology in reptiles. J Exot Pet Med. 16: 210-224.

7. Khosravi, A.R., Shokri, H., Rostami, A., Tamai, I.A., Erfanmanesh, A., Memarian, I. (2012) Severe dermatophytosis due to *Trichophyton mentagrophytes* var. interdigitale in flocks of green iguanas (*Iguana iguana*). J Small Anim Pract. 53: 286-291.

8. Kostka, V.M., Hofmann, L., Balks, E., Eskens, U., Wimmershof, N. (1997) Review of the literature and investigations on the prevalence and consequences of yeasts in reptiles. Vet Rec. 140: 282-287.

9. Krantz, G.W., Walter, D.E. (2009) A Manual of Acarology. (3rd ed.) Texas Tech University Press; Lubbock, Texas, USA.

10. Mancianti, F., Nardoni, S., Cecchi, S., Corazza, M., Taccini, F. (2002) Dermatophytes isolated from asymptomatic dogs and cats in Tuscany, Italy during a 15-year period. Mycopathologia. 156: 13-18.

11. Murgas, D.A., Dutary, S.R., Miranda, R.J. (2013) First report of *Geckobiella stamii* (Acari: Pterygosomatidae) parasitizing *Iguana iguana* (Squamata: Iguanidae) in Panama. Rev Ibér Aracnol. 22: 97-98.

12. Nweze, E.I. (2010) Dermatophytoses in Western Africa: a review. Pakistan J Biol Sci. 13: 649-656.

13. Nweze, E.I. (2011) Dermatophytosis in domesticated animals. Rev Inst Med Trop. 53: 95-99.

14. Pare, J.A., Sigler, L., Rosenthal, K.L., Mader, D.R. (2006) Microbiology: fungal and bacterial diseases of reptiles. In: Reptile Medicine and Surgery. Mader, D.R. (ed.). (2nd ed.) Saunders Elsevier. St Louis, USA. p. 217-238.

15. Paredes-Leon, R., Klompen, H., Perez, T.M. (2012) Systematic revision of the genera Geckobiella Hirst, 1917 and Hirstiella Berlese, 1920 (Acari: Prostigmata: Pterygosomatidae) with description of a new genus for American species parasites on geckos formerly placed in Hirstiella. Zootaxa. 3510: 1-40.

16. Peterson, S. (2006) Skin Diseases of Exotic Pets. Blackwell Science. UK.

17. Schumacher, J. (2003) Fungal diseases of reptiles. Vet Clin North Am Exot Anim Pract. 6: 327-335.

18. Scott, D.W., Miller, W.H., Griffin, C.E. (2001) Parasitic Skin Diseases. Muller & Kirk's Small Animal Dermatology. (6th ed.) WB Saunders Co. Philadelphia, USA.

5

Isolation, phenotypic and molecular characterization of motile *Aeromonas* species, the cause of bacterial hemorrhagic septicemia in affected farmed carp in Iran

Soltani, M.[1*], Moghimi, S.M.[1], Ebrahimzade Mousavi, H.[1], Abdi, K.[2], Soltani, E.[3]

[1]*Department of Aquatic Animal Health, Faculty of Veterinary Medicine, University of Tehran, Tehran, Iran*

[2]*Aquatic Animal Health Expert, Office of Health and Control of Aquatic Animal Diseases, Iranian Veterinary Organization, Tehran, Iran*

[3]*Department of Microbiology, Faculty of Science, University of Tehran, Tehran, Iran*

Key words:

Farmed carp, Motile *Aeromonas* septicemia, 16S rRNA gene

Correspondence

Soltani, M.
Department of Aquatic Animal Health, Faculty of Veterinary Medicine, University of Tehran, Tehran, Iran

Email: msoltani@ut.ac.ir

Abstract:

BACKGROUND: Motile *Aeromonas* species cause heavy mortalities in carp farms during spring and summer in Iran. **OBJECTIVES:** The aim of this study was to detect phenotypic and genotypic characterization of motile *Aeromonas* species isolated from diseased carps in some northern and southern provinces of Iran. **METHODS:** A number of 40 samples from 22 fish farms were collected. The identified motile *Aeromonas* species were sequenced and phylogenetic tree was drawn by MEGA6 using UPGMA analysis. **RESULTS:** A number of 19 bacterial isolates were identified as motile *Aeromonas* sp. by biochemical tests, and the DNA segments of 16S rRNA gene of all these strains gave 1200 bp after running on 1% agarose electrophorus gel. Also, the sequencing results showed that the bacterial samples were determined as *A. hydrophila* and *A. veronii* biovar veronii. **CONCLUSIONS:** Phylogenetic analysis revealed that motile *Aeromonas* strains in this study were separated in two clusters and four genogroups with high similarities.

Introduction

Aeromonas hydrophila and other motile *Aeromonas* species which cause motile *Aeromonas* septicemia are known as the most common bacterial infections in freshwater aquaculture worldwide (Borrell et al., 1997; Leblanc, et al., 1981; Woo et al., 2011; Henebry et al., 1988). The species of *A. hydrophila*, *A. sobria*, *A. caviae* and *A. veronii* are the cause of carp mortalities (Popoff and VéEron, 1976; Garrity et al., 2004). Motile *Aeromonas* species cause some pathologic conditions including acute, chronic and latent infections with different clinical signs (Soltani, 2002). The disease occurrence is common in spring and summer in farmed carp that is related to high temperature, fish metabolism and organic loading rate (Soltani, 2002). According to the Iranian veterinary organization, the most epizootics occur in the north and south regions of Iran where the carp aquaculture is located (Iranian Veterinary Organization, unpublished data, 2011). So far, some epizootics of the disease have occurred in various species of carp in the north and south provinces (Peyghan and Esmaili, 1997; Soltani et al., 1998; Alishahi et al., 2009). Although the morphological and biochemical approaches have been applied to identify the genus *Aeromonas* in Iran, there is no adequate data on the phylogenetic position of the *Aeromonas* species involved in morbidity and mortality of carps. Therefore, the aim of this study was to isolate and characterize the motile *Aeromonas* species involved in carp mortality in the north and south regions of the country. Such data are useful for prevention and control criteria of disease and outbreaks.

Materials and Methods

Collection of bacterial isolates and phenotypic identification: After collecting 40 samples from different carp ponds, a total of 19 *Aeromonas* strains were isolated from common carp (*Cyprinus carpio*) and silver carp (*Hypophthalmichthys molitrix*) with clinical symptoms of bacterial infection such as hemorrhages in skin and gill, exophthalmia and dropsy. The samples were collected from three different geographical locations in Iran during a two-year period (2014 - 2015): 10 samples from Mazandaran province, 14 samples from Gilan province and 16 samples from Khuzestan province. The samples were isolated from kidney, cultivated on blood agar and incubated at 30°C for 72 h. First, the morphological characteristics of the colonies were identified by Gram staining which confirmed the bacterial colonies were Gram negative. Biochemical tests were carried out in all strains including SIM (Sulfide, Indole, and Motility), gelatin and esculin hydrolysis, lysine and ornothine decarboxylase, nitrate reduction, fermentation and gas production of glucose, maltose and inositol, triple sugar iron agar (TSI), methyl red and voges-proskauer (MRVP) tests.

DNA extraction: The DNA Biospin Bacteria Genomic Extraction Kit, Bioflux Co. (Gapan) was used to extract the genomic DNA. Briefly, a volume of 10 ml of culture was collected by centrifugation for 1min at 14000 g and resuspended in 100 µl of EL buffer incubated at 37°C for 40 min. Then RS buffer and PK solution were added, respectively and incubated at 56°C for 15 min. 200 µl of GA buffer was then added and centrifuged at

12,000 x g for 1 min and the supernatant was transferred to a new 1.5ml tube. An aliquot of 400 µl of BA buffer was then added and centrifuged at 10,000 x g for 1 min. A volume of, 500 µl of G binding buffer was then added into the spin column and centrifuged at 10,000 x g for 1 min. A volume of 500 µl of washing buffer was added to the spin column and centrifuged at 10,000 x g for 1 min two times. After transferring the spine column to a sterile 1.5ml micro centrifuge tube, 100 µl of elution buffer was added and the mixture was incubated at room temperature for 1 min, centrifuged at 12,000 x g for 1 min. The spin column was removed with the buffer in the micro centrifuge tube containing the DNA. The analysis of DNA concentration and quality were based on the 260 /280 nm and absorbance ratio using the spectrophotometer (Biophotometer Eppendorf) according to manufacturer's instructions. The solution was kept at -20°C when stored.

Polymerase chain reaction: The polymerase chain reaction was used to detect the presence of the 16S rRNA gene in all isolates. Briefly, the 25 µl PCR mix consisted of 2.5µl 10x reaction buffer, Fermentas Co. (Lithuania), 0.2U Taq polymerase, 1µl of the two primer solutions (forward: 5′-AGA GTT TGA TCA TGG CTC AG -3′; reverse: 5′-GGT TAC CTT GTT ACG ACT T-3′), 4µl mix dNTP (2.5mM each) and 1µl of DNA sample. PCR was carried out on the thermocycler Bio-Rad Co. (USA) performed the following cycles of denaturation at 94°C for 3 min followed by 35 cycles at 94°C for 1 min, annealing at 45°C for 1 min and extension at 72°C for 1/5 min and an extension cycle at 72°C was allowed for 10 min. Negative controls with no template DNA were included. Also, PCR products were electrophoresed in 1% agarose gel in TBE buffer. The gel was stained with GenDireX (Biohelix-USA) and photographed on a UV transilluminator XR-plus, Bio-Rad Co. (USA). The identified *Aeromonas* strains by 16S rRNA PCR analysis on 1% agarose gel electrophoresis were then sequenced directly by

Table 1. Biochemical characteristics of *A. hydrophila* isolates in this study.

Tests	M1	M2	M3	M4	G1	G2	G3	G4	G5	K1	K3	K4	K5	K7	K9
Indole	+	+	+	+	+	+	+	+	+	+	+	+	+	+	+
Motility	+	+	+	+	+	+	+	+	+	+	+	+	+	+	+
H2S	+	-	+	+	+	+	+	+	+	+	+	+	+	+	+
Gelatin hydrolysis	-	-	+	+	+	+	+	+	+	-	+	-	+	+	+
Ornithine decarboxylase	-	-	-	-	-	-	-	-	-	-	-	-	-	-	-
Nitrate reduction	+	+	+	+	+	+	+	+	+	+	+	+	+	+	+
MR	+	+	+	+	+	+	+	+	+	+	+	+	+	+	+
VP	+	+	+	+	+	+	+	+	+	+	+	+	+	+	+
TSI	-/+	-/-	-/-	-/-	-/-	-/+	+/+ Gas	+/+ Gas	+/+ Gas	+/+	+/+ Gas	+/+ Gas	+/+	+/+	+/+ Gas
Lysine decarboxilase	+	+	+	+	+	+	+	+	+	+	+	+	-	-	+
Esculin hydrolysis	+	+	-	-	+	+	+	+	+	+	+	+	+	+	+
Inositol fermentation	-	-	-	-	-	-	-	-	-	-	-	-	-	-	-
Maltose fermentation	+	+	+	+	+	+	+	+	+	-	-	-	-	-	-
Glucose fermentation	+	+	+	+	+	+	+	+	+	+	+	+	+	+	+
Gas production of glucose	+	-	-	-	+	+	-	-	-	-	-	-	-	-	-

Table 2. Biochemical characteristics of *A. veronii* isolates in this study.

Tests	K2	K6	K8	K10
Indole	+	+	+	+
Motility	+	+	+	+
H2S	+	+	+	+
Gelatin hydrolysis	-	+	+	+
Ornithine decarboxylase	-	-	-	-
Nitrate reduction	+	+	+	+
MR	+	+	+	+
VP	+	+	+	+
TSI	+/+	+/-	+/+	+/+
Lysine decarboxilase	+	+	+	+
Esculin hydrolysis	-	-	-	-
Inositol fermentation	-	-	-	-
Maltose fermentation	-	-	-	-
Glucose fermentation	-	+	+	+
Gas production of glucose	-	-	-	-

Takapouzist Co. (Tehran, Iran). The results were aligned by the Finch TV software and then compared with available sequences in GeneBank using BLAST service. The phylogenetic tree was drawn by MEGA6 using UPGMA analysis.

Results

Clinical signs and gross pathology: Fish samples collected from 22 farms showed distinct clinical signs of lethargy, anorexia, loss of balance, exophthalmia, ulcers, hemorrhages in skin and gill and abdominal distention (Figs. 1 and 2). Internally, the spleen was enlarged and hemorrhagic. Petechial hemorrhages were observed on the surface of kidney, intestines and many tissues. Also, accumulation of ascetic fluid was observed in almost all the diseased fish.

Biochemical tests: In primary phenotypic tests, grown colonies were gram negative, cocobacilli shaped, motile and oxidase positive which are supposed to be in genus *Aeromonas*. The results of the biochemical tests were compared with the key table in Bergey's manual systematic bacteriology to determine the species. The results are shown in Tables 1 and 2.

Analysis of 16S rRNA gene PCR: The results of PCR amplification of DNA from bacterial strains showed the expected amplicons of 1200 bp (Fig. 3).

Sequencing and phylogenetic analysis: The sequencing of the PCR products resulted in detection of KT378601, KT378602, KT378603, KT378604, KU201534,

Table 3. The Aeromonas strains isolated from carp ponds (sampling region, number of fish samples, number of isolated strains of motile Aeromonas, laboratory code and accession number).

Region	Number of fish samples	Number of isolates identified as Aeromonas sp.	Laboratory Code	Accession Number
Khuzestan State	16	10	K1, K2, K3,K4, K5,K6, K7, K8, K9, K10	KU201536, KU201537, KU201538, KU201539, KU201540, KU216160, KU216161, KU216162, KU216163, KU216164
Gilan State	14	5	G1, G2, G3 G4, G5	KT378601, KT378602, KU201534, KU201535, KU257639
Mazandaran State	10	4	M1, M2, M3, M4	KT378603, KT378604, KU257637, KU257638

KU201535, KU201536, KU201537, KU201538, KU216160, KU216161, KU216164, KU257637, KU257638 and KU257639 as *A. hydrophila* and KU201539, KU201540, KU216162 and KU216163 as *A. veronii* biovar veronii (Table 3). The MEGA 6 software has been applied to show the phylogenetic relationship between all isolates in this study (Fig. 4). According to the phylogenetic tree, high similarities were observed among motile *Aeromonas* species isolated from carps in Iran. The strains were classified in two clusters, A and B with 1.6% variations. There were two genogroups in cluster A, genogroup A1 and A1. In genogroup A1, the similarity between the strain, KU216163 and the other strains including KU216162, KU257637 and KU201154 was 99.4%. Also, the cluster A was divided to two genogroups, B1 and B2 with 99.3% similarity. In genogroup B1, the similarity between the two strains, KU216160 and KU216164 and the strains, KU216161, KU257637, KU 257638 and KU257639 was 99.5%. Also, the strains in genogroup B2 showed high similarities so that the similarity between the strain, KU201537 and the others strains was 99.5%.

Discussion

Recently, there have been many reports of heavy mortalities in carps during spring and summer in Iran. Although motile *Aeromonas* species are usually known as secondary opportunistic pathogens, they can be as primary pathogens in some conditions. So, there are no effective approaches for control and treatment of disease in carp farms since Aeromons infection is related to the environmental conditions and physicochemical parameters of water. Therefore, isolation and identification of the bacteria would be useful for control and prevention of disease. Today, molecular techniques are used widely since they provide a relatively rapid and highly sensitive method for the detection of bacterial pathogens (Chu and Lu, 2005). In this regard the most commonly used gene for taxonomic and phylogenetic purposes in bacteria is the 16S rRNA which is the most conserved gene in bacteria (Clarridge, 2004; Roy et al., 2013). In the present study, various biochemical tests have been applied to identify 40 clinical isolates of motile *Aeromonas* sp. Also, 19 isolates have been characterized as motile *Aeromonas* sp. by PCR analysis of 16S rRNA gene. Most results from both approaches have shown similarities, however, some discrepancies have been observed. Four strains, KT378602, KU257637, KU257638 and KT378603 that were characterized as *A. veronii* biochemically (esculin hydrolysis negative), were identified by PCR and DNA sequencing as *A. hydrophila*. Also, the gelatin hydrolysis test was negative in five

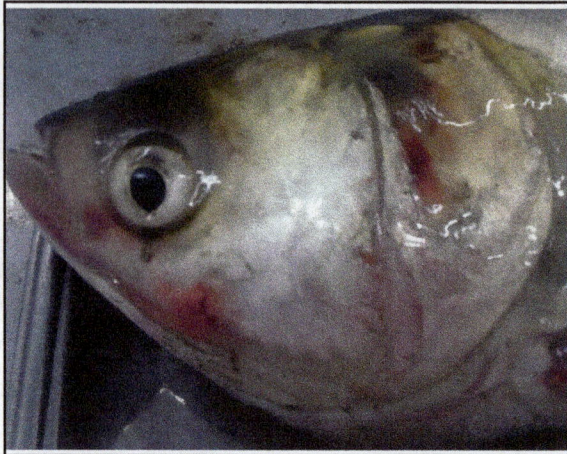

Figure 1. Skin hemorrhage and exophthalmia of silver carp (H. molitrix).

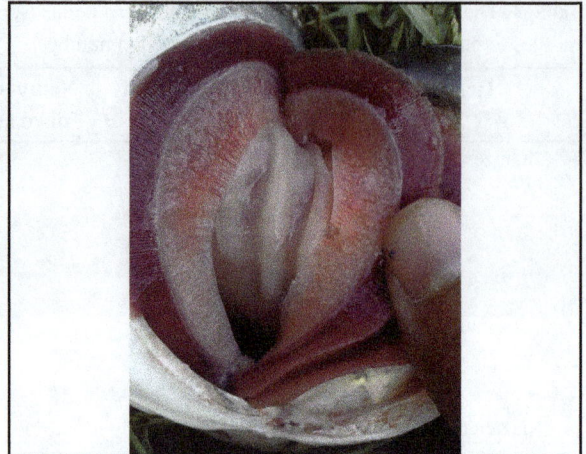

Figure 2. Hemorrhage in gill filaments of silver carp (H. molitrix).

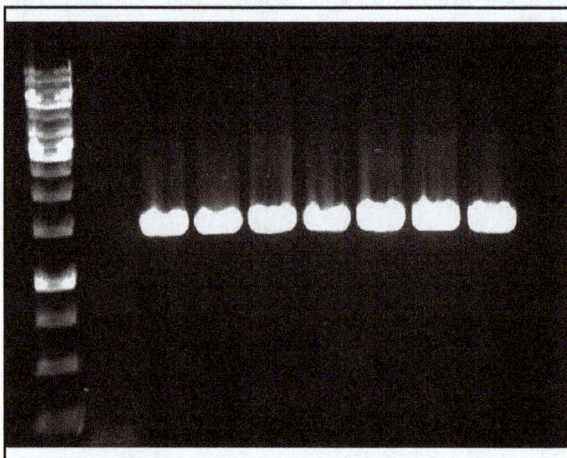

Figure 3. PCR detection of 16S rRNA genes in several Aeromonas recovered from diseased carp in Iran. Lane M= 1 kbp DNA ladder, Lane 1= negative control, Lane 2= positive control (Aeromonas hydrophila - IRTCC1032), Lane 3 to 8= several test samples.

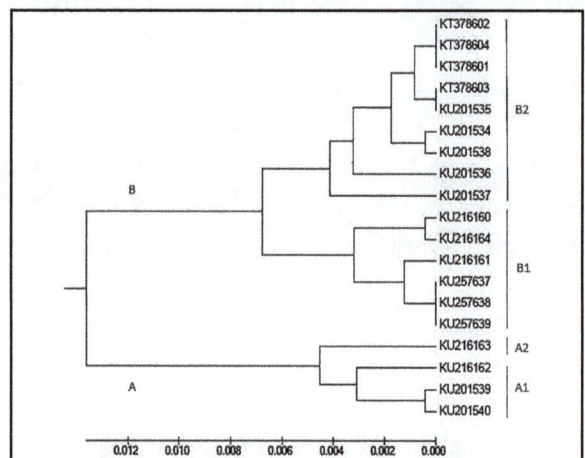

Figure 4. Phylogenetic analysis of Aeromonas strains based on the 16S rRNA sequences using UPGMA method.

strains, KT378601, KT378602, KU216160 and KU201537 and KU201439. But they identified phylogenetically as *A. hydrophila* and *A. veronii*. These results were confirmed by repeating the tests. Such discrepancies may result from the fact that biochemical tests are not reliable for identification of *Aeromonas* sp.. Other strains showed the same results in both biochemical and molecular tests. The phylogenetic tree of 19 bacterial isolates of this study showed 97.2-100% similarity based on the analysis of 16S rRNA gene. Such similarities among the isolates of the country can be applied to promote some prevention methods like vaccination.

Alzahrani (2015) used the 16S rRNA gene to identify and characterize *Aeromonas* species in drinking water since this gene is known as a specific molecular marker for bacterial identification and is useful for the bacterial molecular taxonomy. The results showed that all bacterial samples were *A. veronii* or a new species. Moreover, classical tests as well as molecular studies on the 16S rRNA gene have been applied by Sarkar et al. (2012) for classification of the phylogenetic relationships among *Aeromonas* species isolated from various sources. The biochemical and molecular results were similar to those of the present study and the isolates registered in GeneBank were used for comparison with the isolates of this study by using MEGA6 software. The results showed similarities in 16S rRNA sequences of the strains even though the samples have been collected from different sources. Arora et al. (2006) applied several methods to identify *Aeromonas* species and concluded that both indirect ELISA and duplex-PCR are reliable methods to detect *Aeromonas* species in foods of animal origin due to their specificity and duplex-PCR is the best method among others used in the study on account of its rapidity, sensitivity and specificity. Borrel et al. (1997) used the same gene to identify *Aeromonas* species from different clinical samples such as blood, soft tissue infection and urine. Most results from the biochemical tests and RFLP method were similar but some discrepancies were seen. For instance, some species detected biochemically as *A. veronii* were characterized as *A. hydrophila* and *A. caviae* by RFLP analysis. In conclusion, the RFLP method is proposed as a rapid and reliable method without the need for sequencing to identify *Aeromonas* species. In addition to the 16S rRNA gene, many virulence genes have been detected to identify *Aeromonas* species (Sechi et al., 2002; Yogananth et al., 2009; Uma et al., 2010; Cagatay and Şen, 2014; Hussain et al., 2014). Among the virulence factors of motile *Aeromonas* species, antigen-O, the presence of capsule, S layer, exotoxins such as hemolysins and enterotoxins, exoenzymes such as lipase, amylase and protease and the type III secretion system are well known (Oliveira et al., 2012). Hussain et al. (2014) studied the ahh1, asa1 and 16S rRNA genes by using multiplex PCR to detect the hemolytic strains of *Aeromonas* isolated from fish and fishery products. The results proved the presence of 16S rRNA and asa1 genes in *A. sobria*, 16S rRNA and ahh1 genes in *A. hydrophila* and 16S rRNA gene in *A. liquifaciencs* and provided reliable data to detect the hemolytic strains of *Aeromonas*. In the study of Cagatay and Şen (2014) on the virulence genes of *A. hydrophila* regarding the cause of bacterial hemorrhagic septicemia

in rainbow trout, the AHCYTOEN, Hly and OmpTS genes have been detected. All these genes were detected in the *Aeromonas* strains and are known as specific virulence determinants and genetic markers to identify the bacteria before the disease spread. Biochemical tests as well as PCR for detecting the aerolysin and hemolysin genes of *Aeromonas* strains have been carried out by Yoganath et al. (2009) in which seven strains of 15 strains have been identified as *A. hydrophila*. The PCR assay applied in this study was known as a useful tool to detect the aerolysin and hemolysin genes which can be the genetic virulence markers. A similar study has been done by Uma et al. (2010) that indicated the aerolysin and hemolysin genes are a better indicator of the potential health risk since the pathogenicity of *Aeromonas* strains is associated with such virulence factors. Besides the molecular and biochemical tests, the LD50 determination can be used to identify the virulent *Aeromonas* strains, as Alishahi et al. (2009) applied this method to detect the pathogenic motile *Aeromonas* species. The results showed the presence of *A. hydrophila* (%11), *A. veronii* (%4) and *A. sobria* (%2.7) from a total of 300 samples. Also, *Aeromonas* species were known as the secondary pathogens since they have not presented enough virulence needs for mortalities.

Furthermore, motile *Aeromonas* infection is related to the physicochemical parameters of water quality which can exacerbate the disease outbreaks. In the present study, water temperature was higher than the standard levels and the acidity of water was in the maximum range. Other parameters including dissolved oxygen, carbon dioxide, total hardness as calcium carbonate, nitrite, nitrate and total dissolved solids were in the normal ranges. According to previous studies on detecting *Aeromonas* sp. in carp ponds, this bacteria was known as a secondary pathogen and the disease can occur at stress conditions (Alishahi et al., 2009). Recently, the motile *Aeromonas* species have been isolated from warm water fish in Iran and numerous factors can be associated with the incidence of the disease. Some of these factors were mentioned in the following: The temperature in summer is more than 40 °C as a result of climate change and the ammonia level and the acidity of water occasionally increase in warm weather. Also, the atmospheric pressure decreases in summer and as a result the water capacity to keep oxygen reduces. Another reason of reducing the dissolved oxygen level is toxins produced by algae which increase the organic loading range in water. Further, unsuitable structure of fish ponds leads to an inadequate water exchange and prevent refilling water. Waste water is periodically used for filling the ponds. The organic loading rate increases by the use of animal-based fertilizer in feeding fish. Besides, the owners do not pay attention to the rules and regulations defined by the responsible organizations about the control and prevention of the disease in summer. In this regard, several methods are suggested to prevent the disease such as systematically preparing the ponds before new larva and fish are put into the ponds, water filtration, quarantine process and collecting the dead fish on a daily basis and reporting the mortality rate to the veterinary organization.

In addition, the carp species are sensitive to some viral diseases such as Spring Viremia of Carp (SVC) and Koi Herpes Virus (KHV). Recently, several fresh water ornamental fishes were imported to the country for research aims and experimental studies. SVCV and KHV were detected in the imported ornamental fishes (Soltani, unpublished data, 2012; Zamani et al., 2014). So occurrence of the viral diseases in carp pond is possible and needs further studies.

Acknowledgments

This work was financially supported by Iranian Veterinary Organization, Center of Excellence of Aquatic Animal Health and Research Council of University of Tehran.

References

1. Alishahi, M., Soltani, M., Zargar, A. (2009) Study of the mortality of grass carp (*Ctenopharyngodon idella*) in Khuzestan province. Iran Vet J. 4: 25-34.
2. Borrell, N., Acinas, S.G., Figueras, M.J., Martinez-Murcia, A.J. (1997) Identification of Aeromonas clinical isolates by restriction fragment length polymorphism of PCR-amplified 16S rRNA genes. J Clin Microbiol. 35: 1671-1674.
3. Brenner, D.J., Krieg, N.R., Staley, J.T. (2005) Bergey's Manual of Sustematic Bacteriology (2nd ed.). Baltimore, USA.
4. Cagatay, I.T., Sen, E.B. (2014) Detection of pathogenic *Aeromonas hydrophila* from rainbow trout (*Oncorhynchus mykiss*) farms in Turkey. Intl J Agric Biol. 16: 435-438.
5. Chu, W.H., Lu, C.P. (2005) Multiplex PCR assay for the detection of pathogenic *Aeromonas hydrophila*. J Fish Dis. 28: 437-441.
6. Clarridge, J.E. (2004) Impact of 16S rRNA gene sequence analysis for identification of bacteria on clinical microbiology and infectious diseases. Clin Microbiol Rev. 17: 840-862.
7. Garrity, G.M., Bell, J.A., Lilburn, T.G. (2004) Taxonomic Outline of the Prokaryotes. Bergey's Nanual of Systematic Bacteriology. (2nd ed.). New York, USA.
8. Henebry, M.S., Gorden, R.W., Buck, D.H. (1988) Bacterial populations in the gut of the silver carp (*Hypophthalmichthys molitrix*). Prog Fish Cult. 50: 86-92.
9. Hussain, I., Jeyasekaran, G., Shakila, R.J., Raj, K., Jeevithan, E. (2014) Detection of hemolytic strains of *Aeromonas hydrophila* and *A. sobria* along with other *Aeromonas* spp. from fish and fishery products by multiplex PCR. J Food Sci Technol. 51: 401-407.
10. Leblanc, D., Mittal, K., Olivier, G., Lallier, R. (1981) Serogrouping of motile Aeromonas species isolated from healthy and moribund fish. Appl Environ Microb. 42: 56-60.

11. Oliveira, S.T., Veneroni-Gouveia, G., Costa, M.M. (2012) Molecular characterization of virulence factors in *Aeromonas hydrophila* obtained from fish. Pesquisa Vet Brasil. 32: 701-706.

12. Peyghan, R., Esmaili, F. (1997) Infection of the grass carp with the motile Aeromonas like microrganism. J Fish. 6: 1-8.

13. Popoff, M., VéEron, M. (1976) A taxonomic study of the *Aeromonas hydrophila-Aeromonas punctata* group. J Gen Microbiol. 94: 11-22.

14. Roy, R.P., Bahadur, M., Barat, S. (2013) Isolation, identification and Antibiotic resistance of *Aeromonas* spp. and *Salmonella* spp. from the fresh water loach, *Lepidocephalichthys guntea* and water of Terai River Lotchka, West Bengal, India. Zool Pol. 58: 5-17.

15. Sarkar, A., Saha, M., Roy, P. (2012) Identification and typing of *Aeromonas Hydrophila* through 16S rDNA-PCR finger printing. J Aquacult Res Dev. 3: 1-5.

16. Sechi, L.A., Deriu, A., Falchi, M.P., Fadda, G., Zanetti, S. (2002) Distribution of virulence genes in *Aeromonas* spp. isolated from Sardinian waters and from patients with diarrhoea. J Appl Microbiol. 92: 221-227.

17. Soltani, M. (2002) Fish bacterial diseases. (1st ed.). Published by Iranian Veterinary Oraganization Press, Tehran, Iran.

18. Soltani, M., Mirzargar, S.S., Ebrahimzadeh Maboud, H. (1998) Occurrence of the *Aeromonas septicemia* in the ornamental fish, oscar (*Astronotus ocellatus*), isolation, characterization and pathogenicity. Iran J Vet Med. 53: 62-65.

19. Uma, A., Rebecca, G., Meena, S., Saravanabava, K. (2010) PCR detection of putative aerolysin and hemolysin genes in an *Aeromonas hydrophila* isolate from infected Koi carp (Cyprinus carpio). Tamil J Vet Anim Sci. 6: 31-33.

20. Woo, P.T.K., Leatherland, J.F., Bruno, D.W. (2011). Fish Diseases and Disorders (2nd ed.). Cambridge, UK.

21. Yogananth, N., Bhakyaraj, R., Chanthuru, A., Anbalagan, T., Nila, K.M. (2009) Detection of virulence gene in *Aeromonas hydrophila* isolated from fish samples using PCR technique. Global J Biotech Biochem. 4: 51-53.

22. Zamani, H., Ghasemi, M., Hosseini, S., Karsidani, S.H. (2014) Experimental susceptibility of Caspian white fish, *Rutilus frisii kutum* to Spring viraemia of carp virus. Virus Dis. 25: 57-62.

6

Antibacterial effect of thiazole derivatives on *Rhodoccocus equi*, *Brucella abortus*, and *Pasteurella multocida*

Ghasemi B.[1], Najimi, M.[2*]

[1]*Gratuated from the Faculty of Veterinary Medicine, University of Zabol, Zabol, Iran*
[2]*Department of Pathobiology, Faculty of Veterinary Medicine, University of Zabol, Zabol, Iran*

Key words:

antibacterial activity, *B. abrotus*, *P. multocida*, *R. equi*, thiazole derivatives

Correspondence

Najimi, M.
Department of Pathobiology,
Faculty of Veterinary Medicine,
University of Zabol, Zabol, Iran

Email: najimi.mohsen@gmail.com

Abstract:

BACKGROUND: *Rhodoccocus equi*, *Brucella abortus*, and *Pasteurella multocida* are important veterinary bacterial pathogens that in recent years have been resisted to current antibiotics, and this problem threats the livestock industry. To control this resistant microorganisms, use of new antibacterial compounds, such as thiazole derivatives, in veterinary is necessary. **OBJECTIVES:** In this study, antibacterial effects of thiazole derivatives on *Rhodoccocus equi*, *Brucella abortus*, and *Pasteurella multocida* were evaluated. **METHODS:** Synthesized thiazole derivatives were prepared in DMSO, then the disk diffusion method was used to measure growth inhibition zone diameter and the broth microdilution method was applied to determine the minimum inhibitory concentration (MIC). **RESULTS:** Results showed that thiazole derivatives had no significant inhibitory effects on *B. abrotus*, while they had inhibitory effects on *R. equi* and *P. multocida* with inhibition zone 12.7±0.4 -30.1±0.2 mm and MICs 32- 256 μg/ml. **CONCLUSIONS:** Results of this study indicate that thiazole derivatives have considerable inhibitory effects on *R. equi* and *P. multocida* as veterinary bacterial pathogens.

Introduction

Rhodoccocus equi, *Brucella abrotus*, and *Pasteurella multocida* are important veterinary bacterial pathogens that cause high mortality rates and economic losses in the livestock industry (Adesiyun et al., 2011; Bakavoli et al., 2009; Bakavoli et al; 2011). Development of bacterial resistant in these microorganisms to current antibiotics, such as ciprofloxacin, trimethoprim, and tetracycline have caused serious problems in veterinary in recent years and use of new antibacterial compounds is the best solution for this problem (Bondock et al., 2010; Bondock et al., 2013; Brvar et al., 2010). One of these novel antimicrobials is thiazole derivatives. These derivatives perceive to have multi-therapeutic effects and they have been utilized in treatment of cancer, blood fat, blood pressure, and HIV infection (Chementi et al., 2011). Strong antioxidant and anti-inflammatory effects of thiazoles have been proven (Cheng et al., 2013; Coleman et al., 2010).

In laboratory, thiazoles have shown the ability to kill anopheles insects (Helul et al., 2013). Thiazole derivatives have inhibitory effects on Trypanosoma and *Candida* spp. (Horohov et al., 2011; Jaishree et al., 2013). Thiazole derivatives can inhibit the growth of a variety of gram-positive and gram-negative bacteria, including *Escherichia coli*, *Staphylococcus epidermidis*, *Staphylococcus aureus*,

Streptococcus pyogenes, *Enterococcus faecalis* and *Pseudomonas fluorescens*. Strong and wide range of antibacterial properties of thiazole derivatives has generally made the antibacterial test to be among the initial experiments that is studied after synthesizing these agents in many countries (Juspin et al., 2010; Katsuda et al., 2013. Very few studies on thiazole antibacterial effects against these veterinary bacterial pathogens have been published. In the current study, the antibacterial effects of thiazole derivatives on *R. equi*, *P. multocida*, and *B. abortus* were assessed.

Materials and Methods

Preparation of thiazole derivatives: The number 6a-d of thiazole derivative was incorporated in a three-phase process and its chemical structure was verified with monocrystalline X-ray diffraction, HNMR, CNMR, IR, element decomposition, and spectrometry. Afterwards, this derivative was dissolved in the DMSO solvent with the concentration of 8192 µg/ml (7).

Synthesis of 2-[(E)-(benzo[d]thiazol-2(3H)-ylidene)(cyano)methyl]thiazoles (10a-c); the number 10a-c of thiazole derivative was incorporated in a three-phase process and its chemical structure was verified with monocrystalline X-ray diffraction, HNMR, CNMR, IR, element decomposition, and spectrometry. Afterwards, this derivative was dissolved in the DMSO solvent with the concentration of 8192 µg/ml (Khalil et al., 2009).

Bacterial suspensions: *Rhodococcus equi* ATCC 33701, *P. multocida* ATCC 12948, and *B. abortus* ATCC 23448 were provided by the Faculty of Veterinary Medicine, University of Shiraz. Each bacterium was cultured in Mueller-Hinton agar medium in 37°C for 24 hours. Henceforth, in sterile conditions of Mueller-Hinton medium and in logarithmic growth phase, a concentration of 0.5 McFarland (1.5 × 108 CFU/ml) was obtained with spectropho-

tometer and standard McFarland tube number 0.5 from each bacterium which is assigned as a stock solution (Kofteridis et al., 2009).

Minimum inhibition concentration (MIC): The MIC test was done in a sterile 96-well plates by broth micro dilution as CLSI standard. First, 100 µl of Muller-Hinton broth medium (Merck®, Germany) was added to each well. Then, 100 µl of thiazole derivatives (in control groups, 100 µl of penicillin and gentamycin antibiotics (Sigma®)) were added to the first well and, after mixing, 100 µl of this mixture was embedded into the second well. Similarly, dilution procedure was done in other wells. 10 µl of bacterial suspension was added to each well. For negative control 100 µl of Muller-Hinton broth, 100 µl DMSO and 10 µl of bacterial suspension were added to the last well in each row. The result of incubation was read after 24 hours incubation in 37°C. The lucidity and turbidity in each well indicated lack or existence of bacterial growth, respectively. The last well that did not show any turbidity was reported as MIC (Kofteridis et al., 2009).

Inhibition zone diameter: First, in Muller-Hinton agar medium, the superficial bacterial culture was performed with a swab impregnated to bacterial suspension. 20 µl of obtained MIC thiazole derivatives and also antibiotics was shed on blank sterile disks. For negative control, the DMSO-impregnated disk was used. Then, after 24 hours incubation in 37°C, the growth inhibition zone diameter was measured with particular ruler. The results of growth inhibition zone diameter have been provided as average ± standard deviation and for the aim of analyzing the data, the SPSS statistical software (version 22) was used (Kofteridis et al., 2009).

Results

Thiazole derivatives showed no significant inhibitory effects on *B. abortus*; also 6a-c, 10a and 10c did not have inhibitory effects on any

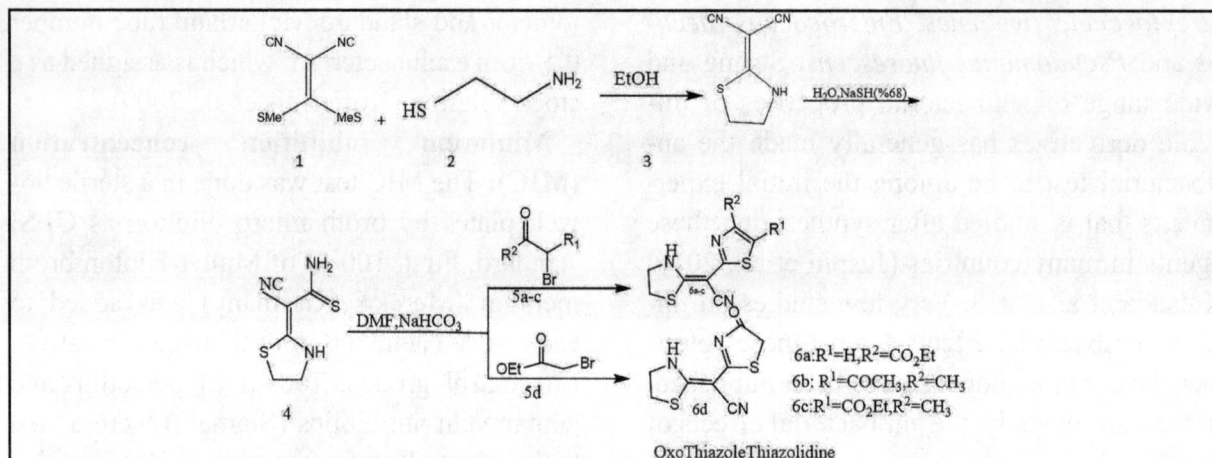

Scheme 1. Synthesis of 2-(E)-cyano(thiazolidin-2-ylidene)thiazoles (6a-d) (derivative from reference No. 7).

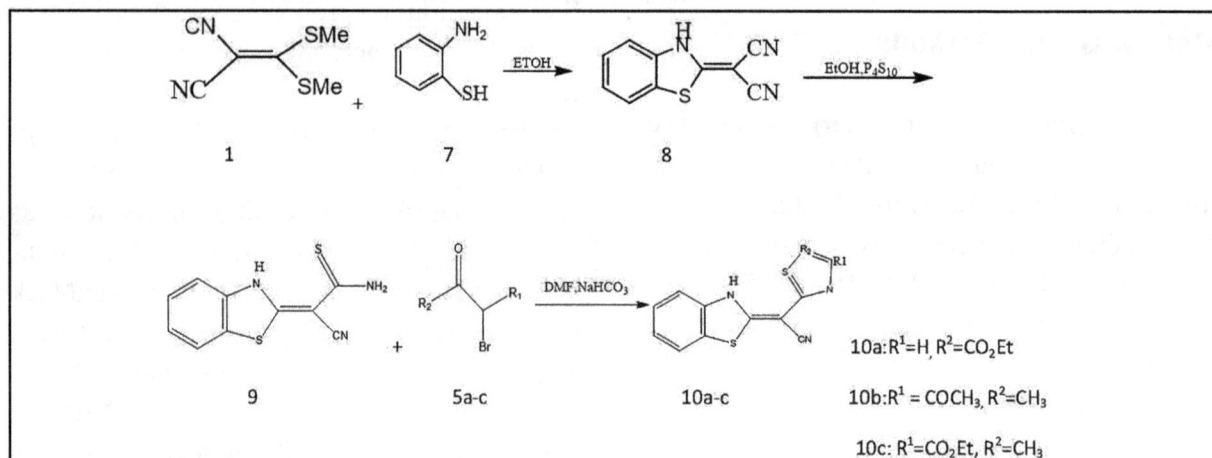

Scheme2. Synthesis of 2-[(E)-(benzo[d]thiazol-2(3H)-ylidene)(cyano)methyl]thiazoles (10a-c) (Bakavoli et al., 2015).

bacterial tested. Just the two derivatives 6d and 10b showed inhibitory effects on *R. equi* and *P. multocida*. The maximum inhibitory effects on *R. equi* and *P. multocida* belonged to derivatives 6d and 10b with MIC of 64 and 32 μg/ml respectively. Ampicillin and neomycin had the maximum and minimum inhibitory effects on *R. equi*, respectively and penicillin and nalidixic acid had the maximum and minimum inhibitory effects on *P. multocida*, respectively. In antibiogram test, the most and the least susceptibility were recorded for *P. multocida* to penicillin with MIC of 0.5 μg/ml and for *B. abortus* to penicillin with MIC of 16 μg/ml (Tables 1 and 2).

Discussion

Thiazole derivatives are novel antibacterial compounds which promise good replacements for some antibacterial drugs. In the current study, inhibitory effects of eight thiazole derivatives have been assessed on three veterinary bacterial pathogens. Results show that the maximum inhibitory effect against *R. equi* belongs to derivative 6d. The structural study of this derivative shows that this compound includes thiazolidine ring as well as thiazole ring. This thiazolidine ring is similar to that of penicillin family of antibiotics. However, this derivative is expected to affect beta-lactamase producing bacteria due to the lack of a beta-lactam ring (Lv et al., 2009).

Thiazolidines are a novel class of antibacterial agents which include inhibitory effects on a broad-spectrum of gram-positive bacteria, such as streptococci and staphylococci. The inhibitory effect of thiazolidine derivatives on *S.*

Table 1. Bacterial growth inhibitory zone (mm) of the thiazole derivatives and antibiotics on studied bcteria. - absence of inhibition effect.

Deriva-tives/Drugs	R. equi ATCC 33701	P. multocida ATCC 12948	B. abortus ATCC 23448
6a-c	-	-	-
6d	25.6±0.1	26.3±0.0	-
10a	-	-	-
10b	12.7±0.4	30.1±0.2	-
10c	-	-	-
Gentamicin	25.4±0.3	21.2±0.0	16.3±0.2
Penicillin	27.2±0.5	30.5±0.3	22.1±0.1

Table 2. MICs (μg/ml) of thiazole derivatives and antibiotics on studied bcteria. - absence of inhibition effect.

Derivatives/ Drugs	R. equi ATCC 33701	P. multocida ATCC 12948	B. abortus ATCC 23448
6a-c	-	-	-
6d	64	64	-
10a	-	-	-
10b	256	32	-
10c	-	-	-
Gentamicin	1	8	2
Penicillin	2	0.5	16

faecalis and *S. aureus* has been proven (Majiduddin et al., 2002). Furthermore, the study of derivatives 6a-c has shown that only derivative 6d contains oxygen bonds with thiazole, resulting in the production of oxothiazole. Moreover, this derivative is the only compound within derivatives 6a-d that includes inhibitory effects on *R. equi* and *P. multocida*. Zaky and Yousef have shown that oxothiazole derivatives are able to inhibit the growth of *E. coli* (Patel et al., 2012).

Benzo[d]thiazole derivative 10b had a powerful inhibition on *P. multocida*. The important structure in this compound is benzothiazole. Antibacterial effect on gram-negtive bacteria, for example *Escherichia coli* and *Salmonella typhi*, were shown from derivatives which have benzothiazole in their structure (Shirharsha 2006). MICs of thiazole derivatives have demonstrated the ability of these compounds

to significantly inhibit the growth of *Pseudomonas aeruginosa*, *S. aureus*, and *B. subtilis*, compared to penicillin G and kanamycin.

Results have also shown that these derivatives have higher inhibition effects with MICs of 12.5-100 μg/ml. Derivatives within the current study possibly include excited Cl and Br in thiazole ring and, therefore, show intensified inhibitory effects (Venugolpa et al., 2013). In a study by Zaky and Yousef (2011), MIC and inhibition zone of thiazole derivatives on *S. aureus* and *P. aeruginosa* were assessed and showed high antibacterial effects, compared to gentamicin as control (Zaky and Yousef, 2011). Furthermore, high inhibitory effects of thiazole derivatives on bacterial pathogens, such as *Bacillus thuringiensis* and *E. coli*, as well as *S. aureus*, *S. pyogenes*, *Proteus vulgaris* and *Klebsiella pneumonia*, have been studied using growth inhibition zone (Zelisko et al., 2013; Zhang et al., 2013).

In recent studies, inhibition of DNA or enzyme has been proposed as the influential mechanism of thiazole derivatives to inhibit bacteria. The inhibition of one enzyme, ecKA-SIII (or FabH) that is essential for synthesis of fatty acids in gram-negative and gram-positive bacteria, and DNA Gyrase, that is needed to replicate DNA, has been studied. Noting that Quinolone family antibiotics and thiazole derivatives could inhibit subunit A and subunit B of DNA Gyrase enzyme, respectively, has increasingly promised the inhibition of Quinolone-resistant bacteria by thiazole derivatives (Zitouni et al., 2003).

Conclusion: Few studies have been published on antibacterial effects of thiazole derivatives against veterinary bacterial pathogens. In this study, antibacterial effect of thiazole derivatives was proved against *R. equi*, *P. multocida*, and clinical use of these compounds needs in vivo studies for detection therapeutic and toxicity effects of them.

Acknowledgments

The authors wish to thank Prof. Zahraei Salehi, Department of Pathobiology, Faculty of Veterinary Medicine, University of Tehran; Dr Tabatabei, Faculty of Veterinary Medicine, University of Shiraz; and Mrs. Sargolzaei within the Microbiology Laboratory of the Faculty of Veterinary Medicine, University of Zabol.

References

1. Adesiyun, A.A., Baird, K., Johnson, A.S. (2011) Antimicrobial resistance, phenotypic characteristics and phage types of *B. abortus* strains isolated from cattle and water buffalo (*Bubalus bubalis*) in Trinidad. Vet Arch. 81: 391-404.

2. Bakavoli, M., Beyzaei, H., Rahimizadeh, M., Eshghi, H., Takjoo, R. (2009) Regioselective synthesis of new 2-(E)-cyano (thiazolidin-2-ylidene) thiazoles. Molecules. 14: 4849-4857.3.

3. Bakavoli, M., Beyzaei, H., Rahimizadeh, M., Eshghi, H. (2011) Regioselective synthesis of 2[(E)(benzo[d]thiazol2(3H)ylidene)(cyano) methyl]thiazoles. Heterocycl Comm. 17: 151-154.

4. Bondock, S., Fadaly, W., Metwally, M.A. (2010) Synthesis and antimicrobial activity of some new thiazole, thiophene and pyrazole derivatives containing benzothiazole moiety. Eur J Med Chem. 45: 3692-3701.

5. Bondock, S., Naser, T., Ammar, Y.A. (2013) Synthesis of some new 2-(3-pyridyl)-4,5-disubstituted thiazoles as potent antimicrobial agents. Eur J Med Chem. 62: 270-279.

6. Brvar, M., Perdih, A., Oblak, M., Masic, L.P., Solmajer, T. (2010) In silico discovery of 2-amino-4-(2,4-dihydroxyphenyl) thiazoles as novel inhibitors of DNA gyrase B. Bioorg Med Chem Lett. 20: 958-962

7. Chementi, F., Bizzarri, B., Bolasco, A., Secci, D., Chimenti, P., Granese, A., Carradori, S., D'Ascenzio, M., Lilli, D., Rivanera, D. (2011) Synthesis and biological evaluation of novel 2,4-disubstituted-1,3-thiazoles anti *Candida* ssp. agents. Eur J Med Chem. 46: 378-382.

8. Cheng, K.,Xue, K.J., Zhu, H.L. (2013) Design, synthesis and antibacterial activity studies o thiazole derivatives as potent eckAS III inhibitors. Bioorg Med Chem Lett. 23: 4235-4238.

9. Coleman, M., Kuskie K., Liu, M., Chaffin, K., Libal, M., Giguere, S., Bernstein, L., Cohen, N. (2010) In vitro antimicrobial activity of gallium maltolate against virulent *Rhodococcus equi*. Vet Microbiol. 146: 175-178.

10. Helul, M.H.M., Salem, M.A., El-Gaby, M.S.A., Aljahdali, M. (2013) Synthesis and biological evaluation of some novel thiazole compounds as potential anti-inflammatory agents. Eur J Med Chem. 65: 517-526.

11. Horohov, D.W., Loynachan, A.T., Page, A.E., Hughes, K., Timoney, J.F., Fettinger, M., Hatch, T., Spaulding, J.G., McMichael, J. (2011) The use of streptolysin O (SLO) as an adjunct therapy for *Rhodococcus equi* pneumonia in foals. Vet Microbiol. 154: 156-162.

12. Jaishree, V., Ramdas, N., Sachin, J., Ramesh, B. (2013) In vitro antioxidant properties of new thiazole derivatives. J Saudi Chem Soc. 16: 371-376.

13. Juspin, T., Laget, M.L., Terme, T., Azas, N., Vanelle, P. (2010) TDAE-assisted synthesis of new imidazol[2,1-b]thiazole derivatives as anti-infectious agents. Eur J Med Chem. 45: 840-845.

14. Katsuda, K., Hoshinoo, K., Ueno, Y., Kohmoto, M., Mikami, O. (2013) Virulence genes and antimicrobial susceptibility in *Pasteurella multocida* isolates from calves. Vet Microbiol. 167: 737-741.

15. Khalil, A., Berghot, M., Gouda, M. (2009) Synthesis and antibacterial activity of some new thiazole and thiophene derivatives. Eur J Med Chem. 44: 4434-4440.

16. Kofteridis, D.P., Christofaki, M., Mantadakis, E., Maraki, S., Drygiannakis, I., Papadakis, J.A., Samonis, G. (2009) Bacteremic community-acquired pneumonia due to *Pasteurella*

multocida. Int J Infect Dis. 13: 81-83.

17. Lv P.C., Wang, K.R., Yang, Y., Mao, W.J., Chen, J., Xiong. J., Zhu, H.L. (2009) Design, synthesis and biological evaluation of novel thiazole derivatives as potent FabH inhibitors. Bioorg Med Chem Lett. 19: 6750-6754.

18. Majiduddin, F.K., Materon, I.C., Palzkill, T.G. (2002) Molecular analysis of beta-lactamase structure and function. Int J Med Microbiol. 292: 127-137.

19. Patel, R., Patel, P.K., Kumari, P., Rajani, D.P., Chikhalia, K.H. (2012) Synthesis of benzimid-azolyl-1,3,4-oxadiazol-2ylthio-N-phenyl (benzothiazolyl) acetamides as antibacterial, antifungal and antituberculosis agents. Eur J Med Chem. 53: 41-51.

20. Sriharsha, S.N., Satish, S., Shashikanth, S., Raveesha, K.A. (2006) Design, synthesis antibacterial activity of novel 1,3-thiazolidine pyrimidine nucleoside analogues. Bioorg Med Chem. 14: 7476-7481.

21. Venugopla, K.N., Krishnappa, M., Nayak, S.K., Subruhmany, B.K., Vaderapura, J.P., Chalannavar, R.K., Gleiser, R.M., Odhav, B. (2013) Synthesis and antimosquito properties of 2,6-substituted benzo[d] thiazole and 2,4-substituted benzo[d]thiazole analogues against anopheles arabiensis. Eur J Med Chem. 65: 295-303.

22. Zaky, R.R., Yousef, T.A. (2011) Spectral, magnetic, thermal, molecular modelling, ESR studies and antimicrobial activity of (E)-3-(2-(2-hydroxybenzylidene) hydrazinyl)-3-oxo-n (thiazole-2-yl) propanamide complexes. J Mol Struct. 1002: 76-85.

23. Zelisko, N., Atamanyuk, D., Vasylenko, O., Grellier, P., Lesyk, R. (2013) Synthesis and antytripanosoma activity of new 6,6,7-trisubstituted thiopyranol [2,3-d][1,3] thiazoles. Bioorg Med Chem Lett. 22: 7071-7074.

24. Zhang, M., Han, X., Liu, H, Tian, M., Ding, C., Song, J., Sun, X., Liu, Z., Yu, S. (2013) Inactivation of the ABC transporter ATPase gene in *Brucella abortus* strain 2308 attenuated the virulence of the bacteria. Vet Microbiol. 164,

322-329.

25. Zitouni, G.T., Demirayak. S., Ozdemir, A., Kaplancikli, Z.A., Yıldız, M.T. (2003) Synthesis of some 2-[(benzazole-2-yl) thioacetylamino] thiazole derivatives and their antimicrobial activity and toxicity. Eur J Med Chem. 39: 267-272.

7

Molecular characterization of canine parvovirus (CPV) antigenic variants from healthy and diarrheic dogs in Urmia region, Iran

Dastmalchi Saei, H.[1*], Javadi, S.[2], Akbari, S.[3], Hadian, N.[3], Zarza, E.[3]

[1]*Department of Microbiology, Faculty of Veterinary Medicine, Urmia University, Urmia, Iran*

[2]*Department of Clinical Sciences, Faculty of Veterinary Medicine, Urmia University, Urmia, Iran*

[3]*Graduated from the Faculty of Veterinary Medicine, Urmia University, Urmia, Iran*

Key words:

antigenic variants, canine parvovirus, dog, PCR-RFLP, sequencing

Correspondence

Dastmalchi Saei, H.
Department of Microbiology, Faculty of Veterinary Medicine, Urmia University, Urmia, Iran

Email: HDSaei561@gmail.com

Abstract:

BACKGROUND: Canine parvovirus (CPV) has been incriminated as a primary pathogen related to acute hemorrhagic enteritis in dogs. Three major antigenic variants of CPV (CPV-2a/2b/2c) have so far been identified. **OBJECTIVES:** This study was carried out to investigate the frequency of CPV-2 and its variants (CPV-2a/2b/2c) in a population of healthy and diarrheic dogs in the northwest of Iran. **METHODS:** A total of 35 stool samples from healthy (n=16) and diarrheic (n=19) dogs were screened for all variants (2a, 2b, and 2c) by polymerase chain reaction (PCR) using primer pair 555for/555rev resulting in a PCR product of 583 bp in length. The resulting fragments were further digested by *Mbo*II endonuclease that selectively recognizes the restriction site "GAAGA" unique to CPV2c only. All undigested samples were subjected to PCR assays with primer pair Pab (which detects both CPV-2a and CPV-2b types) and primer pair Pb (which detects only CPV-2b type) primer pairs. The relationship of health status, breed, age, sex and vaccination status with PCR results was analyzed using statistical tests. **RESULTS:** From a total of 35 samples, 10 samples were found to be positive by 555for/555rev primers that were further analyzed by *Mbo*II digestion of PCR products. One sample was characterized as CPV-2c and nine samples were categorized as CPV-2a or CPV-2b. All nine undigested samples resulted positive by PCR using Pab primers, out of which 7 resulted positive by PCR using Pb primer pairs, indicating that they are of CPV-2b variant. **CONCLUSIONS:** It seems that CPV-2b is prevalent variant circulating in the northwest of Iran. Results also indicated that CPV-2a and CPV-2c are affecting dogs, which suggests constant surveillance and monitoring of CPV variants.

Introduction

Canine parvovirus 2 (CPV-2) remains one of the major etiological agents of highly contagious gastroenteric disease in dogs worldwide (Perez et al., 2012). The virus is a member of the genus Parvovirus of the family Parvoviridae, and it is a non-enveloped DNA virus that contains linear, single-stranded genome of approximately 5.2kb in length. The viral genome containing two major open reading frames (ORFs), one (nt 273 to 2279) encoding two non-structural proteins (NS1 and NS2), while the other (nt 2787 to 4541) encodes the capsid proteins (VP1 and VP2). There is also a third structural protein, VP3, which is a proteolytic cleavage product of VP2, missing a peptide from the amino terminus (Nandi and Kumar, 2010).

In CPV, the genome is surrounded by an icosahedral capsid that is formed by approximately 10 subunits of the larger VP1 protein (84 kDa) and 50 subunits of VP2 (62 kDa). VP1 contains the full-length VP2 sequence plus an additional specific 142 amino acids sequence at its N-terminus (Tattersall et al., 1977). VP2 is the major capsid protein containing the main antigenic determinants and also plays an important role in determining virus pathogenicity (Gallo Calderon et al., 2012).

Soon after its description during the late 1970s, the CPV-2 displayed rapid variation in its sequences compared with the original CPV-2 sequence, giving rise to two different antigenic variants that were termed CPV-2a and CPV-2b (Decaro and Buonavoglia, 2012). CPV-2a and CPV-2b differ from the original type 2 strain in five or six amino acid (aa) substitutions in the VP2 capsid protein, while only two residues differentiated CPV-2a from CPV-2b, i.e., Asn-426 to Asp and Ile-555 to Val (Truyen, 2006). In the year 2001, a new antigenic variant was produced by Asp-Glu substitution of VP2 residue 426 in Italy and now referred to as CPV-2c (Buonavoglia et al., 2001). The Asp-426→ Glu change of CPV-2c strain was due to a change (T → A) in the third codon position at nucleotide 4064, creating

an MboII restriction site (GAAGA) unique to this strain. Therefore, it is possible to distinguish these mutants (types 2c) from the other antigenic types (2a and 2b) by simple digestion using MboII. However, RFLP analysis is not able to differentiate CPV-2b from CPV-2a, since both types remain undigested after MboII digestion (Buonavoglia et al., 2001). These accumulations of aa changes in the VP2 sequences of CPV were associated with genetic adaptation and change in the antigenic and biological properties such as the host range and pathogenicity shift (Carmichael, 2005; Hueffer et al., 2003).

The distribution and genetic diversities of CPV-2 variants fluctuate among countries. Nowadays, CPV-2a and CPV-2b are the predominant types responsible for most CPV infections in Asian countries, although a few CPV-2c strains have been isolated in India (Decaro and Buonavoglia, 2012). In North America and Europe, all three variants are co-distributed in contrast with South America where the most prevalent variant is CPV-2c (Pedroza-Roldan et al., 2015).

Rapid diagnosis of CPV infection is important for design of measures for disease control and study on its antigenic variants is also of particular interest from an epidemiological point of view. Traditional diagnostic methods such as immunochromatographic (IC), hemagglutination (HA) and virus isolation (VI) have been shown to be poorly sensitive (Desario et al., 2005). Moreover, traditional approaches such as hemagglutination inhibition (HI) using monoclonal antibodies (MAbs) also have some limitations in detection of CPV variants (Decaro et al., 2005c; Desario et al., 2005). In comparison with traditional methods, molecular methods such as polymerase chain reaction

(PCR) and restriction fragment length poly-morphism (RFLP) techniques have been developed and have been widely applied for diagnosis of the CPV-2 variants, due to high sensitivity and specificity (Decaro et al., 2005b; Parthiban et al., 2010; Touihri et al., 2009).

In the studied region, dogs are vaccinated against CPV-2 starting at 8 weeks of age, re-vaccination at 12 weeks of age and booster continued every year; the vaccine routinely used (HPRADOG 7, Spain) contains live canine parvovirus C-780916 strain, canine distemper virus, canine adenovirus type 2 Manhattan strain, parainfluenza virus Penn 103/70 strain and inactivated *Leptospira icterohaemorrhagiae* and *Leptospira canicola* microorganisms of each serovar. In Iran, however, reports describing the different variants of CPV circulating in dog populations are scarce. Therefore, the aim of the current study was to provide data about CPV-2 variants in the northwest of Iran.

Materials and Methods

Study population and Collection of samples: A total of 35 rectal swabs were obtained by clinicians from healthy (n=16) and CPV suspected (n=19) dogs in Urmia region located in west Azerbaijan province, Iran. The presence or absence of clinical symptoms characteristic of CPV infection were evaluated to determine the health status of each animal. Clinical symptoms in the dogs included fever, anorexia, depression, gastrointestinal problems, and vomiting. Of the 35 dogs swabbed, 15 were Iraqi (42.9%), 8 Terriers (22.9%), 3 Doberman pinchers (8.6%), 3 Rottweilers (8.6%), 3 German shepherds (8.6%), 1 welsh (2.9%), and there was no breed information regarding 2 other dogs.

Dogs were divided into two age groups (≤6 months and > 6 months). Twenty-seven out of 35 (77.1%) were ≤6 months, and 5 were > 6 months old (14.3%). The samples were submitted to our laboratory for diagnostic purposes during a time span of 8 months from October 2014 to May 2015. In addition, information such as breed, age, gender and vaccination status was also recorded.

DNA extraction: DNA preparation from rectal samples and from a commercial live attenuated vaccine (HIPRADOG 7, HIPRA Co, Spain) was performed as previously described with some modification. In brief, the collected samples were emulsified in 1 ml of 0.1 M PBS of pH 7.4 and clarified by centrifugation at 6000 rpm for 15 min. Next, the collected supernatant was heated at 100°C for 10 min and chilled immediately on crushed ice for 5 min. It was then diluted 1:10 in distilled water to reduce DNA polymerase inhibitors before PCR amplification (Parthiban et al., 2010).

Detection of CPV and its variants by PCR and PCR-RFLP: Confirmation of the presence of CPV in samples was performed by polymerase chain reaction (PCR) amplification of a 583 bp fragment of the VP2 capsid protein-encoding gene of all variants (2a, 2b, and 2c) with the primer pairs 555for 5′-CAG GAA GAT ATC CAG AAG G A-3′ (located at 4003-4022) and 555rev 5′-GGT GCT AGT TGA TAT GTA ATA AAC A-3′ (located at 4585-4561) developed by Buonavoglia et al. (Buonavoglia et al., 2001). The reaction was performed in a total volume of 25 µl consisting of 12.5 µl of 2X master mix (Thermo scientific, Germany), 0.4 µM of primers and 2 µl of template DNA. Amplification was performed with PCR master kit (Thermo scientific, Germany) in a CORBETT thermocycler (Model

CP2-003, Australia). Commercial live attenuated vaccine HIPRADOG 7 (HIPRA Co, Spain) was used as a positive control. For the negative control, sterile water was added instead of nucleic acids. The thermal cycler parameters were as follows: initial denaturation at 94 °C for 5 min, followed by 40 cycles of denaturation at 94 °C for 30 s, annealing at 50 °C for 1 min and extension at 72 °C for 1 min, with the final extension at 72 °C for 10 min. The PCR products were separated by electrophoresis through a 1.2% agarose gel containing ethidium bromide (0.5 µg/ml) and visualized under UV light, and the images were documented in a gel documentation system.

All 583 bp amplicons generated with primer pair 555for/555rev were then digested with the restriction enzyme MboII (Thermo Scientific, Germany) that selectively recognizes the restriction site "GAAGA" (nucleotide 4062-4066 of the VP2 encoding gene) unique to CPV-2c only. In brief, 10 µl of the PCR product was digested with 1U of MboII in the presence of 2µl of 10x FastDigest buffer and 17 µl of distilled water in a final volume of 30 µl. After incubation at 37 °C for 7 min and enzyme inactivation at 65 °C for 5 min, the digested products were analyzed in 2.5% agarose gel. Only, PCR products obtained from CPV-2c are cut by MboII, generating two fragments of 500 and 83 bp, respectively (Buonavoglia et al., 2001; Parthiban et al., 2010).

All undigested samples were then subjected to another PCR using primer pairs Pab sense 5′-GAA GAG TGG TTG TAA ATA ATT-3′ (located at 3025-3045) and Pab antisense 5′-CCT ATA TAA CCA AAG TTA GTA C-3′ (lacated at 3685-3706), which amplify partial VP2-encoding gene (681bp) of both CPV2a and CPV2b types.

The conditions for the Pab PCR assay were initial denaturation step at 94°C for 5 min, followed by 30 cycles of denaturation at 94°C for 30 s, annealing at 55°C for 2 min, and extension at 72°C for 2 min and a final extension at 72°C for 10 min (Senda et al., 1995). Subsequently, a PCR for detection of CPV-2b type utilizing primer pairs Pb sense 5′-CTT TAA CCT TCC TGT AAC AG-3′ (located at 3025-3045) and Pb antisense 5′-CAT AGT TAA ATT GGT TAT CTA C-3′ (located at 4449-4470) with the expected product size of 427 bp (Pereira et al., 2000) was attempted. The PCR products were separated in a 1.2% agarose gel electrophoresis.

Sequencing and phylogenetic analysis of CPV-2c: The amplified PCR product of CPV-2c variant was purified with a commercial kit (GeneJET Gel Extraction and DNA Cleanup Kit, Thermo Scientific, Germany) and the target nucleotide sequence and deduced aa sequence were compared with sequences of prototype CPV strains (M38245-CPV-2; M24003-CPV-2a; M74849-CPV-2b; FJ005264-CPV-2c) using ClustralW.

For phylogenetic analysis, 32 CPV-2c sequences from various parts of the world (China, n = 5; Germany, n = 6, Italy, n = 6; India, n = 4; USA, n = 2; Turkey, n = 1; France, n = 1; Greece, n = 2; Argentina, n = 2; Croatia, n = 1; Thailand, n = 1, Belgium, n = 1) were retrieved from the GenBank and used. The sequences were aligned using ClustalW 1.8 program and .aln file was generated. The .aln file was converted to .meg file using Mega 6 (Tamura et al., 2013) and Neighbor Joining tree (NJ tree) was constructed (bootstrap replicates = 1000) using Kimura 2 parameter method (Kimura, 1980) for pairwise deletion at uniform rates. The GenBank accession numbers for the

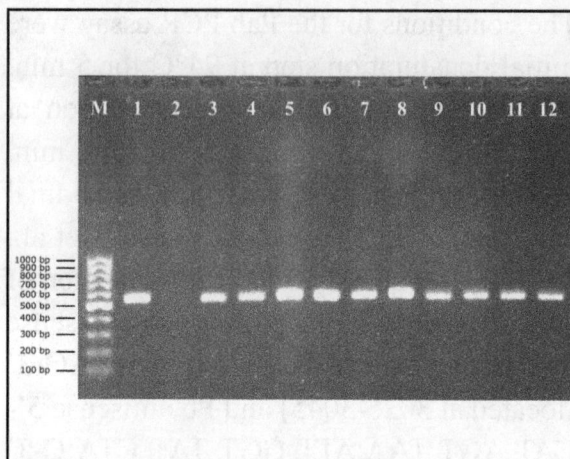

Figure 1. Specific fragment of the VP2 gene (583 bp) was amplified in 10 samples with primers 555for and 555rev. Lane M: Gene Ruler™ 100 bp DNA ladder; Lane 1: positive control (vaccine strain, HIPRADOG 7); Lane 2: negative control; Lanes 3-12: showing amplified fragment of VP2-encoding gene in isolates.

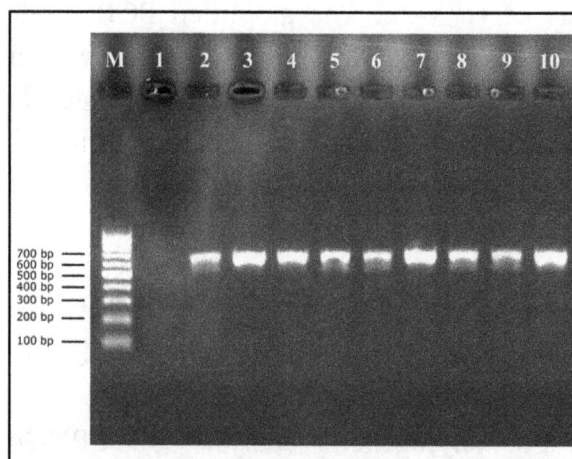

Figure 2. Restriction fragment length polymorphism (RFLP) patterns of 583 bp PCR products from the VP2-encoding gene of 10 CPV strains after digestion with MboII restriction enzyme. Lane M: Gene Ruler™ 100 bp DNA ladder; Lanes 1-4 and 6-10: nine undigested samples (pattern characteristic for CPV-2a and CPV-2b). Lane 5: digested sample (pattern characteristic for CPV-2c).

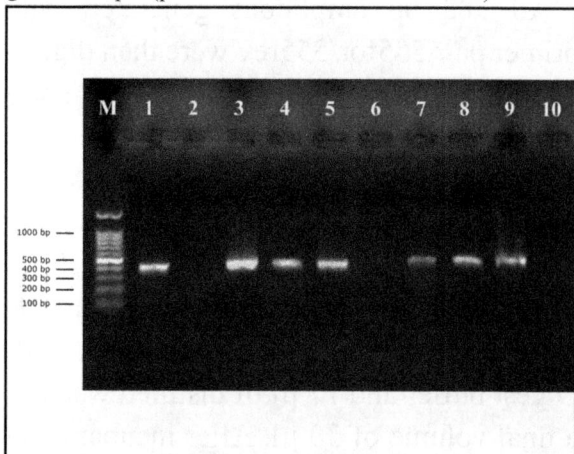

Figure 3. Agarose gel electrophoresis of 681 bp amplicon of samples using Pab primers. Lane M: Gene Ruler™ 100 bp DNA ladder; Lane 1: negative control; Lanes 2-10: samples showed expected product.

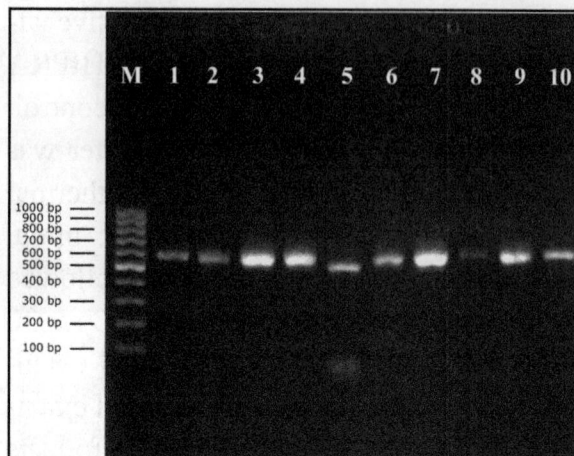

Figure 4. Agarose gel electrophoresis of 427 bp amplicon of clinical samples using Pb primers. M: Gene Ruler™ 100 bp DNA ladder; Lanes 1, 3-5, 7-9: samples showed expected product; Lane 2: negative control; Lanes 6 and 10: samples showed negative result for Pb primers.

reference strains used in the phylogenetic tree construction are shown in Fig. 5.

Statistical analysis: Statistical analysis was performed by SPSS v.20 (IBM Corp., Armonk, NY, USA) using Fischer's exact test and chi square analysis. Differences were considered significant at $p \leq 0.05$.

Results

Among the 35 samples (16 from healthy and 19 from CPV-2 suspected dogs) screened by PCR using primer sets 555for/555rev, 10 samples (28.6%) were found to be positive for CPV and yielded a single DNA amplicon of 583 bp (Fig. 1). In a similar way, the live attenuated vaccine showed a same sized band.

According to the results, CPV was identified in 42.1% (8/19) of the samples originated from CPV-2 suspected dogs and the corresponding percentage for healthy dogs

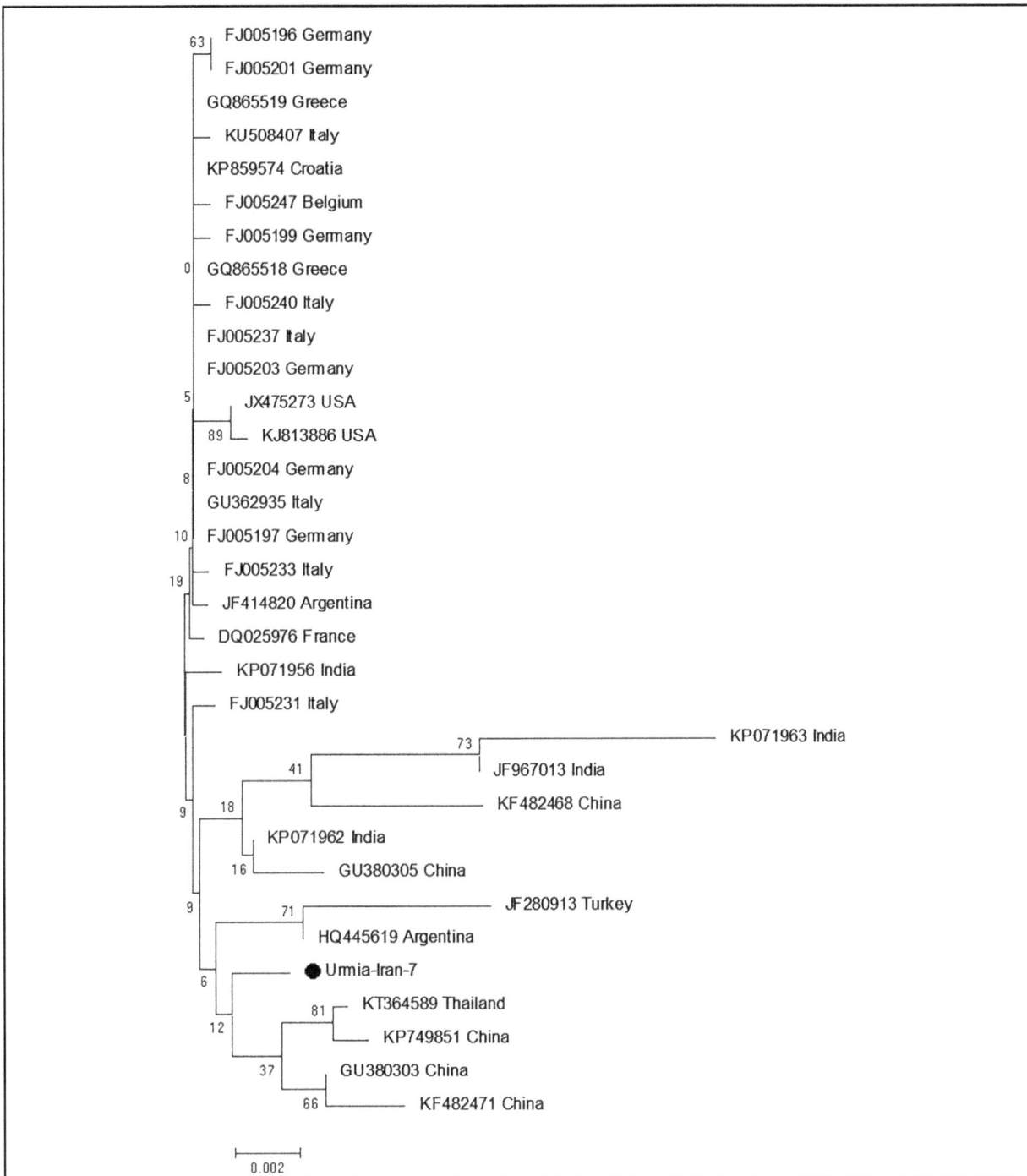

Figure 5. Neighbor Joining tree (Mega-6) constructed using CPV-2c sequence obtained in the current study and the 32 CPV-2c sequences from various parts of the world.

was 12.5% (2/16).

The *Mbo*II digest assay of the 583 bp amplicon showed one out of 10 positive samples had a RFLP pattern associated with the viral variant CPV-2c, which consisted of two bands of 500 and 83 bp (Fig. 2). As shown, nine samples remained undigested

and were subjected to PCR assays using primer pairs Pab and Pb.

The PCR fragment of 681 bp was successfully amplified from all undigested samples using Pab primers (Figure 3), out of which 7 resulted positive by PCR using Pb primer sets, indicating that 7 are of CPV-2b variant

Table 1. Description of breed, age, sex, and vaccination status of the positive sampled animals in the current study.

Isolate	Health status	Breed	Age	Gender	Vaccination status	CPV variant
1	Diarrheic	Terrier	7 month	Male	Vaccinated	2b
2	Diarrheic	Terrier	3 month	Female	Vaccinated	2a
3	Diarrheic	Rottweiller	2 month	Male	None	2c
4	Healthy	Rottweiller	2 month	Male	None	2b
5	Healthy	Rottweiller	2 month	Male	None	2b
6	Diarrheic	Iraqi	4 month	Male	None	2b
7	Diarrheic	NA	NA	NA	NA	2b
8	Diarrheic	Wales	3 month	Female	None	2a
9	Diarrheic	German shepherd	4 month	Male	Vaccinated	2b
10	Diarrheic	Iraqi	2 month	Male	Vaccinated	2b

and 2 are of CPV-2a (Fig. 4).

Table 1 describes the breed, age, sex, and vaccination status of the positive sampled animals. As shown, 80% (8/10) of the diagnosed dogs with CPV were 6 months or younger; 70% (7/10) were male and 20% (2/10) were female; of 10 dogs with confirmed CPV infection, 3 were Rottweillers, 2 were Iraqi, 2 were Terriers, 1 was German shepherd, 1 was Welsh and 1 was nondescript.

In comparison to prototype CPV strains, the nucleotide variation at position 4064 (T → A) with the corresponding amino acid substitution 426-Asp → Glu of the encoded protein led us to type definitively the sequenced strain as CPV-2c. Two additional substitutions in nucleotides 4218 and 4355 from T to G were also observed in CPV-2c sequence under study, which cause non-synonymous (Leu → Val) and synonymous (Thr → Thr) mutations at positions 478 and 523 of the VP2 protein, respectively.

The obtained neighbor-joining tree showed that the sequence CPV-2c from Iran formed a separate lineage and was closely related with the CPV-2c strains of China (KP749851, GU380303 and KF482471) and Thailand (KT364589) (Fig. 5). Interestingly, phylogenetic analysis revealed that most of the CPV-2c sequences obtained from European countries were segregated together.

Discussion

Canine parvovirus type 2 (CPV-2) has spread worldwide and is recognized as an important canine pathogen in all countries (Sutton et al., 2013). CPV-2 was first reported in a 7 month-old male dog in Tehran, Iran in 2002 (Hemmatzadeh and Jamshidi, 2002).

PCR-based methods (conventional and real-time PCR) were demonstrated to be more sensitive than traditional techniques (Desario et al., 2005) in screening of samples for CPV infections in dogs. In the current study, eight out of 19 (42.1%) samples from dogs with diarrhea were found positive for the CPV-2 DNA using PCR and primers 555for/555rev. The results of the PCR assay were in concordance with results obtained by Xu (46.6%) in western China (Xu et al., 2015). The frequency detected in the present study, however, was lower than the 56.0% reported in China (Yi et al., 2014). These discrepancies may be due to differences in sampling season, as a seasonal distribution of disease has been reported in some geographic locations with high prevalence in

July, August, and September (Houston et al., 1996).

CPV-2c variant has been previously identified in many European countries (Decaro et al., 2007; Decaro et al., 2011), Africa and America (Hong et al., 2007) as well as in some Asian countries such as Taiwan (Wang et al., 2005), India (Nandi et al., 2010) and Greece (Ntafis et al., 2010). Digestion assay on 10 PCR positive samples using *Mbo*II restriction endonuclease indicated that only one sample had type 2c RFLP pattern and 9 samples showed the typical profile of CPV-2/2a/b variants. This is the first report demonstrating the presence of CPV-2c DNA in feces of CPV suspected dogs in Iran, which underscores the need for further research examining CPV variants in Iranian dog population. Further sequence analysis can give definite prediction for the presence of type-2c, since *Mbo*II-based identification sometimes gives misleading results. Recently, CPV-2a strains mischaracterized as type 2c have been reported due to a constant mutation in the VP2 gene introducing an *Mbo*II restriction site (Demeter et al., 2010). The results of the aa sequence analysis revealed the amino acid Glu426, which is unique to strain CPV-2c. Host-immunity pressure may contribute to the emergence of this variant. Studies have shown that residue 426 is situated in epitope A, over a threefold spike of the capsid, and a role of antigenic escape has been assigned to the same residue of the VP2 of the parvovirus minute virus of mice (Decaro and Buonavoglia, 2012). According to the Phylogenetic analysis, however, we found that CPV-2c from our study was most closely related to CPV-2c strains of China and Thailand, suggesting that CPV-2c Iranian isolate could have derived from Asian strains rather than from

European strains. Similar finding has been reported from China where a close relationship between the isolates from China, Korea and Thailand has been reported (Xu et al., 2015).

Nucleotide variations at positions 4218 and 4355 were observed in the CPV-2c sequence under study. In particular, residue variations are antigenically important to genetic complexity and might lead to the limitation of vaccine effectiveness on infection control and to other disadvantages (Muz et al., 2012).

Based on PCR analysis of nine undigested samples using primers Pab and Pb, seven samples were characterized as CPV-2b and 2 as CPV-2a. This finding is in agreement with reports from Shiraz, southern Iran, where 39 of 44 positive samples analyzed were CPV-2b (Firoozjaii et al., 2011). It was also found that CPV-2b variants are more common in Ahvaz district in the southwest of Iran (Vakili et al., 2014). This variant is also widely distributed in Tehran, where 32 of 50 (64%) samples from young dogs (less than 2 years-old) with clinical signs of acute gastroenteritis were positive for CPV-2b (Mohyedini et al., 2013). Studies in neighboring countries have shown the high isolation frequencies of the CPV-2b and CPV-2a in Iraq and Turkey, respectively (Ahmed et al., 2012; Timurkan and Oguzoglu, 2015). These variations are likely due to geographical differences. Studies in China have shown that the isolation frequencies of the CPV-2a and CPV-2b differ according to geographic location (Zhong et al., 2014). Viral cross-border dissemination through entering small animals from abroad may be a risk factor for dominant frequency of certain variant in a region. In support of this hypothesis is the finding that the two Iraqi breeds harbored the CPV-2b. Sequence analysis of the complete coding region of VP2 gene and subsequent phylogenetic analysis can clarify the geographical origin of the circulating CPV.

As results, CPV-2 induced disease was significantly observed in dogs less than 4 months old. This is consistent with the results of the previous studies where puppies or dogs less than 6 months of age have a higher predisposition for developing the disease (Lamm and Rezabek, 2008; Pedroza-Roldan et al., 2015). However, CPV infection has recently become an issue in adult dogs also, mostly associated to CPV-2c variant as reviewed by Decaro and Buonavoglia (2012) (Decaro and Buonavoglia, 2012).

Accordingly, two unvaccinated dogs, 2 months of age, that lacked evidence of gastrointestinal signs were found to be positive for the presence of CPV-2b type DNA using PCR assay. False-positive PCR result due to the presence of DNA derived from attenuated live vaccine virus in the feces can be ruled out, since these dogs were unvaccinated. This may suggest a carrier state for the virus between dogs. Host immune status which is affected by various factors such as maternally derived antibodies (MDA) at the moment of infection may contribute to this situation. Subclinical and unapparent infections are frequently detected mainly in pups with intermediate MDA titers and in adult dogs (Decaro et al., 2005a).

In conclusion, the results of the current study reveal that CPV-2b and to lesser extent CPV-2a are the predominant types circulating in Iran, along with the CPV-2c as emerged pathogen of dogs in Iran. Further monitoring and surveillance of large areas will be useful to explore the newer CPV strains/variants.

Acknowledgments

This work was supported by the Research Foundation of Urmia University, Urmia, Iran.

References

Buonavoglia, C., Martella, V., Pratelli, A., Tempesta, M., Cavalli, A., Buonavoglia, D., Bozzo, G., Elia, G., Decaro, N., Carmichael, L. (2001) Evidence for evolution of canine parvovirus type 2 in Italy. J Gen Virol. 82: 3021-3025.

Carmichael, L.E. (2005) An annotated historical account of canine parvovirus. J Vet Med B Infect Dis Vet Public Health. 52: 303-311.

Decaro, N., Buonavoglia, C. (2012) Canine parvovirus--a review of epidemiological and diagnostic aspects, with emphasis on type 2c. Vet Microbiol. 155: 1-12.

Decaro, N., Campolo, M., Desario, C., Elia, G., Martella, V., Lorusso, E., Buonavoglia, C. (2005a) Maternally-derived antibodies in pups and protection from canine parvovirus infection. Biologicals. 33: 261-267.

Decaro, N., Desario, C., Addie, D.D., Martella, V., Vieira, M.J., Elia, G., Zicola, A., Davis, C., Thompson, G., Thiry, E., Truyen, U, Buonavoglia, C. (2007) The study molecular epidemiology of canine parvovirus, Europe. Emerg Infect Dis. 13: 1222-1224.

Decaro, N., Desario, C., Billi, M., Mari, V., Elia, G., Cavalli, A., Martella, V., Buonavoglia, C. (2011) Western European epidemiological survey for parvovirus and coronavirus infections in dogs. Vet J. 187: 195-199.

Decaro, N., Elia, G., Campolo, M., Desario, C., Lucente, M.S., Bellacicco, A.L., Buonavoglia, C. (2005b) New approaches for the molecular characterization of canine parvovirus type 2 strains. J Vet Med B Infect Dis Vet

Public Health. 52: 316-319.

Decaro, N., Elia, G., Martella, V., Desario, C., Campolo, M., Trani, L.D., Tarsitano, E., Tempesta, M., Buonavoglia, C. (2005c) A real-time PCR assay for rapid detection and quantitation of canine parvovirus type 2 in the feces of dogs. Vet Microbiol. 105: 19-28.

Demeter, Z., Palade, E.A., Soos, T., Farsang, A., Jakab, C., Rusvai, M. (2010) Misleading results of the *Mbo*II-based identification of type 2a canine parvovirus strains from Hungary reacting as type 2c strains. Virus Genes. 41: 37-42.

Desario, C., Decaro, N., Campolo, M., Cavalli, A., Cirone, F., Elia, G., Martella, V., Lorusso, E., Camero, M., Buonavoglia, C. (2005) Canine parvovirus infection: which diagnostic test for virus? J Virol Methods. 126: 179-185.

Firoozjaii, H.A., Shoorijeh, S.J., Mohammadi, A., Tamadon, A. (2011) Characterization of Iranian isolates of canine parvovirus in fecal samples using polymerase chain reaction assay. Iran J Biotechnol. 9: 63-68.

Gallo Calderon, M., Wilda, M., Boado, L., Keller, L., Malirat, V., Iglesias, M., Mattion, N., La Torre, J. (2012) Study of canine parvovirus evolution: comparative analysis of full-length VP2 gene sequences from Argentina and international field strains. Virus Genes. 44: 32-39.

Hemmatzadeh, F., Jamshidi, S. (2002) First reportof isolation of canine parvovirus in Iran. Journal of Veterinary Research, University of Tehran. 57: 33-35.

Hong, C., Decaro, N., Desario, C., Tanner, P., Pardo, M.C., Sanchez, S., Buonavoglia, C., Saliki, J.T. (2007) Occurrence of canine parvovirus type 2c in the United States. J Vet Diagn Invest. 19: 535-539.

Houston, D.M., Ribble, C.S., Head, L.L. (1996) Risk factors associated with parvovirus enteritis in dogs: 283 cases (1982-1991). J Am Vet Med Assoc. 208: 542-546.

Hueffer, K., Parker, J.S., Weichert, W.S., Geisel, R.E., Sgro, J.Y., Parrish, C.R. (2003) The natural host range shift and subsequent evolution of canine parvovirus resulted from virus-specific binding to the canine transferrin receptor. J Virol. 77: 1718-1726.

Kimura, M. (1980) A simple method for estimating evolutionary rate of base substitutions through comparative studies of nucleotide sequences. J Mol Evol. 16: 111-120.

Lamm, C.G., Rezabek, G.B. (2008) Parvovirus infection in domestic companion animals. Vet Clin North Am Small Anim Pract. 38: 837-850, viii-ix.

Mohyedini, S., Jamshidi, S., Rafati, S., Nikbakht, G.R., Malmasi, A., Taslimi, Y., Akbarein, H. (2013) Comparison of immunochromatographic rapid test with molecular method in diagnosis of canine parvovirus. Iranian Journal of Veterinary Medicine. 7: 57-61.

Muz, D., Oguzoglu, T.C., Timurkan, M.O., Akin, H. (2012) Characterization of the partial VP2 gene region of canine parvoviruses in domestic cats from Turkey. Virus Genes. 44: 301-308.

Nandi, S., Chidri, S., Kumar, M., Chauhan, R.S. (2010) Occurrence of canine parvovirus type 2c in the dogs with haemorrhagic enteritis in India. Res Vet Sci. 88: 169-171.

Nandi, S., Kumar, M. (2010) Canine parvovirus: current perspective. Indian J Virol. 21: 31-44.

Ntafis, V., Xylouri, E., Kalli, I., Desario, C., Mari, V., Decaro, N., Buonavoglia, C. (2010) Characterization of canine parvovirus 2 variants circulating in Greece. J Vet Diagn Invest. 22: 737-740.

Parthiban, S., Mukhopadhyay, H.K., Antony, P.X., Pillai, R.M. (2010) Molecular typing of canine parvovirus occurring in pondicherry by multiplex PCR and PCR-RFLP. Indian J Virol. 21: 86-89.

Pedroza-Roldan, C., Paez-Magallan, V., Charles-Nino, C., Elizondo-Quiroga, D., Leonel De Cervantes-Mireles, R., Lopez-Amezcua, M.A. (2015) Genotyping of Canine parvovirus in western Mexico. J Vet Diagn Invest. 27: 107-111.

Pereira, C.A., Monezi, T.A., Mehnert, D.U., D'Angelo, M., Durigon, E.L. (2000) Molecular characterization of canine parvovirus in Brazil by polymerase chain reaction assay. Vet Microbiol. 75: 127-133.

Perez, R., Bianchi, P., Calleros, L., Francia, L., Hernandez, M., Maya, L., Panzera, Y., Sosa, K., Zoller, S. (2012) Recent spreading of a divergent canine parvovirus type 2a (CPV-2a) strain in a CPV-2c homogenous population. Vet Microbiol. 155: 214-219.

Senda, M., Parrish, C.R., Harasawa, R., Gamoh, K., Muramatsu, M., Hirayama, N., Itoh, O. (1995) Detection by PCR of wild-type canine parvovirus which contaminates dog vaccines. J Clin Microbiol. 33: 110-113.

Sutton, D., Vinberg, C., Gustafsson, A., Pearce, J., Greenwood, N. (2013) Canine parvovirus type 2c identified from an outbreak of severe gastroenteritis in a litter in Sweden. Acta Vet Scand. 55: 64.

Tamura, K., Stecher, G., Peterson, D., Filipski, A., Kumar, S. (2013) MEGA6: Molecular evolutionary genetics analysis version 6.0. Mol Biol Evol. 30: 2725-2729.

Tattersall, P., Shatkin, A.J., Ward, D.C. (1977) Sequence homology between the structural polypeptides of minute virus of mice. J Mol Biol. 111: 375-394.

Timurkan, M., Oguzoglu, T. (2015) Molecular characterization of canine parvovirus (CPV) infection in dogs in Turkey. Vet Ital. 51: 39-44.

Touihri, L., Bouzid, I., Daoud, R., Desario, C., El Goulli, A.F., Decaro, N., Ghorbel, A., Buonavoglia, C., Bahloul, C. (2009) Molecular characterization of canine parvovirus-2 variants circulating in Tunisia. Virus Genes. 38: 249-258.

Truyen, U. (2006) Evolution of canine parvovirus-A need for new vaccines? Vet Microbiol. 117: 9-13.

Vakili, N., Mosallanejad, B., Avizeh, R., Seyfiabad Shapouri, M.R., Pourmahdi, M. (2014) A comparison between PCR and Immunochromatography assay (ICA) in diagnosis of hemorrhagic gastroenteritis caused by Canine parvovirus. Arch Razi Inst. 69: 27-33.

Wang, H.C., Chen, W.D., Lin, S.L., Chan, J.P., Wong, M.L. (2005) Phylogenetic analysis of canine parvovirus VP2 gene in Taiwan. Virus Genes. 31: 171-174.

Xu, J., Guo, H.C., Wei, Y.Q., Shu, L., Wang, J., Li, J.S., Cao, S.Z., Sun, S.Q. (2015) Phylogenetic analysis of canine parvovirus isolates from sichuan and gansu provinces of china in 2011. Transbound Emerg Dis. 62: 91-95.

Yi, L., Tong, M., Cheng, Y., Song, W., Cheng, S. (2014) Phylogenetic analysis of canine parvovirus VP2 gene in China. Transbound Emerg Dis. 2016 Apr; 63(2):e262-9. doi: 10.1111/tbed.12268. Epub 2014 Sep 11.

Zhong, Z., Liang, L., Zhao, J., Xu, X., Cao, X., Liu, X., Zhou, Z., Ren, Z., Shen, L., Geng, Y., Gu, X., Peng, G. (2014) First isolation of new canine parvovirus 2a from Tibetan mastiff and global analysis of the full-length VP2 gene of canine parvoviruses 2 in China. Int J Mol Sci. 15: 12166-12187.

8

Antifungal activity of the *Trachyspermum ammi* essential oil on some of the most common fungal pathogens in animals

Shokri, H.[1]*, Sharifzadeh, A.[2], Khosravi, A.R.[2]

[1]*Department of Pathobiology, Faculty of Veterinary Medicine, Amol University of Special Modern Technologies, Amol, Iran*

[2]*Mycology Research Center, Faculty of Veterinary Medicine, University of Tehran, Tehran, Iran*

Key words:

antifungal activity, *Aspergillus*, *Candida*, *Trachyspermum ammi*, *Trichophyton*

Correspondence

Shokri, H.
Department of Pathobiology,
Faculty of Veterinary Medicine,
Amol University of Special
Modern Technologies, Amol,
Iran

Email: hshokri@ausmt.ac.ir

Abstract:

BACKGROUND: The increasing resistance to antifungal drugs and the reduced number of available drugs led to the search for therapeutic alternatives among aromatic plants and their essential oils, empirically used by antifungal effects. **OBJECTIVES:** The purpose of the current study was to evaluate the antifungal activity of *Trachyspermum ammi* essential oil (EO) against the most frequent pathogenic fungi including *Candida*, *Aspergillus*, *Chrysosporium* and *Trichophyton* species. **METHODS:** EO from the seeds of the plant was obtained by hydrodistillation. Susceptibility tests were expressed as growth inhibition zone (diameter) using disk diffusion method and minimal inhibitory concentration (MIC) and minimal fungicidal concentration (MFC) using broth microdilution method. **RESULTS:** Results of susceptibility tests showed that *T. ammi* EO was effective against all the tested strains. The diameters of growth inhibition zone of the EO were between 11 mm and 60 mm. The EO was also the most active, with MIC and MFC values ranging from 0.3 to 2.5 mg/ml and 0.6 to 5 mg/ml, respectively. The EO of *T. ammi* showed a significant degree of antifungal activity against different *Candida* species in comparison with other fungi ($p<0.05$). **CONCLUSIONS:** The present study indicated that *T. ammi* EO has considerable antifungal activity, deserving further investigations for its clinical application for treatment of fungal infections.

Introduction

Fungal agents are widespread and can be isolated from a wide range of animals, from the soil and the environment. This makes fungal diseases as a group of transmissible infections in which animals can represent important reservoirs and asymptomatic carriers for people in close contact with them. The important role of farm and pet animals as carriers and spreaders is well known. Fungal infections in animals and immunocompetent individuals are commonly associated with asymptomatic infections or mild and transient local skin or mucosal lesions (Khosravi et al., 2006), but they can represent important risk factors in immunocompromised subjects, due to the impairment of their immune systems. Since the 1960s, when the use of antibiotic therapies has been established, a drastic increase of fungal infections was observed (Vandeputte et al., 2012). Now, emerging fungal pathogens have been described causing severe infections, which include yeasts as azole-resistant *Candida* and non-*Candida* species, and filamentous fungi such as species of the genus *Trichophyton* and *Aspergillus* and some representatives of the hyaline moulds. Therefore, fungal infections are seen as an important threat to global health that needs to receive proper attention (Gauthier and Keller, 2013). Currently, the limited number of antifungals available, the increased multiresistance and the adverse effects are the major obstacles for fungal infection therapy. Additionally, the recent emergence of opportunistic fungal infections reinforced the necessity for discovering novel antifungal agents. For this purpose, molecules with a new mechanism of action and able to escape from the current fungi mechanism of resistance against antifungals are of interest (Vandeputte et al., 2012).

Medicinal plants are usually used in traditional medicine as antimicrobial agents (Hammer et al., 2002). These plants have continued to be used not only for primary health care of the poor in the developing countries, but also in countries where conventional medicine is predominant in the national health care system. According to the World Health Organization (WHO), herbal medicines serve the health needs of about 80% of the world's population, especially for millions of people in the vast rural areas of developing countries (WHO, 2001). Many researchers have shown that secondary plant metabolites, such as essential oil (EO), can exhibit important antifungal activity against yeasts, dermatophyte and *Aspergillus* strains (Pina-Vaz et al., 2004; Salgueiro et al., 2004), and have therapeutic potential, mainly in fungal diseases involving mucosal, cutaneous and respiratory tract infections (Pinto et al., 2003). Major constituents of the EO are phenolic compounds (terpenoids and phenylpropanoids) like thymol, carvacrol or eugenol, of which antimicrobial activity is well documented (Cavaleiro et al., 2006). The limited

occurrence of these phenols in nature is one of the reasons why *Trachyspermum ammi* (*T. ammi*) EO containing thymol has been of great interest for some time (Gandomi et al., 2014). *T. ammi*, known as ajowan, is an annual herbaceous plant belonging to the highly valued medicinally important family, Apiaceae (Gersbach and Reddy, 2002). Ajowan is widely distributed and cultivated in various regions such as Iran, Pakistan, Afghanistan and India (Shojaaddini et al., 2008). Similar to most species of the family Apiaceae, ajowan is famous for its brownish EO. Usually, thymol is the main ajowan EO constituent and may yield 35% to 60% (Ishikawa et al., 2001). The non-thymol fraction (thymene) contains para-cymene, gamma-terpinene, alpha-pinene, beta-pinene, α-terpinene, styrene, delta-3-carene, beta-phyllanderene, terpinene-4-ol and carvacrol (Ranjan et al., 2012). The purpose of this study was to assess the antifungal effect of *T. ammi* EO against important pathogenic fungi for its potential use as a natural antifungal drug.

Material and Methods

Fungal organisms: A total of 16 pathogenic fungi including *Candida albicans* (no. 5), *C. glabrata* (no. 3), *C. tropicalis* (no. 2), *C. krusei* (no. 1), *C. parapsilosis* (no. 1), *Aspergillus niger* (no. 1), *A. fumigatus* (no. 1), *Trichophyton rubrum* (no. 1) and *Chrysosporium farinicola* (no. 1) were used as test microorganisms. Identification of different *Candida* species was performed by germ tube test, CHROM agar, β-glucosidase, chlamydospore production and API20C system (BioMérieux, Paris, France) for sugar assimilation. The macro- and microscopic identifications of filamentous fungi were determined according to the criteria of Klich (2002) and Larone (2002). All fungal isolates were stored in Sabouraud dextrose broth (Merck Co., Darmstadt, Germany) with glycerol at -70°C until used.

Herbal EO: Seeds of *T. ammi* were collected in July 2014 from Isfahan, Iran. Plants were taxonomically identified at the Pharmacognosy Department, Faculty of Pharmacy, Tehran University of Medical Sciences, Tehran, Iran. The vouch¬er herbarium number was 15125. The seeds were thoroughly washed and dried in the shade at room temperature for 24 h. The dried *T. ammi* seeds were submitted to hydrodistillation in a Clevenger-type apparatus at 100oC for 3 h, according to the procedure described in the European Pharmacopoeia (Council of Europe, 1997). The EO was isolated and dried over anhydrous sodium sulfate and then stored in a dark glass bottle at 4oC until needed.

Preparation of fungal inoculum: Filamentous fungi and yeasts were grown on Sabouraud dextrose agar (Merck Co., Darmstadt, Germany) slants at 30oC for 7-21 days and 35oC for 2 days, respectively. Fungal cells were harvested by adding 10 ml of sterile distilled water containing 0.05% Tween 20 (Merck Co., Darmstadt, Germany) and scraping the surface of the culture to free the cells. The fungal suspensions were counted with a hemocytometer and further diluted to give a concentration of $(1-5) \times 10^6$ cell/ml (Naeini et al., 2009; Naeini and Shokri, 2012).

Antifungal susceptibility assay: A) Disk diffusion method): Tests to assess the antifungal activity were performed using disk diffusion based on the M44-A method for yeasts (CLSI, 2004) and the M51-P method for filamentous fungi (CLSI, 2008). *T. ammi* EO (10, 20 and 30 µl) was inoculated to 6-mm-diameter disks and placed on Sabouraud dextrose agar (Merck Co., Darmstadt, Germany) plates inoculated with fungal spore suspension. The plates were incubated at 30oC for 48 h. At the end of the incubation period, the susceptibility of the test organisms was determined by measuring the diagonal of the zone of inhibition around the disk. The results given are an average of two independent experiments.

B) Broth microdilution method: Minimal inhibitory concentration (MIC) and mini-

mum fungicidal concentration (MFC) were performed according to reference documents M27-A3 for yeasts (CLSI, 2008) and M38-A2 for filamentous fungi (CLSI, 2008). Briefly, stock solutions were prepared by dissolving 1 mg dried essential oil in dimethylsulfoxide (DMSO) 5%. The stock solutions were diluted with Roswell park memorial institute (RPMI) 1640 medium containing L-glutamine but no sodium bicarbonate (Sigma Chemical Co., St. Louis, Missouri, USA), buffered to pH 7.0 with 0.165 mol/l MOPS buffer (Sigma Chemical Co., St. Louis, Missouri, USA). Serial two-fold dilutions ranging from 0.1 to 5 mg/ml were tested for EO. One hundred microlitre aliquots of 2-fold diluted EO solution were dispensed into each well of 96-well microtiter plates. Subsequently, 100 µl aliquots of conidial suspensions were added to each well of a microdilution plate, which were incubated at 30°C (for filamentous fungi) and 35°C (for yeasts) for 48 h. The positive control well contained 100 µl of fungal suspension plus 100 µl of RPMI 1640, and the negative one contained 200 µl of RPMI 1640 only. In addition, the reference antifungal compound, fluconazole (Pfizer, New York, USA), was used as the standard antifungal drug. Two-fold serial dilutions ranging from 0.25 to 128 µg/ml for fluconazole were used. MIC90 was defined as the antifungal concentration that inhibited the growth of 90% of the fungal isolates. In addition, MFC was determined by subculturing 100 µl aliquot from all MIC tubes showing no visible growth onto Sabouraud glucose agar plates. All experiments were performed in duplicate.

Statistical analysis: The antifungal activity was analyzed by the two-tailed paired student's t-test. Statistical significance was considered a P value less than 0.05.

Results

Based on disk diffusion method, the diameters of growth inhibition zone of the EO were

Table 1. Antifungal activity of the EO from *Trachyspermum ammi* against different yeasts and filamentous fungi.

Isolates	*Trachyspermum ammi*					Fluconazole	
	Microdilution broth (mg/ml)		Disk diffusion (mm)			Microdilution broth (μg/ml)	
	MIC	MFC	10 μl	20 μl	30 μl	MIC	MFC
Candida glabrata	0.35	0.7	40	52	58	64	128
	0.4	0.8	32	49	55	64	128
	0.45	0.9	39	50	54	64	128
Candida albicans	0.35	0.7	46	50	60	64	128
	0.3	0.6	50	55	60	8	16
	0.4	0.8	40	50	58	32	64
	0.35	0.7	48	49	55	8	16
	0.35	0.7	50	60	60	4	8
Candida tropicalis	0.6	1.2	18	20	22	2	4
	0.5	1	21	22	25	2	4
Candida krusei	0.4	0.8	23	32	41	64	128
Candida parapsilosis	0.5	1	19	22	23	8	16
Aspergillus fumigatus	1	2	10	10.5	12	64	128
Aspergillus niger	1.5	3	9	10	11	64	128
Trichophyton rubrum	2.5	5	13.5	14	15	64	128
Chrysosporium farinicola	2	4	14.5	15	16	32	64

between 11 mm and 60 mm (Table 1, Fig. 1). The EO of *T. ammi* showed a significant degree of antifungal activity against different *Candida* species (mean value: 40.34 mm) in comparison with other fungi (mean value: 13.5 mm) ($p<0.05$). The EO showed little ability to inhibit *Chrysosporium farinicola*, *T. rubrum* and *Aspergillus* strains.

Evaluation of MICs and MFCs showed that *T. ammi* EO was effective against all the tested strains (Table 1). Data from the present study suggested that the conidia of filamentous fungi were comparatively less susceptible to *T. ammi* EO than yeast cells ($p<0.05$). The results showed that MIC values ranged from 0.3 to 0.6 mg/ml and 1 to 2.5 mg/ml against *Candida* isolates and filamentous fungi, respectively. Among different *Candida* isolates, *C. albicans* showed the highest susceptibility (mean value: 0.35 mg/ml) to *T. ammi* EO, followed by *C. glabrata* and *C. krusei* (mean value: 0.4 mg/ml), *C. parapsilosis* (mean value: 0.5 mg/ml) and *C. tropicalis* (mean value: 0.55 mg/ml). Among filamentous fungi, *Aspergillus* species

were more susceptible than *Chrysosporium farinicola* and *T. rubrum* against the tested EO. For yeasts and filamentous strains, MFC values were higher than MIC values, ranging from 0.6 to 1.2 mg/ml for yeasts and 2 to 5 mg/ml for moulds.

As shown in Table 1, the MIC values of fluconazole ranged from 2 to 64 μg/ml for *Candida* species and from 32 to 64 μg/ml for filamentous fungi.

Discussion

Fungi are increasingly important causes of acute or chronic deep-seated animal infections, especially recurrent mucosal and cutaneous infections that may be severe in debilitated or immunocompromised animals (Shokri et al., 2010). The small number of drugs available for their treatment (most of them fungistatic) and emerging resistance permanently encourage the search for alternatives and led us to find them among low cost and low toxicity traditional therapies and natural products. Up

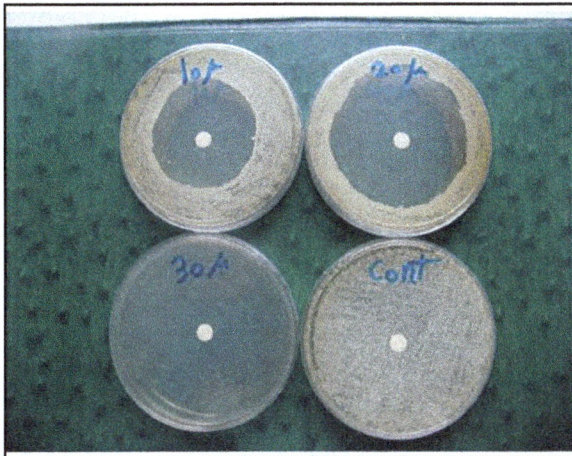

Figure 1. The photo of fungal cultures in disk diffusion method (the diameters of growth inhibition zone of *T. ammi* EO against C. albicans at different concentrations 10, 20 and 30 µl and control [without EO]).

to now, no previous studies have comprehensively investigated the activity of *T. ammi* EO against pathogenic yeasts and filamentous fungi. This study revealed that this EO has both fungistatic and fungicidal activities. *T. ammi* EO disk diffusion method showed the diameters of growth inhibition zone ranging from 11 to 60 mm. There was a statistically significant difference on antifungal activity of *T. ammi* EO against different *Candida* species (mean value: 40.34 mm) in comparison with other fungi (mean value: 13.5 mm) ($p<0.05$). The EO showed little ability to inhibit *Chrysosporium farinicola*, *T. rubrum* and *Aspergillus* strains.

Evaluation of MICs and MFCs showed that *T. ammi* EO was effective against all the tested strains (Table 1). Data from the present study suggested that the conidia of filamentous fungi were comparatively less susceptible to *T. ammi* EO than yeast cells ($p<0.05$). As reported by Pinto et al. (2003), the thickness, composition and density of the conidial wall may be responsible for the reduced susceptibility of conidia to tested EO. Our results showed MIC values ranging from 0.3 to 0.6 mg/ml and 1 to 2.5 mg/ml against *Candida* isolates and filamentous fungi, respectively. The highest susceptibility to *T. ammi* EO was related to *C. albicans* (mean value: 0.35 mg/ml) to *T. ammi* EO, fol-

lowed by *C. glabrata* and *C. krusei* (mean value: 0.4 mg/ml), *C. parapsilosis* (mean value: 0.5 mg/ml) and *C. tropicalis* (mean value: 0.55 mg/ml). Among filamentous fungi, *Aspergillus* species were more susceptible than *Chrysosporium farinicola* and *T. rubrum* against the tested EO. For yeasts and filamentous strains, MFC values were higher than MIC values, ranging from 0.6 to 1.2 mg/ml for yeasts and 2 to 5 mg/ml for moulds. The studies on the EO of *T. ammi* have been reported to inhibit some of the dermatophytes (Tiwari et al., 2003), *Candida* (Ranjan et al., 2012), *Aspergillus* (Murthy et al., 2009) and *Chrysosporium* (Soni et al., 2014) species. Gandomi et al. (2014) showed that *T. ammi* EO contained a mixture of components, mainly thymol together with a small amount of other volatile compounds. Seven components were identified, which represented thymol (63.4%), p-cymene (19%) and g-terpinene (16.9%) as the major components. Totally, it is difficult to attribute the activity of a complex mixture to particular constituents. Nevertheless, it is reasonable to speculate that the activity of this EO can be related to the presence of thymol. The importance of the phenolic hydroxyl groups for the antifungal activity of the monoterpenoids has previously been reported (Aligiannis et al., 2001; Nostro et al., 2004). In agreement with our results, previous studies have also indicated that thymol as a major component of other herbal plants including *Zataria multiflora* (Ebrahimzadeh et al., 2003) and *Thymus vulgaris* (Soković et al., 2009) was responsible for the strong antifungal activity against a variety of pathogenic yeasts and filamentous fungi, especially fungi with decreased susceptibility to fluconazole (Pinto et al., 2003; Shokri et al., 2012).

As shown in Table 1, the MIC values of fluconazole ranged from 2 to 64 µg/ml for *Candida* species and from 32 to 64 µg/ml for filamentous fungi. It should be noted that the EO tested by the disk diffusion method appeared less active than in the test carried out in a liquid medium and these facts might be explained by the more limited diffusion of the EO in a solid medium.

Ergosterol is the major sterol component of the fungal cell membrane, and is responsible for maintaining cell function and integrity. The primary mechanism of action of azole antifungal drugs, such as fluconazole, is to inhibit the fungal cell growth and disruption of normal sterol biosynthetic pathways, leading to a reduction in ergosterol biosynthesis (Alcazar-Fuoli et al., 2013). Pinto et al. (2003) demonstrated that the large spectrum of activity of this EO acting on *Candida*, *Aspergillus* and dermatophyte agrees with the mechanism of fluconazole action, representing a considerable impairment of the biosynthesis of ergosterol and a marked reduction of the ergosterol content. This effect is also superior to the effect of most azole antifungals, as most of them are fungistatic.

In conclusion, the findings of the present study indicated that *T. ammi* EO had considerable antifungal activity. The oil inhibited the filamentous fungi including dermatophyte, *Chrysosporium* and *Aspergillus* species and different *Candida* species. It is necessary to mention that *T. ammi* exhibited remarkable inhibitory effect against fluconazole-resistant *Candida* isolates such as C. krusei and C. glabrata, which were intrinsically resistant to fluconazole or whose resistance was easily inducible. The results presented should stimulate studies on toxicity, improved formulations and the determination of optimal concentrations for clinical applications, as well as comparative studies alongside currently used drugs of the therapeutic efficacy of EO to control fungal infections.

Acknowledgements

This study was funded by Research Council of Faculty of Veterinary Medicine, Amol University of Special Modern Technologies, Amol, Iran.

References

1. Alcazar-Fuoli, E. (2013) Ergosterol biosynthesis in *Aspergillus fumigatus*: its relevance as an antifungal target and role in antifungal drug resistance. Front Microbiol. 3: 1-6.

2. Aligiannis, N., Kalpoutzakis, E., Mitaku, S. (2001) Composition and antimicrobial activity of the essential oils of two Origanum species. J Agric Food Chem. 38: 4168-4170.

3. Cavaleiro, C., Pinto, E., Goncalves, M.J. (2006) Antifungal activity of Juniperus essential oils against dermatophyte, *Aspergillus* and *Candida* strains. J Appl Microbiol. 100: 1333-1338.

4. Clinical and Laboratory Standards Institute (CLSI) (2008) Reference method for broth dilution antifungal susceptibility testing of yeasts; Approved standard. (3rd ed.) CLSI document M27-A3, Clinical and Laboratory Standards Institute, Wayne, PA, USA.

5. Clinical and Laboratory Standards Institute (CLSI) (2008) Reference method for broth dilution antifungal susceptibility testing of filamentous fungi; Approved standard. (2nd ed.) CLSI document M38-A2, Clinical and Laboratory Standards Institute, Wayne, PA, USA.

6. Clinical and Laboratory Standards Institute (CLSI) (2004) Method for antifungal disk diffusion susceptibility testing of yeasts; Approved guideline. CLSI document M44-A, Clinical and Laboratory Standards Institute, Wayne, PA, USA.

7. Clinical and Laboratory Standards Institute (CLSI) (2008) Method for antifungal disk diffusion susceptibility testing of filamentous fungi; Proposed guideline. CLSI document M51-P, Clinical and Laboratory Standards Institute, Wayne, P, USA.

8. Council of Europe (1997) Methods of Pharmacognosy. In: European Pharmacopoeia. (3rd ed.) European Department for the Quality of Medicines. Strasbourg, France. p. 121-122.

9. Ebrahimzadeh, H., Yamini, Y., Sefidkonc, F. (2003) Chemical composition of the essential oil and supercritical CO2 extracts of Zataria multiflora Boiss. Food Chem. 83: 357-361.

10. Gandomi, H., Abbaszadeh, S., Jebellijavan, A. (2014) Chemical constituents, antimicrobial and antioxidative effects of *Trachyspermum ammi* essential oil. J Food Process Pres. 38: 1690-1695.

11. Gauthier, G.M., Keller, N.P. (2013) Crossover fungal pathogens, the biology and pathogenesis of fungi capable of crossing kingdoms to infect plants and humans. Fungal Genet Biol. 8: 1-12.

12. Gersbach, P.V., Reddy, N. (2002) Non-invasive localization of thymol accumulation in *Carum copticum* (Apiaceae) fruits by chemical shift selective magnetic resonance imaging. Ann Bot. 90: 253-257.

13. Hammer, K., Carson, C., Riley, T. (2002) In-vitro activity of *Melaleuca alternifolia* (tea tree) oil against dermatophytes and other filamentous fungi. J Antimicrob Chemother. 50: 195-199.

14. Ishikawa, T., Sega, Y., Kitajima, J. (2001) Water-soluble constituents of Ajowan. Chem Pharmaceut Bull. 49: 840-844.

15. Khosravi, A.R., Shokri, H., Yahyaraeyat, R. (2006) Veterinary mycology. (1st ed.) Tehran University Press. Tehran, Iran.

16. Klich, M.A. (2002) Identification of common *Aspergillus* species. (1st ed.) Centraalbureau voor Schimmelcultures. Utrecht, The Netherlands.

17. Larone, D.H. (2002) Medically Important Fungi. A guide to Identification. (4th ed.) ASM Press. Washington D.C., USA.

18. Murthy, P.S., Borse, B.B., Khanum, H. (2009) Inhibitory effects of Ajowan (*Trachyspermum ammi*) ethanolic extract on *A. ochraceus* growth and ochratoxin production. Turk J Biol. 33: 211-217.

19. Naeini, A., Khosravi, A.R., Chitsaz, M. (2009) Anti-*Candida* albicans activity of some Iranian plants used in traditional medicine. J Mycol

Méd. 19: 168-172.

20. Naeini, A., Shokri, H. (2012) Chemical composition and in vitro antifungal activity of the essential oil from *Cuminum cyminum* against various *Aspergillus* strains. J Med Plants Res. 6: 1702-1706.

21. Nostro, A., Blanco, A.R., Cannatelli, M.A. (2004) Susceptibility of methicillin-resistant staphylococci to oregano essential oil, carvacrol and thymol. FEMS Microbiol Lett. 230: 191-195.

22. Pina-Vaz, C., Rodrigues, A.G., Pinto, E. (2004) Antifungal activity of Thymus oils and their major compounds. J Eur Acad Dermatol. 18: 73-78.

23. Pinto, E., Palmeira, A., Salgueiro, L. (2003) Antifungal activity of oregano oils (*Lippia graveolens* and *Origanum virens*) on dermatophyte species. Clin Microbiol Infect. 9: 222-230.

24. Ranjan, B., Manmohan, S., Singh, S.R. (2012) Medicinal uses of *Trachyspermum ammi*: a review. Pharmacogn Rev. 6: 56-60.

25. Salgueiro, L.R., Pinto, E., Gonc alves, M.J. (2004) Chemical composition and antifungal activity of the essential oil of *Thymbra capitata*. Planta Med. 70: 572-575.

26. Shojaaddini, M., Moharramipour, S., Sahaf, B. (2008) Fumigant toxicity of essential oil from *Carum copticum* against Indian meal moth, Plodia interpunctella. J Plant Prot Res. 48: 411-419.

27. Shokri, H., Khosravi, A.R., Rad, M.A. (2010) Occurrence of *Malassezia* species in Persian and domestic short hair cats with and without otitis externa. J Vet Med Sci. 72: 293-296.

28. Shokri, H., Sharifzadeh, A., Ashrafi Tamai, I. (2012) Anti-*Candida* zeylanoides activity of some Iranian plants used in traditional medicine. J Mycol Méd. 22: 211-216.

29. Soković, M.D., Vukojević, J., Marin, P.D. (2009) Chemical composition of essential oils of *Thymus* and *Mentha* species and their antifungal activities. Molecul. 14: 238-249.

30. Soni, S., Soni, U.N. (2014) In-vitro anti-bacterial and anti-fungal activity of select essential

oils. Int J Pharm Pharm Sci. 6: 586-591.

31. Tiwari, T.N., Chansouria, J.P.N., Dubey, N.K. (2003) Antimycotic potency of some essential oils in the treatment of induced dermatomycosis of an experimental animal. Pharm Biol. 41: 351-356.

32. Vandeputte, P., Selene, F., Coste, A.T. (2012) Antifungal resistance and new strategies to control fungal infections. Int J Microbiol. 2012: 1-26.

33. World Health Organization (WHO). (2001) General Guidelines for Methodologies on Research and Evaluation of Traditional Medicine, WHO, Geneva, Switzerland.

9

Fasciola gigantica of Ruminants: The phylogenetic analysis based on COX1 sequence

Jahani, Z., Meshgi, B.*, Amininia, N.

Department of Parasitology, Faculty of Veterinary Medicine, University of Tehran, Tehran-Iran (Center of Excellent of Ecosystem and Ultrastructural Changes of Helminthes)

Key words:

COX1, *Fasciola gigantica*, phylogenetic, ruminants, sequence

Correspondence

Meshgi, B.
Department of Parasitology, Faculty of Veterinary Medicine, University of Tehran, Tehran-Iran (Center of Excellent of Ecosystem and Ultrastructural Changes of Helminthes)

Email: Bmeshgi@ut.ac.ir

Abstract:

BACKGROUND: Fasciola species are parasitic trematode with world wide distribution that infects wild and domesticated herbivores, particularly ruminants. **OBJECTIVES:** The aim of the present study was to investigate the intra species variations of *F. gigantica*, from goats and buffalo isolates in two common geographic climates of Iran. **METHODS:** *Fasciola* species were collected from goat, buffalo, sheep, and cattle in different regions. Cytochrome c oxidase I (COX1) of mitochondrial DNA (mt-DNA) was amplified from individual trematodes by polymerase chain reaction (PCR), using universal primers, and the amplicons were consequently sequenced and sequencing data were analyzed, using Clutal W software against the GenBank database. **RESULTS:** A monomorphic DNA segment of approximately 499bp was seen in Fasciola isolates. The results of the amino acid sequence alignment defined strictly conserved amino acid residues in buffalo isolates of *F. gigantica* and partially conserved residues for goat isolates of *F. gigantica*. There are four tandem amino-acid replacements in the goat isolates at the position of 135-138, where Leucine (L), F (Phenylalanine), T (Threonine), and D (Aspartate) sequences changed into S (Serine), L (Leucine), H (Histidine), and L (Leucine), respectively. Furthermore, a replacement in the sequence of amino acid was found in isolates from buffalo at the position of 154, where Serine (S) was transformed into Leucine (L). **CONCLUSIONS:** The findings of our study indicate that the variants of goat and buffalo can be responsible for persistence of Fasciola infection in the endemic areas of Iran. It seems that biological differences could occur by considering a variety of *F. gigantica*-hosts in Iran. Thus, suitable approaches are required for effective treatments and useful control strategies.

Introduction

Fasciolosis is one of the most common zoonotic diseases in different regions of Iran (16). It has been reported that 32% of sheep, 17% of cattle, and 50% buffalos are infected by *Fasciola* spp. in Bandar Anzali, as well as 9.5%, 32.5%, and 50% of sheep, cattle, and horses in Guilan province, north of Iran, respectively (8, 13). Two species, *F. hepatica* and *F. gigantica*, are common causative agents of fasciolosis in ruminants and humans. *F. hepatica* is found in Europe, the Americas, as well as Oceania, while *F. gigantica* is distributed in Africa and Asia (14, 15). Although morphological characterization clearly determines the differentiation between *F. hepatica* and *F. gigantica* and separates them in to two distinct species, it is difficult to accurately differentiate the two species due to the numerous variations in their morphological parameters (10). Previous studies indicated that the ribosomal and mitochondrial DNA sequences are useful for phylogenetic studies and analysis (7, 10). However, some researchers suggested that r-DNA sequences are suitable for molecular identification of plathyhelminthes (3). It is likely that cytochrome c oxidase 1 subunit could be a potential candidate for taxo-molecular studies such as *D. dendriticum*. Therefore, the mitochondrial genome was applied to discriminate between the sub species or strains, and COX1 provided valuable information for the identification of Fasciola strains in Egypt (2). The second nuclear internal transcribed spacer (ITS-2) rDNA of Schistosoma japonicum has been previously applied to determine the genetic diversity (20). The findings of the mentioned studies indicated that ITS2 region is not a suitable marker for assessing inter- and intra- population variation in S. japonicum, while mitochondrial genes are suitable resources for molecular taxonomic studies. Recent investigations have shown that mt-genome can be considered as a useful molecular marker in the population genetic and phylogenic studies of trematoda such as *S. japonicum* (21) and *F. hepatica* (18). Nowadays, the drug treatment against fasciolosis in Iran is carried out with various anthelminthes combinations such as triclabendazol and albendazol, as well as

monitoring of performance which is based on fecal examination for EPG (egg per gram) and slaughterhouse inspection. The purpose of this study was to determinate the molecular characterization of Iranian *F. gigantica* from goats buffalos, sheep and cattle isolates using PCR on COX1-mtDNA fragment.

Materials and Methods

Parasite collection: Adult flukes of Fasciola species were obtained from livers of naturally infected cattle, sheep, buffalos, and goats from local slaughterhouses of two geographical origins, Guilan and Tehran Provinces, Iran. Fresh worms were washed in phosphate-buffered saline (pH=7.2).

Two Fasciola species were differentiated from each other based on their morphological and morphometric characteristics. The samples were labeled and preserved immediately in a 70% ethanol solution until DNA extraction. The hosts and localities of the specimens are shown in Table 1.

DNA extraction, Amplification, and Sequencing: One hundred adult *F. gigantica* and *F. hepatica* from four hosts and two geographical origins were considered in the present molecular study. Total genomic DNA was extracted from individual flukes, using a DNA extraction kit (MBST, Iran) according to the manufacturer's instructions

DNA was extracted from a small portion of anterior end of the worm that lacked eggs (16). DNA fragments of mitochondrial COX1 gene were amplified by the specific primers. The primer sets which were employed in amplifying the fragments were F-COX: (forward; 5́-ACGTTGGATCATA-AGCGTG-3́) and (reverse; 5́-CCTCATC-CAACATAACCTC-3́). The polymerase chain reaction (100 µl) was performed using master mix (Amplicon, USA), 2 µl of each forward and reverse primers and 4 µl of genomic template in an automated thermocycler (Biorad-Italia) with the following procedure: 95°C for 5 min, 37 cycles of denaturation at 95°C for 45 sec, annealing at 54°C for 45 sec, extension at 72°C for 45 sec, and final extension at 72°C for 5 min as the final step. Samples without any genomic DNA were included as negative controls in each PCR run. All amplicons were subjected to 1.5% agarose gel containing Sybersafe staining (Cinaclone, Iran) and were visualized under UV, and their size was compared with 100 bp DNA ladder (Vivantis- Malaysia) as well. Consequently, the PCR products were purified, using a quick PCR purification kit (MBST, Iran) according to the manufacturer's protocol and 10 PCR products from goat (Guilan), 10 PCR products from buffalo (Guilan), 10 PCR products from cattle (Guilan) for *F. gigantica* and 10 PCR products from cattle (Tehran) for *F. hepatica* were considered for sequencing analysis (Takapouzist, Iran). The obtained sequences were then analyzed using the Chromas software (version 2.1.1) and subsequently aligned with the ClustalW software for nucleotide and T-COFFEE software for amino acid (version-11). Sequences available in the National Center for Biotechnology Information (www.ncbi.nlm.nih.gov/) were included in the final alignment for comparing the obtained sequences. The aligned sequences were analyzed with Neighbor Joining Analysis, using MEGA 7 software (version 7.0).

Results

PCR amplification: DNA amplification

Table 1. *Fasciola* species in Iran based on isolates and origin Subtitle: FGGG: *F. gigantica*-Goat Guilan isolate, FGBG: *F. gigantica*-Buffalo Guilan isolate, FGCG: *F. gigantica*-Cattle Guilan isolate, FGST: *F. gigantica*-Sheep Tehran isolate, FGCT: *F. gigantica*-Cattle Tehran isolate, FGGT: *F. gigantica*-Goat Tehran isolate, FHGG: *F. hepatica*-Goat Guilan isolate, FHCG: *F. hepatica*-Cattle Guilan isolate, FHSG: *F. hepatica*-Sheep Guilan isolate, FHCT: *F. hepatica*-Cattle Tehran isolate, FHST: *F. hepatica*-Sheep Tehran isolate, FHGT: *F. hepatica*-Goat Tehran.

Species (host)	Trematode code	N. of worms	Isolate origin
F. gigantica (goat)	FGGG	38	Gilan
F. gigantica (buffalo)	FGBG	26	Gilan
F. gigantica (cattle)	FGCG	26	Gilan
F. gigantica (sheep)	FGST	33	Tehran
F. gigantica (cattle)	FGCT	21	Tehran
F. gigantica (goat)	FGGT	14	Tehran
F. gigantica (goat)	FHGG	40	Gilan
F. hepatica (cattle)	FHCG	30	Gilan
F. hepatica (sheep)	FHSG	19	Gilan
F. hepatica (cattle)	FHCT	33	Tehran
F. hepatica (sheep)	FHST	29	Tehran
F. hepatica (goat)	FHGT	12	Tehran

of COX1-mtDNA showed a single fragment of 499 bp in all Fasciola species from different isolates. Moreover, the negative controls produced no bands in any experiments. Agarose gel electrophoresis of COX1 PCR product of *F. gigantica* and *F. hepatica* from different hosts and localities are shown in Figs 1 and 2, respectively.

Sequence analysis and phylogenetic: Sequences of 499 bp COX1 of the Fasciola species were aligned with those of available sequences in GenBank (acces-

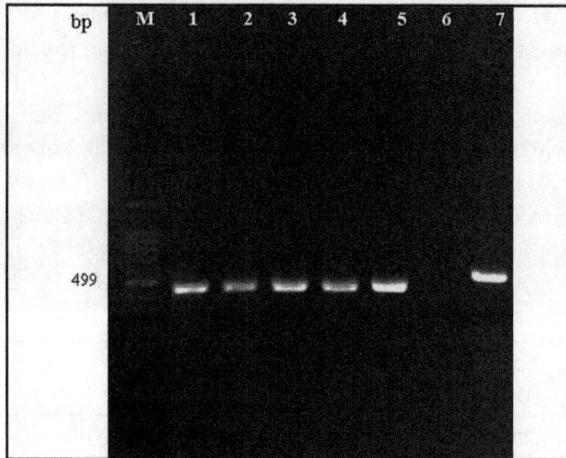

Figure 1. Agarose gel electrophoresis of COX1 PCR product of *F. gigantica* from Goats- Guilan (Lane 1), Buffalos-Guilan (Lane 2), Cattle- Guilan (Lane 3), Cattle-Tehran (Lane 4), Sheep-Tehran (Lane 5), Negative DNA control (Lane 6), Goats-Tehran (Lane 7), M: DNA marker.

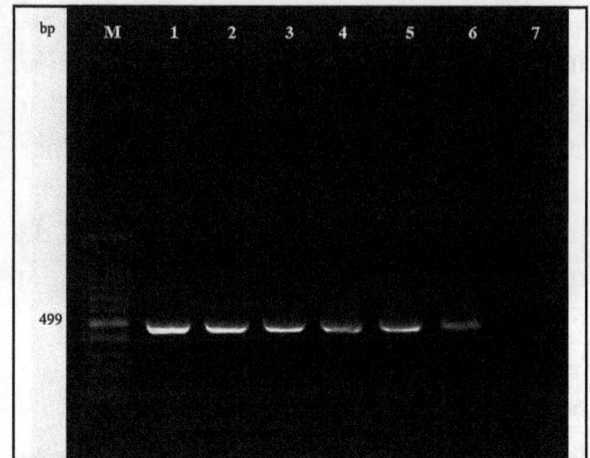

Figure 2. Agarose gel electrophoresis of COX1 PCR product of *F. hepatica* from Cattle- Guilan (Lane 1), Sheep-Guilan (Lane 2), Goats- Guilan (Lane 3), Cattle-Tehran (Lane 4), Sheep-Tehran (Lane 5), Goats-Tehran (Lane 6), Negative DNA control (Lane 7), M: DNA marker.

sion no. GQ398051.1, AB536898.1 and AB385622.1 for *F. hepatica* from cattle, Iran; *Fasciola* spp. from cattle-Vietnam and *F. gigantica* from cattle, Vietnam, respectively). Although COX1 nucleotid sequences of different isolates of *F. gigantica* showed 96-100% similarity, findings demonstrated 91% similarity between isolates of goat and cattle isolates from Iran ,while 81% similarity was observed between the goat isolates of Iran and cattle isolates from Vietnam.

The sequences were sub¬mitted to GenBank (accession no. KX423725 for *F. gigantica*- Guilan cattle isolate, KX395645 for *F. gigantica*- Guilan buffalo isolate, KX458034 for *F. gigantica*- Guilan goat isolate and KX423726 for *F. hepatica*-Tehran cattle isolate,).

Furthermore, nucleotide sequence was translated into amino acids. Consequently, *F. hepatica* and *F. gigantica* nucleotide sequences were aligned with sequences released in GenBank, which were similar to each other. In addition, host diversity was observed in *F. gigantica*.

Phylogenetic tree was plotted based on partial sequences of COX1 gene of Fasciola isolates in Iran using neighbor joining analysis. This phylogenetic tree indicates that *F. gigantica* isolates clustered in a separate cluster, in accordance with the specific host variations. *F. gigantica* isolates of goats are placed in the separate cluster, while those of buffalos and cattle are placed in the same cluster and different branches. Moreover, *F. gigantica* isolates of cattle in two different geographical regions of Tehran and Guilan are placed in the same cluster (Fig. 3).

Our findings suggested that the isolate of *F. gigantica* and *F. hepatica* from Iran (GQ398050.1 and GQ398056.1, respectively) are located at the same cluster together with Fasciola species.

Amino acids sequence of *F. gigantica* isolates from goats showed noticeable difference as compared to submitted sequences of *F. hepatica* in GenBank (Accession numbers: AB300704, AB207170, KJ716921, GQ398054.1, GQ398056.1, and FJ895606.1).

Amino acid sequence of *F. gigantica* isolates from buffalo and the sequence of *F. gigantica* isolated from cattle in GenBank were quite similar. The sequences of *F. gi-*

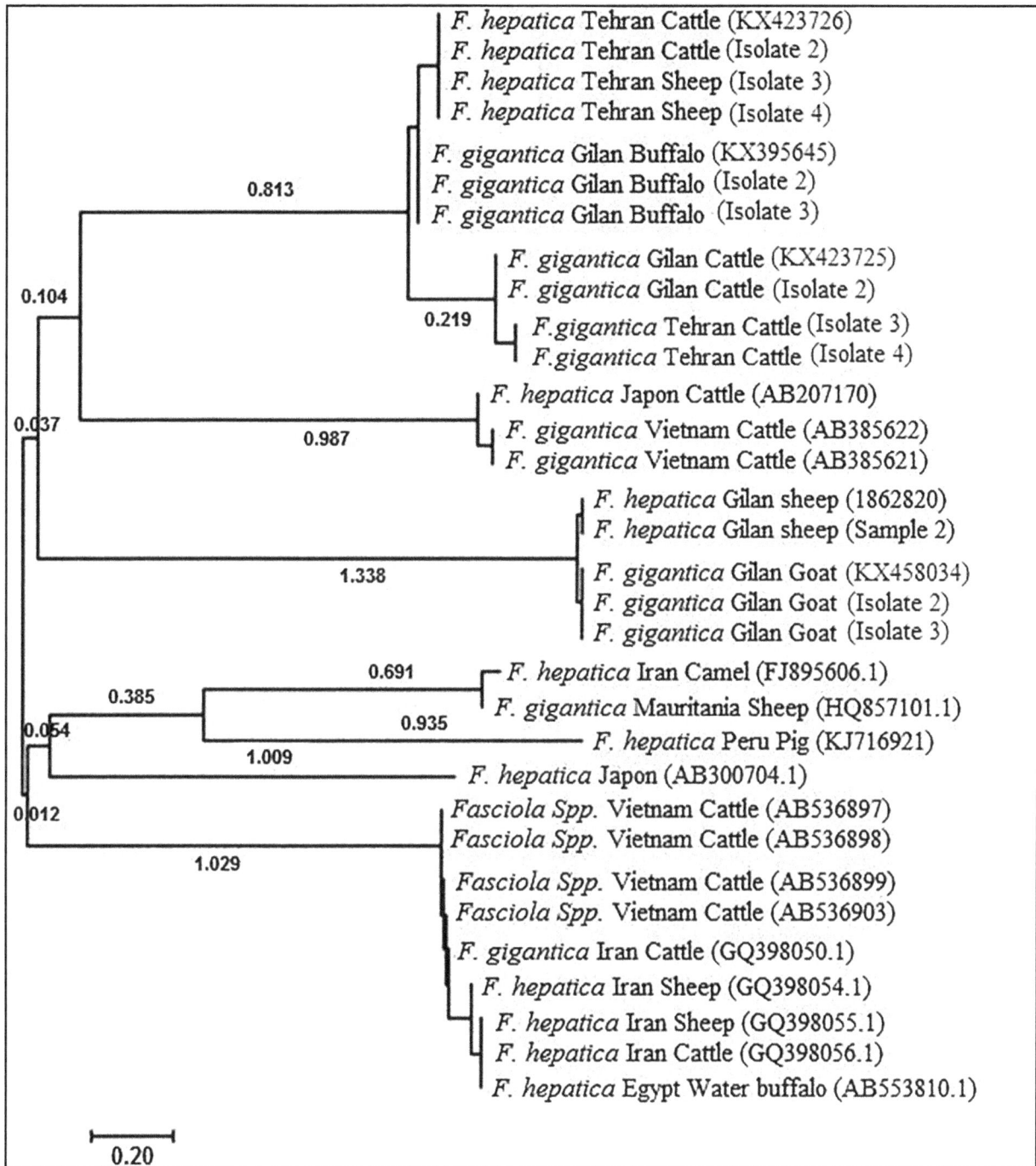

Figure 3. Phylogenetic relationships of Iranian *Fasciola* species derived from different isolates based on COX1 amino acids sequences in comparison with other isolates (Phylogenetic analyses were conducted in MEGA 7).

gantica isolates from goats were not in Gen-Bank database and they had the least difference from *F. gigantica* isolates of cattle in four amino acids. Amino acids of Serine, Leucine, Histidine, and Leucine in the sequence of GenBank changed into Leucine, Phenylalanine, Threonine, and Aspartate in Iranian goats isolates (Fig. 4).

Discussion

The liver flukes of *F. hepatica* and *F. gigantica* are the two most important helminthes, causing substantial economic loss in ruminants worldwide mainly due to loss of weight, fertility, and liver condemnation

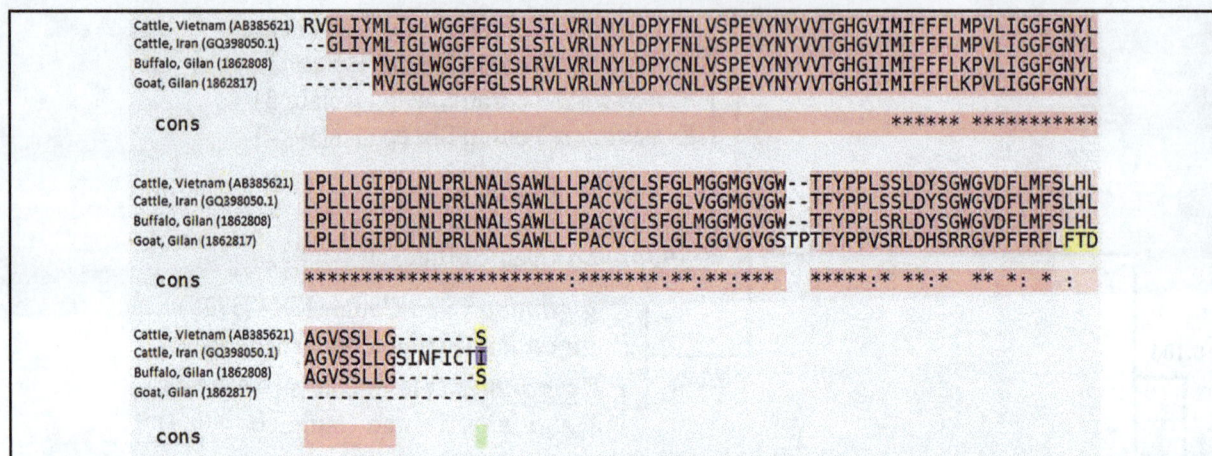

Figure 4. Amino acid alignment of Fasciola species by T-COFFEE software.

(9).

F. hepatica and *F. gigantica* infections have generally occurred in temperate and tropical zones, respectively, both species may overlap in subtropical areas (6, 11). Both species have been reported in cattle, sheep, goats, buffalos, and camels in Iran (5, 9, 16).

During the past fifty years, high prevalence rate of fasciolosis has been documented, especially in southern and northern areas of Iran. Recent studies indicated that prevalence rates of fasciolosis in northern provinces of Guilan and Mazandaran are higher compared with other parts of the country. On the other hand, the prevalence rate of fasciolosis in livestock has decreased in the southern part of Iran. It is worth noting that two *Fasciola* species, *F. hepatica* and *F. gigantica*, are prevalent in both animal and human. Recent studies determined that *F. hepatica* transmission occurs in the mountainous area of Guilan and *F. gigantica* transmission takes place in the lowlands. However, overlap distribution of *F. hepatica* and *F. gigantica* are involved in other parts of Iran (4).

Molecular approaches are the powerful tools to determine the diversity of inter and intra-species as well as intermediate forms of micro and macro organisms, particularly in helminth populations. Among all targets of DNA makers, genomic sequencing of different regions is a useful technique for specific identification of species and molecular variation studies for a wide range of parasitic flat worm.

Mitochondrial and nuclear DNA sequences have been previously used for molecular studies of Fasciola species (2, 10). The molecular characterization of human Fasciola samples from Guilan, the coastal Caspian Sea of Iran, based on ITS1 and COX1 genes, indicated that human Fasciola specimens were represented as *F. hepatica* (19). It has been previously reported that host association and geographical origin are not likely to be useful indicators for Fasciola molecular classification based on COX1 fragment (17).

Itagaki et al. (2005) studied genetic characterization of parthenogenic Fasciola on the basis of the sequences of ribosomal and mitochondrial DNA (12, 14). Their findings suggested that 2 major and 3 minor distinct forms of Fasciola occurred in Japan. Heterozygosis in mitochondrial DNA of Japanese form may be originated from interspecific cross hybridization between paternal *F. hepatica* and maternal *F. gigantica*.

Previous study by Agatsuma et al. (2000) reported that COX1 and NADH dehydrogenase subunit 1 (Nicotinamide adenine dinucleotide) fragments are monomorphic in the Korean fasciolid and similar to those of *F. gigantica* (1).

Most of the molecular variations of *F. gigantica* have been explained by specific variation within host-associated populations of ruminants. In other words, *F. gigantica* tends to be relatively host-specific in ruminants. However, it is not an individual variation related to common geographic location. Semyenova et al. (2006) revealed that single cattle may be concurrently harbored with more than one genotypes of the trematode (18). It must be said that intermediate forms of two Fasciola species are present in Iran. But in the present study, the used samples were quite identifiable in terms of morphological characteristics.

In the present study, genomic DNA was extracted from *F. gigantica* isolates in goats, buffalos, cattle, and sheep in two geographical locations of Guilan and Tehran Provinces, Iran. COX1 fragments were amplified from each sample, using universal primers, and fragments with 499 bp in length were amplified and consequently sequenced. The sequencing results showed that goat isolates are different from the other amino acid sequences in a consecutive sequence with 4 amino acids. Goat sequence was LFTD (Leucine: hydrophobic-nonpolar, Phenylalanine: hydrophobic-nonpolar, Threonine: hydrophilic-nonpolar and Aspartate: hydrophilic-negatively charged polar) but all other sequences contained SLHL (Serine: hydrophilic-nonpolar, Histidine: hydrophilic-positively charged polar) and were similar to each other. The amino acid sequences of buffalo isolates were different

from cattle isolates only in one amino acid. Amino acid of S was replaced with L in cattle isolates of Iran, but it was similar to cattle isolates from Vietnam that had S at this position. The identification of amino acid substitutions showed the least variability in the buffalo isolates. The results of phylogenetic tree defined the separate cluster that was associated with particular host species. *F. gigantica* of goat isolates were placed in separate cluster, while buffalo and cattle isolates were clustered in the same cluster, although they were placed in the separate branches.

Acknowledgments

Project support was provided by the Iran National Science Foundation (Grant no. 93023576).

References

Agatsuma, T., Arakawa, Y., Iwagami, M., Honzako, Y., Cahyaningsih, U., Kang, S.Y., Hong, S.J. (2000) Molecular evidence of natural hybridization between *Fasciola hepatica* and *F. gigantica*. Parasitol Int. 49: 231-238.

Amer, S., Dar, Y., Ichikawa, M., Fukuda, Y., Tada, C., Itagaki, T., Nakai, Y. (2011) Identification of Fasciola species isolated from Egypt based on sequence analysis of genomic (ITS1 and ITS2) and mitochondrial (NDI and COI) gene markers. Parasitol Int. 60: 5-12.

Amor, N., Halajian, A., Farjallah, S., Merella, P., Said, K., Slimane, B.B. (2011) Molecular characterization of *Fasciola* spp. from the endemic area of northern Iran based on nuclear ribosomal DNA sequences. Exp Parasitol. 128: 196-204.

Ashrafi, K., Massoud, J., Holakuei Naieni, K., Mahmoodi, M., Jo-Afshani, M.A., Valero, M.A., Fuentes, M.V., Khoubbane, M., Artigas, P., Bargues, M.D., Mas-Coma, S. (2004) Evidence suggesting that *Fasciola gigantica* might be the most prevalent causal agent of fascioliasis in the endemin province of Guilan, northern Iran. Iran J Public Health. 33: 31-37.

Ashrafi, K., Valero, M.A., Panova, M., Periago, M.V., Massoud, J., Mas-Coma, S. (2006) Phenotypic analysis of adult of *Fasciola hepatica*, *Fasciola gigantica* and intermediate forms from the endemic region of Guilan, Iran. Parasitol Int. 55: 249-260.

Choi, I.W., Kim, H.Y., Quan, J.H., Ryu, J.G., Sun, R., Lee, Y.H. (2015) Monitoring of Fasciola species contamination in water dropwort by COX I mitochondrial and ITS-2 rDNA sequencing analysis. Korean J Parasitol. 53: 641-645.

Cwiklinski, K., Allen, K., LaCourse, J., Williams, D.J., Paterson, S., Hodgkinson, J.E. (2015) Characterisation of a novel panel of polymorphic microsatellite loci for the liver fluke, *Fasciola hepatica*, using a next generation sequencing approach. Infect Genet Evol. 32: 298-304.

Eslami, A., Hosseini, S.H., Meshgi, B. (2009) Animal Fasciolosis in North of Iran. Iran J Pub Health. 38: 132-135.

Eslami, A., Ranjbar-Bahadori, Sh., Eskandari, A., Sedaghet, R. (2004) Prevalence and pathology of camel fasciolosis in Iran. J Vet Res, University of Tehran. 58: 97-100.

Farjallah, S., Ben-Slimane, B., Piras, C.M., Amor, N., Garippa, G., Merella, P. (2013) Molecular characterization of *Fasciola hepatica* from Sardinia based on sequence analysis of genomic and mitochondrial gene markers. Exp Parasitol. 135: 471-478.

Furst, T., Keiser, J., Utzinger, J. (2012) Global burden of human food-borne trematodiasis: a systematic review and meta-analysis. Lancet Infect Dis. 12: 210-221.

Huang, W.Y., He, B., Wang, C.R., Zhu, X.Q. (2004) Characterization of Fasciola species from Mainland China by ITS2 ribosomal DNA sequence. Vet Parasitol. 120: 75-83.

Hosseini, S. H., Meshgi, B., Abbassi, A., Eslami, A. (2012) Animal fascioliasis in coastal regions of the Caspian Sea, Iran. Iran J Vet Res. 13: 64-67.

Itagaki, T., Kikawa, M., Sakaguchi, K., Shimo, J., Terasaki, K., Shibahara, T., Fukuda, K. (2005) Genetic characterization of parthenogenic Fasciola sp. in Japan on the basis of the sequences of ribosomal and mitochondrial DNA. Parasitology. 131:679-685.

Liu, G.H., Gasser, R.B., Young, N.D., Song, H.Q., Ai, L., Zhu, X.Q. (2014) Complete mitochondrial genomes of the 'intermediate form' of Fasciola and *Fasciola gigantica*, and their comparison with *F. hepatica*. Parasit Vectors. 31: 150.

Meshgi, B., Eslami, A., Shayan, P. (2007) Evaluation of Dot-ELISA for serodiagnosis of fasiolosis in naturally infected sheep. J Appl Anim Res. 31: 89-91.

Moazeni, M., Sharifiyazdi, H., Izadpanah, A. (2012) Characterization of *Fasciola hepatica* genotypes from cattle and sheep in Iran using cytochrome C oxidase gene (CO1). Parasitol Res. 110: 2379-2384.

Semyenova, S.K., Morozova, E.V., Chrisanfova, G.G., Gorokhov, V.V., Arkhipov, I.A., Moskvin, A.S., Movsessyan, S.O., Ryskov, A.P. (2006) Genetic differentiation in eastern European and western Asian populations of the liver fluke, *Fasciola hepatica*, as revealed by mitochondrial NDI and COI genes. J Parasitol. 92: 525-530.

Sharifiyazdi, H., Moazeni, M., Rabbani, F. (2011) Molecular characterization of human Fasciola samples in Guilan province, Northern Iran on the basis of DNA sequences of ribosomal and mitochondrial genes. Comp

Clin Pathol. 10: 1193-1198.

Zhao, G.H., Li, J., Mo, X.H., Li, X.Y., Lin, R.Q., Zou, F.C., Weng, Y.B., Song, H.Q., Zhu, X.Q. (2012) The second transcribed spacer rDNA sequence: an effective genetic marker for inter-species phylogenetic analysis of trematodes in the order Strigeata. Parasitol Res. 10: 210-215.

Zhao, G.H., Mo, X.H., Zou, F.C., Li, J., Weng, Y.B., Lin, R.Q., Xia, C.M., Zhu, X.Q. (2009) Genetic variability among Schistosoma japonicum isolates from different endemic regions in China revealed by sequences of three mitochondrial DNA genes. Vet Parasitol. 162: 67-74.

10

Detection of *eaeA*, *hlyA*, *stx1* and *stx2* genes in pathogenic *Escherichia coli* isolated from broilers affected with colibacillosis

Jamshidi, A.[1*], Razmyar, J.[2], Fallah, N.[1]

[1]Department of Food Hygiene, Faculty of Veterinary Medicine, Ferdowsi University of Mashhad, Mashhad, Iran

[2]Department of Clinical Sciences, Faculty of Veterinary Medicine, Ferdowsi University of Mashhad, Mashhad, Iran

Key words:

chicken colibacillosis, *Escherichia coli*, STEC

Correspondence

Jamshidi, A.
Department of Food Hygiene,
Faculty of Veterinary Medicine,
Ferdowsi University of Mashhad, Mashhad, Iran

Email: ajamshid@um.ac.ir

Abstract:

BACKGROUND: Foodborne outbreaks associated with shiga toxin-producing *Escherichia coli* (STEC) have been well documented worldwide. STECs are major causative agents of gastroenteritis in humans that may be complicated by hemorrhagic colitis (HC), hemolytic uremic syndrome (HUS), and thrombotic thrombocytopenia purpura (TTP). OBJECTIVES: The aim of this study was to investigate the presence of virulence-associated genes including eaeA, hlyA, stx1 and stx2 in *Escherichia coli* strains isolated from broiler's Colibacillosis in the northeast of Iran. METHODS: From a total of 78 *E.coli* strains isolated from yolk sac infection, hepatitis and pericarditis, that were referred to educational veterinary clinic during 2011-2014, subculturing of the isolates was performed using selective media and a typical colony from each sample was subjected to multiplex PCR assay for identification of the presence of STEC important virulence-associated genes (eaeA, hlyA,stx1 and stx2) causing shiga toxin-mediated diseases. RESULTS: Of 78 *E.coli* isolates, one isolate was positive for both eaeA and hlyA genes while negative for stx1 and stx2 genes. CONCLUSIONS: The results showed low prevalence of STEC virulence genes associated with human infections in avian pathogenic *E.coli* (APEC) strains isolated from different flocks of broilers affected with colibacillosis.

Introduction

Shiga toxin-producing *Escherichia coli* (STEC) or verotoxin-producing *Escherichia coli* remains a major cause of foodborne-related gastrointestinal diseases in humans (Wani et al., 2004), particularly since these infections may result in life-threatening sequel such as hemorrhagic colitis (HC), hemolytic uremic syndrome (HUS), and thrombotic thrombocytopenia purpura (TTP) (Best et al., 2005; Dhanashree and ShrikarMallya., 2008; Feng, 2013; Mohammadi et al., 2013; Paton and Paton., 1998; Paton and Paton., 2002; Paton and Paton., 2005; Wani et al., 2004). Ruminants are considered to be the main reservoir of STECs (Paton and Paton., 1998). Other domestic animals, such as pigs, poultry, cats and dogs can also harbor STECs (Dhanashree and Shrikar-Mallya, 2008; Kobayashi et al., 2002; Wani et al., 2004). The pathogenicity of these bacteria is mainly mediated by shiga toxins(Stx1,

Stx2 and their variants) encoded by stx1 and stx2 genes. Within human disease-associated strains, those producing Shiga toxin type 2 appear to be more commonly responsible for serious complications such as HUS than those producing only Shiga toxin type 1 (Feng, 2013; Fode-Vaughan et al., 2003; Paton and Paton., 1998). In addition, a subset of STEC strains considered to be highly virulent for humans has the capacity to produce attaching and effacing lesions on intestinal mucosa, a property encoded on a pathogenicity island termed the locus for enterocyte effacement (LEE). LEE encodes a type III secretion system and *E. coli* secreted proteins, which deliver effector molecules to the host cell and disrupt the host cytoskeleton. LEE also carries eaeA, which encodes an outer membrane protein (intimin) required for intimate attachment to epithelial cells. The eaeA gene has been used as a convenient diagnostic marker for LEE-positive STECs (Mohammadi et al., 2013; Paton and Paton., 1998; Paton and Paton., 2002; Paton and Paton., 2005; Wani et al., 2004). Another putative accessory virulence factor produced by STEC strains (both LEE positive and LEE negative) is plasmid-encoded enterohemolysin (hlyA) (Paton and Paton., 1998; Paton and Paton., 2002; Wani et al., 2004). This haemolysin seems to have an important role in complex diseases (HC and HUS) in humans. (Beutin et al., 1994). Accordingly, the capacity to rapidly determine the STECs virulence profile associated with the mentioned serious diseases is important to ensure the public safety. As chicken products are suspected to be a source of foodborne pathogenic *Escherichia coli* infections in humans (Heuvelink et al., 1999; Mellata, 2013; Tabatabaei et al., 2011), we have described using multiplex PCR assays for detection of the important marker genes associated with major STEC-outbreaks, eaeA and hlyA in the first step, then stx1 and stx2 in isolates harboring eaeA and/or hlyA. *Escherichia coli* strains isolated from chicken visceral organs suffering from clinical colibacillosis were screened to analyze their potential hazard for public health.

Materials and Methods

Sampling and bacterial culture: A total of 78 *E.coli* isolates were obtained from broiler chickens belonging to different flocks which were diagnosed as affected with systemic Colibacillosis. These isolates of *E.coli* were swabbed from affected organs of birds harboring lesions of Colibacillosis such as hepatitis and pericarditis, each isolate represented one flock. They were sampled during the years of 2011 to 2014 in the northeast of Iran. The strains were isolated from liver, blood (heart) and egg yolk sac. The respective specimens were plated on MacConkey agar (Merck, Germany) and suspected colonies were confirmed as *E.coli* using biochemical tests, afterwards a loopful of typical colonies on overnight culture were inoculated on Brain Heart Infusion (BHI) broth (Hi-Media, India) to transport to the food microbiology laboratory. The samples were incubated at 37°C for 24h and were then cultured on Sorbitol-MacConkey agar(Hi-Media, India) supplemented with cefexime 0.05mg/l and potassium tellurite 2.5mg/l. After incubating overnight at 37°C, both sorbitol fermenting and non-fermenting colonies were chosen separately for DNA extraction.

DNA extraction: Crude DNA extracts were prepared by using boiling method, in brief, bacterial colonies were suspended in 200µl of sterile distilled water, then microtubes were vortexed and the bacterial suspensions were lysed by boiling in a water bath at 100°C for 10 min. The lysates were centrifuged at 15000 rpm for 15 min. The supernatants were transferred to sterile nuclease free microtubes and frozen at -18 °C until used as templates for PCR assay.

PCR analysis: Extracted DNA was subjected to multiplex polymerase chain reaction (m-PCR) for detection of eaeA and hlyA genes. Strains that were positive for eaeA and/or hlyA were further tested in another m-PCRassay for the presence of the genes encoding shiga toxins (Stx1 and Stx2). Amplifications were carried out in single-tubes, 25µl reaction mixture in an automated thermal cycler (TC-512, Techne, England). The PCR cocktail consisted of 3µl DNA template, 11.5µl of 2x Taq premix (consists of ParstousTaq DNA polymerase, reaction buffer, dNTPs mixture, protein stabilizer and 2x solution of loading dye) and 1.25µl of each primer(10 pm/µl, AccuPower PCR PreMix, Bioneer). Deionized distilled water was added to make a final volume of 25 µl. Details of the primers nucleotide sequences, the specific gene region amplified and the predicted size of PCR products are listed in Table1, according to Paton and Paton (Paton and Paton., 1998). Amplification reactions were performed in duplicate for 35 cycles. For all reactions the mixture was heated at 94°c for 5 min prior to thermocycling for initial denaturation. Each cycle consisted of 1 min for denaturation at 94°c, 1min of annealing at 54°c and 1 min of extension at 72°c. This was followed by final extension of 10 min at 72°c. Both duplex PCRs had the same temperatures and conditions (Hosseini et al., 2013). In addition, the E.coli O157:H7 reference strain (ATCC35150) was used as positive control for detection of virulence genes and sterile distilled water as negative control in all PCR runs.

The amplified products were visualized by standard gel electrophoresis using 3 µl of the final reaction mixture on 1.5% agarose gel in TAE buffer (89 mMTris, 89 mM glacial Acetic acid, 0.5 M EDTA) for 45 min at 100 V. A 100 bp DNA ladder molecular weight marker (Fermentas, UK.) was included in each electrophoretic run to allow identification of the amplified products. The agarose gel was stained with DNA Green Viewer and photographed using a gel documentation system (Stratagene EE 2, Germany).

Results

Among 78 isolates of *E. coli* isolated from chicken colibacillosis, only one strain (1.28%) harbored eaeA and hlyA genes simultaneously. This strain was screened for the presence of stx1 and stx2 genes by m-PCR and was found to be negative for these genes.

Discussion

Despite the fact that most avian pathogenic Escheichia coli (APEC) infections are extra intestinal, some APECs contain traits associated with the intestinal *E.coli* pathotypes, including enteropathogenic *E.coli* (EPEC), enterotoxigenic *E.coli* (ETEC), enteroinvasive *E.coli* (EIEC) and enterohemorragic *E.coli* (EHEC) (Barnes et al., 2008). However, information on *E.coli* isolates genotypes in poultry as a food source is of considerable importance in the food safety or public health's viewpoint. In this investigation the possible pathogenicity of APECs in producing human shiga toxin-mediated disease including HC and HUS was addressed by screening the important virulence associated genes.For the rapid and sensitive detection, PCR has proven to be of great diagnostic value (Mohammadi et al., 2013, Paton et al., 1996). Cultivation in liquid medium (BHI broth in this study) and then plating on CT-SMAC may increase the number of bacteria and therefore assist in the detection of STECs which are present in low numbers or in a physiologically stressed state (Mohammadi et al., 2013). It should be noted that STEC include both sorbitol fermenting and non-fermenting strains (Harrigan., 1998), therefore all colonies (sorbitol-positives and negatives) were picked from SMAC for DNA extraction.

Target virulence factors in the present study were as follow: 1-chromosomal eaeA gene (Gerrish et al., 2007), 2-plasmid hlyA gene (Dhanashree and Shrikar Mallya, 2008,

Table 1. Sequence of used primers and the size of amplified products.

Primer	Sequence(5′-3′)	Specificity	Amplicon size (bp)
stx1F	ATAAATCGCCATTCGTT GACTAC	nt 454–633 of A subunit coding region of stx1	180
stx1R	AGAACGCCCACTGAGATCATC		
stx2F	GGCACTGTCTGAAACTGCTCC	nt 603–857 of A subunit coding region of stx2 (including stx2 variants)	255
stx2R	TCGCCAGTTATCTGACATTCTG		
eaeAF	GACCCGGCACAAGCATAAGC	nt 27–410 of eaeA (this region is conserved between EPEC and STEC)	384
eaeAR	CCACCTGCAGCAACAAGAGG		
hlyAF	GCATCATCAAGCGTACGTTCC	nt 70–603 of EHEC hlyA	534
hlyAR	AATGAGCCAAGCTGGTTAAGCT		

Gerrish et al., 2007, Paton and Paton, 2002) 3-phage stx1 and stx2genes (Dhanashree and ShrikarMallya, 2008, Gerrish et al., 2007). Testing for eaeA and hlyA genes confirms the presence of the LEE pathogenicity island and the large virulence plasmid, respectively, and detection of either stx1 or stx2 genes confirms the presence of STECs (Boerlin et al., 1999; Paton and Paton., 2002). Upon transit through the stomach, STEC must adhere to the luminal surface of the large intestine in order to effectively colonize the host and compete with normal microbiota. The best-characterized adhesion and an absolutely essential virulence factor, is the ~94-kDa outer-membrane protein intimin, encoded by the eaeA gene (Vanaja et al., 2013) as many of the STEC strains that do not produce putative accessory virulence factors such as intimin and enterohemolysin have a low degree of virulence in humans (Paton and Paton., 1998). It should be noted that though a number of sporadic cases of HUS were caused by eaeA-negative STECs (Beutin et al., 1999, Mohammadi et al., 2013, Paton et al., 1999), harboring the hlyA gene is a significant contributor to shiga toxin-mediated disease, as there is increasing evidence of hemolysin gene being the marker for STECs (Dhanashree and ShrikarMallya., 2008, Schroeder et al., 2002). For this reason we have assayed both eaeA and hlyA in all isolates simultaneously. In the following, isolates harboring eaeA and/or hlyA were tested for the presence of other principal virulence factors for human infections, stx1 and stx2.

Results obtained in our study revealed none of the 78 E.coli strains can be regarded as important carriers of zoonotic E.coli. However, one (1.28%) eaeA and hlyA positive isolate was found which did not produce shiga toxins (stx1 or stx2). The absence of stx genes in this isolate could be due to the fact that stx gene is bacteriophage coded and the isolate would have lost the same during preservation (Dhanashree and Shrikar Mallya, 2008, Schroeder et al., 2002).

Our results are in agreement with the earlier findings of Wani et al. (2004) who reported none of 426 E.coli isolates from fecal samples originating from chickens and pigeons in India was positive for stx1 and stx2 and the percentage rate of eaeA and hlyA was 2.74% and 1.74%, respectively (Wani et al., 2004). Janben et al. (2001) also did not find any STEC virulence factors (stx1, stx2, eaeA and hlyA genes) in 80 E.coli strains of poultry internal organs having died from colibacillosis (Janben et al., 2001). Other research findings indicating prevalence level similar to our results are as follow: Krause et al. (2005) who have reported 2.3% eaeA positive while all their screened isolates were negative for stx gene (Krause et al., 2005); Mellata et al. (2001) in Algeria who observed none of the 50 studied intestinal avian E.coli strains harbored eaeAand hlyAgenes(Mellataet al., 2001) and the study of Schroeder et al. (2003) that also did not reveal any STEC in retail chicken and turkey obtained from Washington, DC, USA (Schroeder et al., 2003). In contrast, Kobayashi et al.

(2002) detected a high percentage (57%) of fecal samples of contaminated chicken flocks in Finland bearing eaeA gene, while they lacked stx and hlyA genes (Kobayashi et al., 2002).

Low prevalence rate of STEC virulence genes associated with human infections in this research corroborate the fact that most APECs isolated from poultry are specific clonal types that are pathogenic only for birds and represent a low risk of disease for people or other animals (Barnes et al., 2008; Cayaet al., 1999; Ron., 2006). APECs also are much less toxigenic than pathogenic *E.coli* in mammals and human beings (Barnes et al., 2008; Blanco et al., 1997; Janben et al., 2001; Mellataet al., 2001). Moreover, infection with STEC in chicken requires flagella but not intimin, the surface adhesion responsible for attachment of the organism to epithelial cells in mammals (Barnes et al., 2008; Best et al., 2005; La Ragioneet al., 2005). In summary, the data presented in this study show a low presence of infective STECs occurrence in colibacillosis cases of chicken flocks in the northeast of Iran. The results are in contrast with Tabatabaei et al. (2011) who have isolated STEC from 4% chicken fecal samples in Iran (Tabatabaei et al., 2011). Therefore, further investigations are required to evaluate the role of poultry as a putative vehicle of infective STEC to human. Furthermore, knowledge in distribution of the virulence-associated genes may be a useful instrument to design comprehensive epidemiological studies.

Acknowledgments

This study was supported by Faculty of Veterinary Medicine, Ferdowsi University of Mashhad. The authors are grateful to Samira Khajenasiri and Ali Kargar for their technical assistance.

References

1. 1-Barnes, H. J., Nolan, L. K., Vaillancourt, J. P. (2008) Colibacillosis. In: Diseases of Poultry. Y., Saif, M.(eds.). (12th ed.). Iowa State Press. A Blackwell Publishing Company. Iowa, USA. p. 691-737.

2. Best, A., La Ragione, R.M., Sayers, A.R., Woodward, M.J. (2005) Role for flagella but not intimin in the persistent infection of the gastrointestinal tissues of specific-pathogen-free chicks by shiga toxin-negative *Escherichia coli* O157:H7. Infect Immun. 73: 1836-1846.

3. Beutin, L. (1999) *Escherichia coli* O157 and other types of Verocytotoxigenic *E.coli* (VTEC) Isolated from Humans, Animals and Food in Germany. *Escherichia coli* O157 in Farm Animals. Ed. CS Stewart, HJ Flint. CABI Publishing. UK. p. 121-145.

4. Beutin, L., Aleksic, S., Zimmermann, S., Gleier, K. (1994) Virulence factors and phenotypical traits of verotoxigenic strains of *Escherichia coli* isolated from human patients in Germany. Med Microbiol Immunol. 183: 13–21.

5. Blanco, J.E., Blanco, M., Mora, A., Blanco, J. (1997) Production of toxins (enterotoxins, verotoxins, and necrotoxins) and colicins by *Escherichia coli* strains isolated from septicemic and healthy chickens: relationship with in vivo pathogenicity. J Clin Microbiol. 35: 2953-2957.

6. Boerlin, P., McEwen, S.A., Boerlin-Petzold, F., Wilson, J.B., Johnson, R.P., Gyles, C.L. (1999) Associations between virulence factors of Shiga toxin-producing *Escherichia coli* and disease in humans. J Clin Microbiol. 37:497–503.

7. Caya, F., Fairbrother, J. M., Lessard, L., Quessy, S. (1999) Characterization of the risk to human health of pathogenic *Escherichia coli* isolates from chicken carcasses. J Food Prot. 67: 741-746.

8. Dhanashree, B., ShrikarMallya, P. (2008) Detection of shiga-toxigenic *Escherichia coli* (STEC) in diarrhoeagenic stool & meat samples in Mangalore, India. Indian J Med Res. 128: 271-277.

9. Feng, P. (2013) *Escherichia coli* (ETEC, EPEC, EHEC, EIEC). In: Bad Bug Book. Hand book of Foodborne Pathogenic Microorganisms

and Natural Toxins. (3rd ed.) Food and Drug Administration. USA.

10. Fode-Vaughan, K.A., Maki, J.S., Benson, J.A., Collins, M.L.P. (2003) Direct PCR detection of *Escherichia coli* O157:H7. Lett Appl Microbiol. 37: 239–243.

11. Gerrish, R.S., Lee, J.E., Reed, J., Williams J., Farrell, L.D., Spiegel, K.M., Sheridan P.P., Shields, M.S. (2007) PCR versus Hybridization for Detecting Virulence Genes of Enterohemorrhagic *Escherichia coli*. Emerg Infect Dis. 13: 1253-1255.

12. Harrigan, W.F. (1998) Detection and Enumeration of Pathogenic and Toxigenic Organisms. In: Laboratory Methods in Food Microbiology. (3rd ed.) Academic Press. Harcourt Brace and Company. San Diego, California, USA.

13. Heuvelink, AE., Zwartkruis-Nahuis, JT., van den Biggelaar, FL., van Leeuwen, WJ., de Boer, E. (1999) Isolation and characterization of verocytotoxin-producing *Escherichia coli* O157 from slaughter pigs and poultry. Int J Food Microbiol. 1;52:67-75.

14. Hosseini, H., Jamshidi, A., Bassami, M.R., Khaksar, R., Zeynali, T., MousaviKhaneghah, A., Khanzadi, S. (2013) Isolation, Identification and virulence gene profiling of *Escherichia coli* O157:H7 in retail donor kebabs, Iran. j Food Safety 33: 489-496.

15. Janben, T., Schwarz, C., Preikschat, P., Voss, M., Philipp, H.C., Wieler, L.H. (2001) Virulence-associated genes in avian pathogenic *Escherichia coli* (APEC) isolated from internal organs of poultry having died from colibacillosis.Int J Med Microbiol. 291: 371-378.

16. Kobayashi, H., Pohjanvirta, T., Pelkonen, S. (2002) Prevalence and characteristics of intimin-and Shiga toxin-producing *Escherichia coli* from gulls, pigeons and broilers in Finland. J Vet Med Sci. 64: 1071-1073.

17. Krause, G., Zimmermann, S., Beutin, L. (2005) Investigation of domestic animals and pets as a reservoir for intimin-(eae) gene positive *Escherichia coli* types. Vet Microbiol. 106: 87-95.

18. La Ragione, R.M., Best, A., Springings, K.,

Liebana, E., Woodward, G.R., Sayers, A.R., Woodward, M.J. (2005) Variable and strain dependent colonization of chickens by *Escherichia coli* O157. Vet Microbiol 107: 103-113.

19. Mellata, M., Bakour, R., Jacquemin, E., Mainil, J.G. (2001) Genotypic and phenotypic characterization of potential virulence of intestinal avian *Escherichia coli* strains isolated in Algeria. Avian Dis. 45: 670-679.

20. Mellata, M. (2013) Human and avian extraintestinal pathogenic *Escherichia coli*: Infections, zoonotic risks, and antibiotic resistance trends. Foodborne Pathol Dis. 10: 916-932.

21. Mohammadi, P., Abiri, R., Rezaei, M., Salmanzadeh A.S. (2013) Isolation of Shiga toxin-producing *Escherichia coli* from raw milk in Kermanshah, Iran. Iran J Microbiol. 5: 233-238.

22. Paton, A.W., Paton, J.C. (1998) Detection and characterization of shiga toxigenic *Escherichia coli* by using multiplex PCR assays for stx1, stx2, eaeA, Enterohemorrhagic *E. coli* hlyA, rfbO111, and rfbO157. J Clin Microbiol. 36: 598–602.

23. Paton, A.W., Paton, J.C. (2002) Direct detection and characterization of shiga toxigenic *Escherichia coli* by multiplex PCR for stx1, stx2, eae, ehxA, and saa. J Clin Microbiol. 40: 271–274.

24. Paton, A.W., Paton, J.C. (2005) Multiplex PCR for direct detection of shiga toxigenic *Escherichia coli* strains producing the novel subtilase cytotoxin. J Clin Microbiol. 43: 2944–2947.

25. Paton, A.W., Ratcliff, R.M., Doyle, R.M., Seymour-Murray, J., Davos, D., Lanser, J.A. (1996) Molecular microbiological investigation of an outbreak of hemolytic-uremic syndrome caused by dry fermented sausage contaminated with Shiga-like-producing *Escherichia coli*. J Clin Microbiol. 34: 1622-1627.

26. Paton, A.W., Woodrow, M.C., Doyle, R.M., Lanser, J.A., Paton, J.C. (1999) Molecular characterization of a Shiga toxigenic *Escherichia coli* O113:H21 strain lacking eae responsible for a cluster of cases of hemolytic-uremic syndrome. J Clin Microbiol. 37: 3357-3361.

27. Ron, E.Z. (2006) Host specificity of septice-micEscherichia coli; human and avian pathogens. Current Opin Microbiol. 9: 28-32.

28. Schroeder, C.M., Meng, J., Zhao, S., DebRoy, C., Torcolini, J., Zhao, C. (2002) Antimicrobial resistance of *Escherichia coli* O26, O103, O111, O128 and O145 from animals and humans. Emerg Infect Dis. 8: 1409-1414.

29. Schroeder, C.M., White, D.G., Zhang, Ge. B., McDermott, Y., Ayers, P.F., Zhao, S., Meng, J. (2003) Isolation of antimicrobial-resistant *Escherichia coli* from retail meats purchased in Greater Washington, DC, USA.Int J Food Microbiol. 85: 197–202.

30. Tabatabaei, M., Mokarizadeh, A., Foad-Marashi, N. (2011) Detection and molecular characterization of sorbitol negative shiga toxigenic *Escherichia coli* in chicken from northwest of Iran. Vet Res Forum. 2: 183-188.

31. Vanaja, S.K., Jandhyala, D.M., Mallick, E.M., Leong, J.M., Balasubramanian, S. (2013) Enterohemorrhagic and other Shigatoxin-producing *Escherichia coli*. In: *Escherichia coli* pathotypes and principle of pathogenesis. Donnenberg, M. (ed.). (2nd ed.) Academic Press. London, UK. p.121-182.

32. Wani, S.A., Samanta, I., Bhat, M.A., Nishikawa, Y. (2004) Investigation of shiga toxin-producing *Escherichia coli* in avian species in India. Lett Appl Microbiol. 39: 389-394.

11

Molecular and serological detection of *Neospora caninum* in multiple tissues and CSF in asymptomatic infected stray dogs in Tehran, Iran

Pouramini, A.[1], Jamshidi, Sh.[1*], Shayan, P.[2], Ebrahimzadeh, E.[2], Namavari, M.[3], Shirian, S.[5]

[1]*Department of Internal Medicine, Faculty of Veterinary Medicine, University of Tehran, Tehran, Iran*

[2]*Department of Parasitology, Faculty of Veterinary Medicine, University of Tehran, Tehran, Iran*

[3]*Razi Vaccine and Serum Research Institute, Agricultural Research,Educationanl Extention Organization (AREEO),Shiraz, Iran*

[4]*Department of Pathology, School of Veterinary Medicine, Shahrekord University, Shahrkord, Iran*

[5]*Shefa Neuroscience Research Center, Khatam-Al-Anbia Hospital, Tehran, Iran*

Key words:

dog, indirect ELISA, *Neospora caninum*, neosporosis, nested-PCR

Correspondence

Jamshidi, Sh.
Department of Internal Medicine, Faculty of Veterinary Medicine, University of Tehran, Tehran, Iran

Email: shjamshidi@ut.ac.ir

Abstract:

BACKGROUND: *Neospora caninum* is an Apicomplexan parasite. It causes paralysis and neuromuscular disorders in dogs and abortion in cattle. Although contamination with *N. caninum* is common in stray dogs, most of the dogs are infected with subclinical neosporosis. **OBJECTIVES:** The objective of this study was to evaluate the presence of *N. caninum* in multiple tissues and cerebrospinal fluid (CSF) using Nested-PCR technique. Furthermore, the *N. caninum* specific antibody was detected in serum of examined dogs by indirect enzyme-linked immunosorbent assay (ELISA). **METHODS:** Forty-two stray dogs of mixed breeds captured from districts of Tehran, Iran, were examined physically and euthanized. A commercially indirect ELISA kit was used to detect the anti-*N. caninum* antibodies in sera. Nested PCR was applied to analyze the extracted DNA from brain, skeletal muscle, CSF, liver, spleen and mandibular lymph nodes for Nc5 gene. **RESULTS:** Indirect ELISA assay for *N. caninum* antibody was positive in a seven year-old male dog (2.22%). Out of 42 stray dogs whose multiple organs were examined using Nested PCR, 15 samples (35%) were positive. The highest presence of *N. caninum* was found in skeletal muscle with 30% (13/42) frequency, followed by CSF (26.2%) (11/42), brain (19%) (8/42), liver (7.14%) (3/42), lymph node (4.62%) (2/42) and spleen samples (0/42). **CONCLUSIONS:** These results suggest that the highest presence of *N. caninum* is seen in skeletal muscle, CSF and brain in asymptomatic infected dogs respectively. Nested-PCR could be considered a sensitive method to detect *N. caninum* in subclinical infected dogs.

Introduction

Neospora caninum is a pathogen protozoan from Apicomplexan phylum. *N. caninum* is morphologically very similar to *Toxoplasma gondii*. Domestic dogs and some wild canids are definitive hosts and the cattle are the intermediate host. The Oocysts are shed by infected dogs after ingestion of infected tissues with *N. caninum* cysts (1-5).

Serologic assays in serum or in CSF are the main methods of *N. caninum* diagnosis and include indirect fluorescent antibody test (IFAT) and ELISA (6), Direct Agglutination Test (DAT) or Neospora agglutination test (NAT) (7). Nevertheless, serology is an indirect diagnosis test, has considerable variations and also in case of early or chronic infection with cysts formation, the serology could be negative even if the parasite is present in the dog. Furthermore, some weak serologic cross-reactivity may occur between *T. gondii* and *N. caninum* antigens. Therefore, direct diagnosis and highly sensitive methods such as immunohistochemistry or PCR can be used (6). In comparison, PCR has been reported to be more sensitive to immunohistochemistry as some cross-reactivity could occur with immunocytochemistry depending on the antibodies used (6). Besides Classical PCR, Semi-nested or nested PCR was also developed to increase the sensitivity. (8-10).

N. caninum infection causes paralysis and neuromuscular disorders in dogs. Although *N. caninum* contamination is common in stray dogs, clinical manifestation is uncommon and most of the dogs are infected with subclinical and asymptomatic neosporosis (11, 12). Chemotherapy or immunosuppressive drugs can reactivate subclinical form of the disease to clinical neosporosis (13-15). Subclinically infected dogs can transmit the parasite to their pups (16-19). Detection of the infection in asymptomatic dogs, especially in females is crucial for prevention of vertical transmission to newborns; therefore, diagnosis of the asymptomatic dogs

remains essential and the results of this study can be used for proper diagnosis of this parasite.

The aim of this study was to determine the levels of *N. caninum* infection in some organs/tissues of asymptomatic stray dogs using Nested-PCR and ELISA, in order to compare the positive results in different infected organs.

Materials and Methods

Sample collection: This study was performed under dog population control program and under permission and guidelines of the ethic committee of the University of Tehran. Forty-two stray dogs (22 male /20 female) of mixed breeds, ranging from one to seven years old, were captured from districts of Tehran, Iran, from November 2014 to September 2014. The captured dogs were first physically examined and their details were recorded. None of the dogs had any clinical symptoms associated with neosprosis. Blood samples (10ml) were then drawn from jugular vein. The samples were centrifuged at 3000×g for 10 min. Separated sera were stored at -20 oC until testing. The stray dogs were then euthanized and necropsies were performed. Samples were collected from individual organs using sterile scalpels, to minimize potential contamination of the tissues. Collected samples consisted of brain (from left hemisphere, 5-10 g), skeletal muscle (Biceps femoris), CSF (foramen magnum space), liver, spleen and mandibular lymph nodes were removed and the organs were stored at -20 °C until DNA extraction. Samples were maintained in PBS buffer containing 2% antibiotic (Penicillin and Streptomycin)-antimycotic (Amphotericin B) solution (Gibco BRL, Paisley, UK) and stored at −20 °C until being used for

DNA extraction and PCR amplification. The DNA obtained from cultured tachyzoites (Nc1) was used as positive control.

ELISA assay: For serological analysis, a commercially indirect multi-species ELISA kit (IDvet Co., France) for the detection of anti-*N. caninum* antibodies in serum was used according to the manufacturer's instructions. S/P of 0.5 was considered as cut-off based on the instructions of the manufacturer.

DNA Extraction: Each of the brain, skeletal muscle, liver, spleen and mandibular lymph nodes samples was first finely chopped using a sterile blade, and then powdered by being crushed in liquid nitrogen in a mortar. Furthermore, the powdered tissues were diluted in distilled water and homogenized.

DNA was extracted from the homogenized tissues and CSF samples using DNA extraction kit (MBST, Iran). The extraction procedure was performed according to the manufacturer's protocol.

DNA amplification by Nested-PCR: The sequence of the primer pair used in this study to amplify Nc5 gene of *N. caninum* was adapted from that used in a research carried out by Müller and colleagues (1996). Np6+ (5' gggtgtgcgtccaatcctgtaac3') and Np21+ (5' ctcgccagtcaacctacgtcttct3') primers were used to amplify a 328bp fragment of Nc5 gene (20). The product of the fist PCR reaction using Np6+ and Np21+ primers was then used as a template to run the second PCR reaction using Np7 (5'gggtgaaccgagggagttg3') and Np10(5'tcgtccgcttgctccctatgaat3'). The PCR product the size of the second reaction was 198bp.

The PCR reaction mixture consisted of 1μg template DNA, 2mM MgCl2, 5μl 10×reaction buffer, 10pmol of each reverse and forward primer, 200μM dNTP and 1U of Taq DNA polymerase. The thermal steps of the PCR reaction was as follows: 5 min incubation at 95 °C to denature double strand DNA, 35 cycles of 45s at 95 °C (denaturing step), 45s at 64 °C (annealing step) and 45s at 72 °C (final extension step). The PCR product of the first reaction was diluted 1:10 in distilled water prior to being used as the template in the second reaction (Nested-PCR). The thermal steps of the second PCR reaction using Np7/Np10 primers were similar to the first reaction.

PCR products were electrophoresed on 2% agarose gel followed by ethidium bromide staining. PCR products were visualized using UV illuminator.

Sequencing and Nucleotide sequence analysis: To confirm the specificity of the primers used in this study, Nc5 Nested-PCR specificity, amplicons of the second PCR reaction were sent to be sequence by Takapouzist Co, Iran. The obtained sequences were analyzed and edited using Finch TV software (GeospizaInc, Seattle, USA) and Bioedit software version 7.7.9 (mBio, Inc., North Carolina, USA), respectively.

The obtained nucleotide sequences (Nc5 gene) were blasted and compared with those already registered in the GenBank™ database (http://blast.ncbi.nlm.nih.gov/Blast.cgi).

Results

ELISA assay: From 42 serum samples of stray dogs that were tested by indirect ELISA kit, 1 (2.22%) of them (a seven year old male) was positive for antibodies (IgGs) against *N. caninum*.

Gene Expression of *N. caninum* Nc5 in stray dogs: The data obtained from PCR

Table 1. Summary of PCR and ELISA test carried out on various samples obtained from stray dogs.

Sample number	Age (year)	Sex	ELISA assay(S/P)	Brain	Muscle	CSF	Liver	Spleen	Mandibular lymph nodes
1	2	Female	-(0.24)	+	+	+	-	-	-
2	7	Male	+(1.01)	+	+	-	-	-	-
3	3	Female	-(0.16)	-	+	-	-	-	-
4	3	Male	-(0.18)	-	+	-	-	-	-
5	3	Female	-(0.16)	+	+	+	-	-	-
6	3	Female	-(0.16)	-	+	+	-	-	-
7	4	Female	-(0.18)	+	+	+	+	-	+
8	5	Male	-(0.17)	-	+	+	-	-	-
9	3	Male	-(0.18)	+	-	+	+	-	-
10	3	Male	-(0.20)	-	-	+	-	-	-
11	2	Male	-(0.17)	-	+	+	-	-	-
12	4	Male	-(0.19)	-	+	+	-	-	-
13	2	Female	-(0.22)	+	+	-	-	-	-
14	6	Male	-(0.20)	+	+	+	+	-	+
15	1	Male	-(0.17)	+	+	+	-	-	-

analysis are illustrated in Fig. 1. *N. caninum* Nc5 gene was expressed in brain, skeletal muscle, CSF, liver, spleen and mandibular lymph nodes samples obtained from 15 out of 42 stray dogs (35%).

The presence of *N. caninum* was highest in skeletal muscle with 30% (13/42) positive PCR test. In the other organs, 19% of brain (8/42) and 26.2% of CSF (11/42) samples tested positive. The numbers of liver and mandibular lymph nodes samples were relatively lower, 7.14% (3/42) and 4.76% (2/42), respectively. None of the spleen samples (0/42) tested positive for Nc5 gene expression. The data obtained from Nested-PCR are presented in Table 1.

Sequencing and nucleotide sequence BLAST (BLASTn): Sequencing the amplified fragment confirmed the specificity of the used primers. Quality of the sequenced Nc5 gene fragment was confirmed by Finch TV software (Geospiza Inc., Seattle, USA). No variations of intra population were observed for the Nc5 sequences of *N. caninum*

samples. Nucleotide sequences of partial Nc5 gene of *N. caninum* were used as the entry data to NCBI BLAST search to compare and verify with the existing paralogues in the GenBank. The fragment of the Nc5 gene sequenced in this study was 96% identical to the homologous sequences from *N. caninum* (Sequence ID: GQ899206, AJ271354, U17345, U16159, L24380 and U03069).

Discussions

This study aimed to estimate the serological prevalence of *N. caninum* infection in serum and the molecular prevalence in some organs/tissues of asymptomatic stray dogs in Tehran province, Iran.

Serological assays show widespread exposure to the *N. caninum* in Asia, Europe, Africa and America (11). Several studies have reported the prevalence of *N. caninum* by serological methods in Iran. In Meshkin-Shahr District (Northwestern Iran) from 171 domestic dogs, 52 cases (30.4%) had antibodies against *N. caninum* in their sera

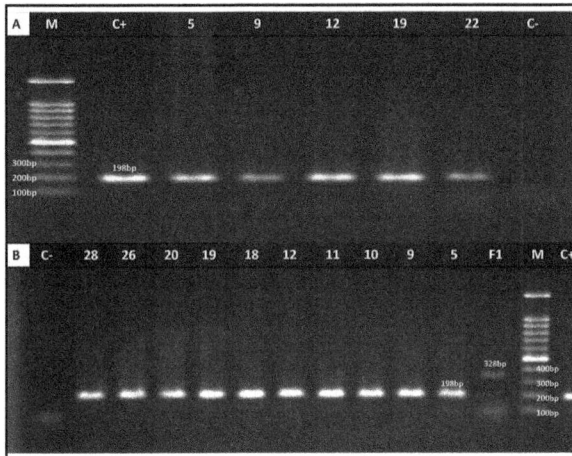

Figure 1. Detection of *Neospora caninum* using Nested-PCR. The applied primers targeted the Nc5 gene (A: Brains, B:Muscle) at -198bp. M, marker of 100bp ladder; C+, positive control; C-, negative control, Numbers (lanes 3-8 (A)& 4-14(B)); samples; F1, a sample of first round Nested-PCR.

which was detected by indirect ELISA (21). Furthermore, antibodies against *N. caninum* were detected in 36 (27%) of 135 dogs in Urmia, Iran using IFAT (22). Haddadzadeh et al., found that 20 of 103 (19.4%) cases they studied in Tehran were seropositive using IFAT. They have also reported that the infection rate in farm dogs was higher (28%) than in urban dogs (11.3%) (23). In household dogs and dogs living in dairy and beef cattle farms of Tehran, antibodies against *N. caninum* were detected in 10 (20%) of 50 household dogs and in 23 (46%) of 50 farm dogs using IFAT (24). The present study is the first study to investigate the presence of *N. caninum* in some organs of asymptomatic stray dogs in Iran using molecular technique (Nested-PCR) alongside serological detection method (ELISA). In the present study, only 1 of 42 stray dogs was seropositive using indirect ELISA. This dog was one of the 15 dogs (6.67%) that was positively assessed by Nested-PCR. Furthermore, the other 27 dogs that tested negative for Nested-PCR were also seronegative. Therefore, Nested-PCR might indicate a better sensitivity compared to ELISA for *N. caninum* detection in asymptomatic stray dogs. Serology is an indirect diagnosis test that has several variations. Moreover, in case of early or chronic infection with cysts formation, serology test could be negative even if the parasite is present in the dog (25). Furthermore, some weak serologic cross-reactivity may occur between *T. gondii* and *N. caninum* antigens. Therefore, direct diagnosis and highly sensitive methods such as immunohistochemistry or PCR based detection methods can be more suitable (6). In comparison, PCR has been reported to be more sensitive to immunohistochemistry as some cross-reactivity could occur in immunocytochemistry depending on the antibodies used (6).

In our study, as previously mentioned, 15 dogs from 42 dogs that were examined with Nested-PCR method had positive results at least in one tissue sample for each dog. Skeletal muscle (13/15), CSF (11/15) and brain (8/15) had significant higher positive results than liver (3/15) and mandibular lymph nodes (2/15). As confirmed by the results obtained using Nested-PCR in this study, skeletal muscle and brain are the major site of *N. caninum* infection and are suitable organs to detect the parasite (26-28).

Ghalmi et al. detected *N. caninum* in liver and spleen of 28 (32.2%) of 87 asymptomatic pound dogs in Algeria using PCR technique. From 28 dogs tested for Nc5 gene expression, 14 (50%) expressed Nc5 in both organs, 11 (39.28%) in spleen and 3 (10.72%) in liver. 19 of these dogs were seronegative using IFAT and only 8 seropositive dogs were seen in PCR positive dogs (25). Although Ghalmi et al. only tested liver and spleen using PCR which were shown to have the lowest infection in present study.

Therefore, it is possible that the other organs such as brain and muscle were infected and underestimated in the study reported by Ghalmi et al. Therefore, the organ/tissue chosen to be tested using PCR might be critical in making the correct diagnosis. Similarly, all the positive samples in PCR test did not test positive using ELISA technique in present study. Also, the study of Castaneda-Hernandez shows that the results of Nested-PCR were significantly greater than serology results in asymptomatic sheep. The seroprevalence was 5.5% and the prevalence of the *N. caninum*'s DNA in sheep's blood was 25% using Nested-PCR (29).

Ferroglio et al. showed that in samples obtained from 233 wild rodents 19 muscle, 6 kidney and 4 brain samples tested positive for Nc5 expression using PCR. Their study demonstrated that results obtained only based on the brain samples may potentially lead to an underestimation of the levels of infection as the majority of positive PCR samples were skeletal muscle, similar to the finding of present study (30).

Moreover, with respect to the presence of *N. caninum* in brain, CSF and muscle, this parasite should be considered in the differential diagnosis of neuromuscular disorders of dogs. The present study demonstrated that based on the Nested-PCR results and the data obtained using ELISA, the stray dogs in Tehran province are infected with *N. caninum* without any symptoms.

Serology can underestimate the real carrier of *N. caninum* in asymptomatic dogs. The main benefit of PCR technique to detect *N. caninum* in comparison with serology tests is to directly detect the presence of the DNA. However, incapacity to perform the test on living dogs is the main disadvantage of this technique (31).

In conclusion, Serology tests can underestimate the carrier of *N. caninum* in asymptomatic dogs compared to PCR. However, cross-reactivity between Leishmania species or *T. gondii* and *N. caninum* antigens may occur. Skeletal muscle, CSF and brain are the most infected tissues in dogs with *N. caninum* respectively. Nested-PCR is a potential alternative for the serology methods to detect *N. caninum* in asymptomatic infected dog.

Acknowledgements

The study was supported financially by the Faculty of Veterinary Medicine, University of Tehran.

References

Barber, J.S., Trees, A. (1996) Clinical aspects of 27 cases of neosporosis in dogs. Vet Rec. 139: 439-443.

Baszler, T.V., Gay, L.J., Long, M.T., Mathison, B.A. (1999) Detection by PCR of *Neospora caninum* in fetal tissues from spontaneous bovine abortions. J Clin Microbiol. 37: 4059-4064.

Buxton, D., Maley, S.W., Wright, S., Thomson, K.M., Rae, A.G., Innes, E.A. (1998) The pathogenesis of experimental neosporosis in pregnant sheep. J Comp Pathol. 118: 267-279.

Castaneda-Hernandez, A., Cruz-Vazquez, C., Medina-Esparza, L. (2014) *Neospora caninum*: Seroprevalence and DNA detection in blood of sheep from Aguascalientes, Mexico. Small Rumin Res. 119: 182-186.

Dubey, J.P., Jenkins, M.C., Rajendran, C., Miska, K., Ferreira, L.R., Martins, J., Kwok, O.C.H., Choudhary, S. (2011) Gray wolf (*Canis lupus*) is a natural definitive host for *Neospora caninum*. Vet Parasitol. 181: 382-387.

Dubey, J.P., Lindsay, D.S. (1996) A review of *Neospora caninum* and neosporosis. Vet Parasitol. 67: 1-59.

Dubey, J.P., Schares, G. (2006) Diagnosis of bovine neosporosis. Vet Parasitol. 140: 1-34.

Dubey, J.P., Schares, G. (2011) Neosporosis in animals-The last five years. Vet Parasitol. 180: 90-108.

Dubey, J.P., Vianna, M.C.B., Kwok, O.C.H., Hill, DE, Miska, K.B., Tuo, W., Velmurugan, G.V., Conors, M., Jenkins, M.C. (2007) Neosporosis in Beagle dogs: Clinical signs, diagnosis, treatment, isolation and genetic characterization of *Neospora caninum*. Vet Parasitol. 149: 158-166.

Ferroglio, E., Pasino, M., Romano, A., Grande, D., Pregel, P., Trisciuoglio, A. (2007) Evidence of *Neospora caninum* DNA in wild rodents. Vet Parasitol. 148: 346-349.

Fry, D.R., McSporran, K.D., Ellis, J.T., Harvey, C. (2009) Protozoal hepatitis associated with immunosuppressive therapy in a dog. J Vet Intern Med. 23: 366-368.

Galgut, B.I., Janardhan, K.S., Grondin, T.M., Harkin, K.R., Wight-Carter, M.T. (2010) Detection of *Neospora caninum* tachyzoites in cerebrospinal fluid of a dog following prednisone and cyclosporine therapy. Vet Clin Pathol. 39: 386-390.

Garosi, L., Dawson, A., Couturier, J., Matiasek, L., de Stefani, A., Davies, E., Jeffery, N., Smith, P. (2010) Necrotizing cerebellitis and cerebellar atrophy caused by *Neospora caninum* infection: magnetic resonance imaging and clinicopathologic findings in seven dogs. J Vet Intern Med. 24: 571-578.

Georgieva, D.A., Prelezov, P.N., Koinarski, T.S. (2006) *Neospora caninum* and neosporosis in animals-a review. Bulg J Vet Med. 9: 1-26.

Ghalmi, F., China, B., Kaidi, R., Daube, G., Losson, B. (2008) Detection of *Neospora caninum* in dog organs using real time PCR systems. Vet Parasitol. 155: 161-167.

Gondim, L.F.P., McAllister, M.M., Pitt, W.C., Zemlicka, D.E. (2004) Coyotes (*Canis latrans*) are definitive hosts of *Neospora caninum*. Int J Parasitol. 34: 159-161.

Habibi, G.R., Hashemi-Fesharki, R., Sadrebazzaz, A., Bozorgi, S., Bordbar, N. (2005) Seminested PCR for diagnosis of *Neospora caninum* infection in cattle. Arch Razi Ins. 59: 55-64.

Haddadzadeh, H.R., Sadrebazzaz, A., Malmasi, A., TaleiArdakani, H., KhazraiiNia, P., Sadreshirazi, N. (2007) Seroprevalence of *Neospora caninum* infection in dogs from rural and urban environments in Tehran, Iran. Parasitol Res. 101: 1563-1565.

Heckeroth, A.R., Tenter, A.M. (2007) Immuno analysis of three litters born to a Doberman bitch infected with *Neospora caninum*. Parasitol Res. 100: 837-846.

King, J.S., Šlapeta, J., Jenkins, D.J., Al-Qassab, S.E., Ellis, J.T., Windsor, P.A. (2010) Australian dingoes are definitive hosts of *Neospora caninum*. Int J Parasitol. 40: 945-950.

Lindsay, D.S., Dubey, J.P. (2000) Canine neosporosis. Vet Parasitol. 14: 1-11.

Lindsay, D.S., Dubey, J.P., Duncan, R.B. (1999) Confirmation that the dog is a definitive host for *Neospora caninum*. Vet Parasitol. 82: 327-333.

Malmasi, A., Hosseininejad, M., Haddadzadeh, H., Badii, A., Bahonar, A. (2007) Serologic study of anti-*Neospora caninum* antibodies in household dogs and dogs living in dairy and beef cattle farms in Tehran, Iran. Parasitol Res. 100: 1143-1145.

McAllister, M.M., Dubey, J.P., Lindsay, D.S., Jolley, W.R., Wills, R.A., McGuire, A.M. (1998) Rapid communication: Dogs are definitive hosts of *Neospora caninum*. Int J Parasitol. 28: 1473-1479.

Müller, N., Zimmermann, V., Hentrich, B., Gottstein, B. (1996) Diagnosis of *Neospora caninum* and *Toxoplasma gondii* infection by PCR and DNA hybridization immunoassay. J Clin Microbiol. 34: 2850-2852.

Okeoma, C.M., Williamson, N.B., Pomroy, W.E., Stowell, K.M., Gillepsie, L. (2004) The use of PCR to detect *Neospora caninum* DNA in the blood of naturally infected cows. Vet Parasitol. 122: 307-315.

Ordeix, L., Lloret, A., Fondevila, D., Dubey, J. P., Ferrer, L., Fondati, A. (2002) Cutaneous neosporosis during treatment of pemphigus foliaceus in a dog. J Am Anim Hosp Assoc. 38: 415-419.

Packham, A.E., Sverlow, K.W., Conrad, P.A., Loomis, E.F., Rowe, J.D., Anderson, M.L., Marsh, A.E., Cray, C., Barr, B.C. (1998) A modified agglutination test for *Neospora caninum*: development, optimization, and comparison to the indirect fluorescent-antibody test and enzyme-linked immunosorbent assay. Clin Diagn Lab Immunol. 5: 467-473.

Peters, M., Wagner, F., Schares, G. (2000) Canine neosporosis: clinical and pathological findings and first isolation of *Neospora caninum* in Germany. Parasitol Res. 86: 1-7.

Sharifdini, M., Mohebali, M., Keshavarz, H., Hosseininejad, M., Hajjaran, H., Akhoundi, B., Foroushani, A.R., Zarei, Z., Charehdar, S. (2011) *Neospora caninum* and *Leishmania infantum* co-infection in domestic dogs (*Canis familiaris*) in Meshkin-Shahr district, Northwestern Iran. Iranian Journal of Arthropod Born Disease. 1: 60-68.

Yakhchali, M., Javadi, S., Morshedi, A. (2010) Prevalence of antibodies to *Neospora caninum* in stray dogs of Urmia, Iran. Parasitol Res. 106: 1455-1458.

12

Comparison of *Leptospira interrogans* infection in the goats and sheep

Rezaei, S.[1], Haji Hajikolaei, M.R.[1*], Ghadrdan Mashhadi, A.R.[1], Ghorbanpour, M.[2], Abdollahpour, G.[3]

[1]*Department of Clinical Sciences, Faculty of Veterinary Medicine, Shahid Chamran University of Ahvaz, Ahvaz, Iran*

[2]*Department of Pathobiology, Faculty of Veterinary Medicine, Shahid Chamran University of Ahvaz, Ahvaz, Iran*

[3]*Department of Internal Medicine, Faculty of Veterinary Medicine, University of Tehran, Tehran, Iran*

Key words:

goat, leptospirosis, seroprevalence, sheep,

Correspondence

Haji Hajikolaei, M.R.
Department of Clinical Sciences,
Faculty of Veterinary Medicine,
Shahid Chamran University of
Ahvaz, Ahvaz, Iran

Email: mhajih@scu.ac.ir

Abstract:

BACKGROUND: Most leptospiral infections in sheep and goat are asymptomatic but may result in high fever, abortion, stillbirth, agalactiae. There is a different foraging behavior between sheep and goat that may cause the different prevalence of Leptospira interrogans infection in sheep and goats. OBJECTIVES: The purpose of the present study was to compare the prevalence of *L. interrogans* antibodies in sheep and goats. METHODS: Blood samples were taken from 246 sheep and 210 goats in 12 herds from 8 areas of Ahvaz where the animals were kept together. Sera were initially screened at dilution of 1:100 against 8 live serovars of *L. intrrogans*: pomana, canicola, hardjo, ballom, ictrohaemorrhagiae, grippotyphosa, tarasovi and australis using the microscopic agglutination test (MAT). RESULTS: The prevalence of leptospiral infection was 8.53% in sheep and 10.95% in goats. The highest reacting leptospira in both species was *L.i.* Pomona with a reactor rate of 68.18% in sheep and 56% in goats, followed in descending order by ictrohaemorrhagiae (18.8%), canicula, hardjo and grippotyphosa (each of them 4.54%), in sheep and ictrohaemorrhagiae (28%), canicula (16%) in goats. Statistical analysis showed that were no significant differences between sheep and goat (P=0.428). There were no significant differences among age groups in sheep (p=0.301) and goats (p= 0.363), but there was a tendency in adults sheep and goats (≥3years) to be more seropositive than young sheep and goats. Seroprevalence of leptospiral infection among various areas in sheep (p= 0.464) and goats (p= 0.710) was also not significantly different. CONCLUSIONS: It is concluded that there is no difference between sheep and goats in terms of leptospiral infection when they are kept together in the same herd and husbandry condition.

Introduction

Leptospirosis is a reemerging zoonotic disease of human and animals worldwide. It is presumed to be the most widespread zoonosis in the world. The disease is caused by pathogenic species of spirochetes of the genus leptospira (Samir et al., 2015). Among sheep and goats, most of the outbreak goes unnoticed due to lack of proper clinical signs and they usually react asymptomatically to the infection (OIE, 2000). The clinical manifestation of leptospires ranges from mild to severe life threatening disease with jaundice, renal failure or abortion during pregnancy (Shivaraj et al. 2009). Unfortunately, a definitive diagnosis of leptospirosis is difficult to make. Most diagnostic laboratories do not try to isolate leptospires because of their fragile nature, cost and complexity of the isolation media, and prolonged incubation period. Therefore, recognition of leptospiral infection has generally been based on serological evidence. Two tests have a role in veterinary diagnosis: the Microscopic Agglutination Test (MAT) and the Enzyme Linked Immunosorbent Assay (ELISA) (OIE, 2000)

Previous serological surveys of leptospiral infection in Ahvaz were carried out on cattle, horse and donkey (Hajikolaei et al., 2006, 2005a, 2005b) and two studies have been conducted to determine seroprevalence of leptospiral infection in goats and sheep, separately (Hajikolaei et al., 2007a, 2007b). A big different between sheep and goats is their foraging behavior and diet selection. Goats are natural browsers, preferring to eat leaves, twigs, vines and shrubs. They are very agile and will stand on their hind legs to reach vegetation. Goats like to eat the tops of plants. Sheep are grazers, preferring to eat short, tender grasses and clover. Their dietary preference is forbs and they like to graze close to the soil surface. These differences between sheep and goats may be responsible for the difference in prevalence of leptospiral infection in sheep and goats (Bojkovski et al., 2014). As there has been no study on comparison of leptospiral infection in sheep and goats in similar region, this study was undertaken to compare the prevalence of *L. interrogans* antibodies in sheep and goats in different areas of Ahvaz, the center of Khouzestan province in the southwest of Iran.

Materials and Methods

Blood samples were taken from 246 sheep and 210 goats from 8 areas of Ahvaz, in the southwest of Iran, during May to July of 2015. None of these animals had been vaccinated against leptospires and there was no history of leptospirosis-related symptoms or sign of the disease at the time of sampling. According to dental formula, these goats and sheep were divided into 5 ages groups ($\leq$ 1, 1, 2, 3 and $\geq$4 years old). The number of samples of goats from area A to H were 40(A), 40(B), 40(C), 24(D), 14(E), 13(F), 16(G), 20(H) and those numbers of sheep were 40(A), 40(B), 40(C), 40(D), 20(E), 14(F), 21(G), 30(H), respectively.

The blood samples were allowed to clot and were centrifuged for 8 min at 3000g. After centrifugation, the sera were removed and stored at -20 °C until ready for test. The sera were tested for antibodies to 8 live antigens of *leptospira interrogans* (*L.introgans* serovars pomona, canicola, hardjo, ballum, ictrohemorrhagiae, grippotyphosa, tarasovi, australis) using the microscopic agglutination Test (MAT), in leptospiral research laboratory in faculty of veterinary medicine, university of Tehran. According to the methods of OIE, sera were initially screened at a dilution of 1:100 against these antigens. At first, serum dilution of 1:50 was performed and a volume of each serovar, equal to the diluted serum volume, was added to each well of microtitrations plates, making the final serum dilution 1:100. The microtitrations plates were incubated at 29 °C for 2h. The plates were examined by dark-field microscopy. Results were considered positive when 50% or more of agglutination of leptospires was found (OIE, 2000). Sera with positive result were titrated against reacting antigens in serial two-fold dilution from 1:100 to 1:800.

Statistical analysis was achieved using Chi-Square and Fisher's exact test which aimed to

Table 1. The Results of MAT on sheep and goats in some areas of Ahvaz-Iran.

Animals	No. positive (%)	No. negative (%)	No. exam
Sheep	21 (8.53)	225(91.47)	246
Goats	23 (10.95)	187(89.05)	210

detect differences between all variables.

Results

Out of 246 sheep and 210 goats tested, 21 (8.53%) and 23 (10.95%), were seropositive and antibodies against one or more serovars were detected (Table 1). One goat (4.76%) and two sheep (8.69%) were positive for more than one serovar. Significant difference (p= 0.428) between the sheep and goats as reactors to leptospires were not found. The highest number of reactors in sheep (68.2%) and goats (56%) was due to *L.introgans* serovar pomona, followed in descending order by icterohaemorrhagiae (18.2%), hardjo (4.5%), canicola (4.5%), and grypothyphosa (4.5%) in sheep and icterohaemorrhagiae (28%), and canicola (16%), in goats (Table 2). With the exception of one sample that had a titer level of 200, the other samples had a titer level of 100.

There was no significant difference among age groups in sheep (p=0.301) and goats (p= 0.363), but there was a tendency in adult sheep and goats (≥3years) to be more seropositive than the younger animals (Table 3 and 4). Distribution of leptospiral infection in sheep (p= 0.464) and goats (p= 0.710) among various areas was also not significantly different (Table 5 and 6). In area F, none of the examined sheep and goats have shown antibodies against various serovars of *L.interrogans* (Table 5, 6).

Discussion

Leptospirosis is an infectious zoonotic disease caused by different serotypes of the leptospires in any geographical area and infor-

mation about the serotypes in one region may help the epidemiology and pathogenesis of this bacteria. Cattle are maintenance host for many serotypes of this bacteria. Sheep and goats are not naturally maintenance hosts for some of the serotypes such as pomona or hardjo and are likely to have infection of relatively short duration and produce severe pathologic effects. However, persistent leptospiruria and high seroprevalence rates of infection in sheep and goat where no contact with cattle have occurred suggest that sheep and goat may be a maintenance host for some serovars. This could complicate control of the infection in cattle, sheep and goat. Infected sheep and goat are a potential zoonotic risk to humans such as abattoir workers, sheep and goat farmers and shearers which previously had not been considered (Radostits et al., 2007). Long-term survival of pathogenic leptospires outside the host requires a warm, moist environment with a near natural pH (Miller et al., 1991). According to different foraging behavior in sheep and goats it is suspected that leptospiral infection in these animals has substantial differences but in this study there were no significant differences of the seroprevalence infection between sheep and goats in similar regions and situations. However, it may be due to the fact that neither of them like to get their feet wet and both prefer upland grazing to lowland that results in less exposure to leptospires (Bojkovski et al., 2014). We found that the seroprevaalence of leptospiral infection in goat and sheep in Ahvaz was 10.95% and 8.53%, respectively. The prevalence of leptospiral infection in goats and sheep from other countries based on serological survey has been reported to be 1.2%, 12.3%, 13.1, 14.3%, 16.8%, 32%, 40%, 42%, 42.1%, 55.2% and 70% in France, Italy, Nigeria, Bolivia, Greece, Croix, Belize, Australia, Egypt, India and New Zealand (Agunloye, 2002; Ciceroni et al., 1997; Flint et al., 1988; Maronpot and Barsoum, 1972; Sratnam, 1992; Trap and Gaumont, 1983) and

Table 2. The Prevalence of leptospiral antibody titer to different serovars in sheep and goats in some areas of Ahvaz-Iran. G-grypo-thyphosa, P-ponnona, I-icterohaemorrhagiae, C-canicola, H-hardjo, B-ballum, T- tarasovi, A-australis.

Animals	G	P	I	C	H	B	T	A
Sheep	1 (4.5%)	15 (68.2%)	4 (18.2%)	1 (4.5%)	1 (4.5%)	0 (0%)	0 (0%)	0 (0%)
Goats	0 (0%)	14 (56%)	7 (28%)	4(16%)	0 (0%)	0 (0%)	0 (0%)	0 (0%)

Table 3. Age distribution in leptospiral seroprevalence of sheep in some areas of Ahvaz-Iran.

Age (year)	No. positive (%)	No. negative (%)	Total (%)
<2	0 (0)	10 (100)	10 (4.06)
2	1 (2.7)	36 (97.29)	37 (15.04)
3	8 (13.33)	52 (86.66)	60 (24.39)
≥4	12 (8.63)	127 (91.37)	139 (56.50)
Total	21 (8.53)	225 (91.47)	246

Table 4. Age distribution in leptospiral seroprevalence of goat in some areas of Ahvaz-Iran.

Age (year)	No. positive (%)	No .negative (%)	Total(%)
<2	3 (5.36)	56 (94.64)	59 (28.09)
2	3 (13.04)	20 (86.96)	23 (10.95)
3	5 (13.51)	32 (86.49)	37 (17.61)
≥4	12 (13.18)	79 (86.82)	91 (43.33)
Total	23 (10.95)	187 (89.04)	210

14.3%, 19.7%, 4.2%, 60.4%, 6.1% and 16.8% in Bolivia, Argentina, Egypt, India, Italy and Greece, respectively (Ciceroni et al., 1997; Draghi et al., 1984; Maronpot and Barsonm, 1972; Stratname et al., 1992; Ciceroni et al., 2000 and Burriel et al., 2002).

There are some reports of leptospiral infection in goat and sheep from Iran (Hajikolaei et al., 2007a; 2007b; Hassanpour et al., 2012; Zainali et al., 1997; Ramin, AG and Azizza-deh, F., 2013). According to these reports, the seroprevalence of leptospiral infection in goat was 27.5%, 10.46% and 13.3% in Ahvaz, Uremia and Khoy, respectively and in sheep 14.9% and 19.3% respectively in Ahvaz and Uremia. The results of these reports confirm that prevalence of leptospiral infection in goat and sheep is different from region to region or country to country. These differences may be the consequence of environmental factors and control efforts (Maleki et al., 2014 and Milller et al., 1991). The results of this study showed that the serological infection rate in goat and sheep in Ahvaz is relatively high and

consequently the preventive methods must be applied to stop the spread of disease and its transmission to the human and other farm animals and the important role of goat and sheep on the epidemiology of the infection must be emphasized. The predominant leptospire serovars in serological reaction varies somewhat among countries. For example, *L. interrogans* serovars poi and pommona in Bolivia (Ciceroni et al., 1997), wollfi, pomona and ballum in Argentina (Draghi et al, 1984), pomona in India (Manickavel et al., 1991), autumnalis in Egypt (Maronpot and Baarsoum, 1972) and pomona in Malaysia (Bahaman et al., 1987) were the predominant serovars in sheep and automnalis, pomona, automnalis, poi, bratislava and ictrohemorrhagiae were the common serovars in goats in Egypt, Nigeria, India, Bolivia, Italy and France, respectively (Agunloye, 2002; Cerri, 2003; Ciceroni et al., 1997; Maronpot and Barsoum, 1972 and Trap and Gaumont, 1983).

In this study, *L. interrogans* serovars pomona and icterohaemorrhagiae were detected as the

Table 5. Distribution of leptospiral infection in sheep from various areas of Ahvaz-Iran.

Area	No. positive (%)	No. negative (%)	Total
A	2 (5)	38 (95)	40
B	6 (15)	34 (85)	40
C	3 (7.5)	37 (92.5)	40
D	3 (7.5)	37 (92.5)	40
E	1 (5)	19 (95)	20
F	0 (0)	14 (100)	14
G	2 (9.09)	20 (90.9)	22
H	4 (13.33)	26 (86.67)	30
Total	21	225	246

Table 6. Distribution of leptospiral infection in goats from various areas of Ahvaz-Iran.

Area	No. positive (%)	No. negative (%)	Total
A	4 (10)	36 (90)	40
B	7 (17.5)	33 (82.5)	40
C	3 (7.5)	37 (92.5)	40
D	4 (16.66)	20 (83.33)	24
E	1 (6.66)	14 (93.33)	15
F	0 (0)	14 (100)	14
G	2 (11.76)	15 (88.23)	17
H	2 (10)	18 (90)	20
Total	23	187	210

most prevalent serovars with 68.18%, 18.8% and 56%, 28% in sheep and goats, respectively. In previous studies in Tehran, Tabriz, Ahvaz and Khorramabad, the predominant serovars in cattle were Pomona; Pomona; grippotyphosa and Pomona; canicola and grippotyphosa, respectively, respectively (Hajikolaei et al., 2007; Hassanpour et al., 2012; Maleki et al., 2013). It is probable that this serovar may be adapted to and maintained by these farm animals in Ahvaz. There is a need for futher investigation on clinical cases of leptospirosis to determine whether this serovar is the main cause of leptospirosis in this region.

Percentage of seropositive for more than one serovar was 8.6% and 4.76% in seropositive goats and sheep, respectively. In serological tests for leptospirosis such as MAT, the results often indicate infection with more than one serovar (Egan and Yearly, 1989; Hajikolaei et al, 2005, Hataway et al., 1981). This may be the result of mixed serovar infection but the exis-

tence of cross reactivity in the MAT among the serovars is well known and can be excluded from this interpretation. The high prevalence of infection and dominant titre of 1:100 reveal that leptospiral infection in goats and sheep in Ahvaz (in the southwest of Iran) is endemic and occurs mostly in subclinical form. There were no significant differences among the ages and areas groups in sheep and goats, but there was a tendency in adult sheep and goats (≥3 years) to be more seropositive than young sheep and goats that is in agreement with the other studies (Hassanpour et al., 2008 and 2012 and Maleki et al., 2014).

These results confirm that leptospiral infection may exist in the goat and sheep population in Ahvaz area and the presence of antibodies in the absence of infection indicates the exposure to the organism and must be acknowledged. In addition, these results confirm that the majority of leptospiral infections is asymptomatic. Because of the importance of leptospira interrogans as an abortifacient agent in goat and sheep, it will be considered as one of the possible causes of abortion in goat and sheep in Ahvaz, southwestern Iran.

Acknowlegments

The authors would like to acknowledge the research vice chancellor of Shahid Chamran University of Ahvaz for financial support.

References

1. Agunloye, C.A. (2002) Leptospiral agglutination antibodies in sheep and goat in southwest Nigeria. Israel Vet Med Assoc. 57: 2.
2. Bahaman, A.R., Ibrahim, A.L., Adam, H. (1987) Serological prevalence of leptospiral infection in domestic animals in west Malaysia. Epidemiol Infect. 99: 379-392.
3. Bojkovski, D., Stuhee, I., Kompan, D., Zupan, M. (2014) The behavior of sheep and goats co-grazing on pasture with defferent types of vegetation in the karst region. J Anim Sci. 92: 2752-278.
4. Burriel, A.R., Vougiouka, D.M., Butsini, S., Nomikou, K., Patakakis, M. (2002) A serological investigation of some causes of reproductive failure among small ruminants in Greece. Online J Vet Res. 6: 57-63.
5. Cerri, D., Ebani, V.V., Fratini, F., Pinzauti, P., Andreani, E. (2003) Epidemiology of leptospirosis: observation on serological data obtained by a diagnostic laboratory for leptospirosis from 1995 to 2001. New Microbiol. 26: 383-389.
6. Ciceroni, L., Bartoloni, A., Pinto, A., Guglielmetti, P., Vasquez, C.V. (1997) Serological survey of leptospiral infection in sheep, goats and dogs in Cordillera province, Bolivia. New Microbiol. 20: 77-81.
7. Ciceroni, L., Lombordo, D., Pinto, A., Ciarrocchi, S., Simeoni, J. (2000) Prevalence of antibodies to leptospira serovars in sheep and goats in Alto Adige-South Tyrol. J Vet Med. 47: 217-223.
8. Draghi de Benitez, M.G., Zubriggen, M.A., Vanzini, V.R. (1984) Serological survey for ovine leptospirosis in Correentes province, Argentina. Vet Argent. 1: 336-340.
9. Egan, J., Yearley, D.A. (1989) Serological survey of leptospiral infection in Republic of Irland. Vet Rec. 119: 306.
10. Flint, S.H., Corner, R.J., Marshall, R.B. (1988). Leptospirosis in farmed goats. New-Zealand. Vet J. 36: 156-158.
11. Haji Hajikolaei, M.R., Ghorbanpour, M., Keshavarzi-Yangabadi, M., Abdollapour, G.R. (2007a) Seroprevalence of leptospiral infection in goats of Ahvaz. Iran J Vet Res. 4: 93-96.
12. Haji Hajikolaei, M.R., Ghorbanpour, M., Gharibi, D., Abdollapour, G.R. (2007b) Serologic study on leptospiral infection in sheep of Ahvaz, southwestern Iran. J Vet Res. 8: 333-336.
13. Haji Hajikolaei, M.R., Ghorbanpour, M., Abdollapour, G.R. (2005a) Serological study of leptospirosis in cattle in Ahvaz. J Vet Res (University of Tehran). 60: 7-14.
14. Haji Hajikolaei, M.R., Ghorbanpour, M., Haidari, M., Abdollapour, G.R (2005b) Comparison of leptospiral infection in the horse and donkey. Bull Vet Inst Pulawy. 49: 175-178.
15. Hasanpor, A., Asgarloo, S., Imandar, M., Mashayekhi, M., Abdollhapour, G.R., Safarmashaei, S. (2012) Seroepidemiologic study of Goats leptospirosis in Khoy-Iran. J Anim Vet Adv. 11: 229-233.
16. Maleki, S.H., Abdollapour, G.R., Bahonar, A.R. (2013) Serological and bacteriological study of leptospirosis in dairy herds and feedlot in Tehran areas. Iran J Vet Med. 7: 177-183.
17. Maleki, S.H. (2014) Serological study on leptospiral infection in goats in Khorramabad. Bull Georg Natl Acad Sci. 8: 553-558.
18. Manickavel, K., Kalyanasundaram, C.K., Venkataraman, K.S., Rao, V.N.A., Thanagavelu, S. (1991) Reports on leptospirosis in sheep in Tamil Nadu. Indian Vet J. 68: 503-505.
19. Maronpot, R.R., Barsoum, I.S. (1972) Lepto-

spiral Microscopic agglutination antibodies in sera of man and domestic animals in Egypt. Am J Tropic Clinic Microbiol. 30: 2219-2224.

20. Miller, D.A., Wilson, M.A., Beran, G.W. (1991) Relationship between prevalence of *Leptospira introgans* in cattle and regional climatic and seasonal factors. Am J Vet Res. 52: 1761-1768.

21. O.I.E. (2000) Manual of standards of diagnostic tests and vaccines, leptospirosis, part 2, section 22: chapter 2.2.4., Paris, France.

22. Radostits, O.M., Gay, C.C., Hinchcliff, K.W., Constable, P.D. (2007) Veterinary Medicine: A Textbook of the Disease of Cattle, Horses, Sheep, Pigs and Goats. (10th ed.) Saunders Elsevier, Philadelphia, PA, USA.

23. Ramin, A.G., Azizzadeh, F. (2013) Seroepidemiological detection of antibodies against leptospiral spp using microscopic agglutination test in uremia cows and sheep. Acta Vet. 63: 53-61.

24. Saglama, Y.S., Yenerb, Z., Temurc, A., Yalcinc, E. (2007) Immonohistochemical detection of leptospiral antigens in cases of naturally occurring abortion in sheep. Small Rumin Res. 74: 119-122.

25. Samir, A., Soliman, R., El-Hariri, M., Abdel-Moein, K.H., Hatem, M.E. (2015) Leptospirosis in animal and human contacts in Egypt: broad range surviilance. Rev Soc Bras Med Trop. 48: 272-727.

26. Shivaraj, M.D., Venkatesha, Rajkumari, S., Sripad, K., Sanjeevkumar, B., Chandranaik, M., Renukapraasad, C. (2009) Leptopriosis in sheep and its diagnosis. Vet World. 2: 263-264.

27. Sratnam, K.L. (1992) Leptospiral antibodies among sheep and goat. Indian J Anim Sci. 62: 1041-1043.

28. Zainali, A., Vand-yousefi, J., Ahoraei, P. (1997) The survey of leptospiral infection in Uremia. J Pajouhesh Va Sazandegi (In Persian). 37: 76-78.

13

The first study of bovine immunodeficiency virus (BIV) and brucellosis co-infection in west-central Iran

Mokhtari A.[1*], Mahzounieh M.[1], Frossard J.P.[2]

[1]Department of Pathobiology, Faculty of Veterinary Medicine, University of Shahrekord, Shahrekord, Iran
[2]Department of Virology, Veterinary Laboratories Agency, Addlestone, United Kingdom

Key words:

Bovine immunodeficiency virus, Brucella, seroprevalence

Correspondence

Mokhtari A.
Department of Pathobiology, Faculty of Veterinary Medicine, University of Shahrekord, Shahrekord, Iran

Email: a.mokhtari@alumni.ut.ac. ir

Abstract:

BACKGROUND: BIV is a well-known bovine immunosuppressive cause, but its pathogenesis has not been well characterized. In recent years, it has been hypothesized that infection with BIV might predispose cattle to be infected by other agents. **OBJECTIVE:** This study was performed to investigate of BIV and Brucella co-infection so that in the future more studies will be done on the issue of predisposing cattle to other microorganisms like Brucella after BIV infection. **METHODS:** Blood samples were collected from a total of 2290 cattle in Iran (490 and 1800 cattle in non-industrial and industrial dairy farms, respectively from Isfahan and Chaharmahal and Bakhtiari provinces). The BIV-positive animals were detected by Lab-ELISA and nested PCR tests. **RESULTS:** In this study, the overall prevalence of BIV in Iran was 1.61% (4.5% and 0.83% in non-industrial and industrial dairy farms, respectively). **CONCLUSIONS:** There was a statistically significant relationship between BIV status and Brucella infection using Chi square and Pearson's correlation coefficient test for all of the samples (p=0.0001, r=0.24), samples from Chaharmahal and Bakhtiari (p=0.044, r=0.13) and from industrial farms in Isfahan (p=0.001, r=0.074).

Introduction

Bovine immunodeficiency virus (BIV) is a lentivirus of the family Retroviridae. BIV infections are lifelong and generally subclinical (Amborski et al., 1989; Belloc et al., 1996). Serological investigations have shown wide distribution with differing prevalence (1.4% to 80%) of BIV infections around the world (Amborski et al., 1989; Belloc et al., 1996; Baron et al., 1998; Burkala et al., 1999). Serologic evidence for BIV infection has been reported in many countries around the world such as the Netherlands, France, Japan, Canada, Australia, Brazil, Costa Rica, Venezuela, and Turkey (Baron et al., 1998; Gonda et al., 1987; Gonda et al., 1994; Horzinek et al., 1991; McNab et al., 2010; Meas et al., 2003; Polack et al., 1996; Usui et al., 2003). The impact of BIV is controversial due to the difficulty in culturing new isolates in vitro and the complexity in identifying BIV-infected animals (Evermann et al., 1997; Gradil et al., 1999; Lew et al., 2004). Although several pathological changes, including monocyte dysfunction, encephalopathy, lymphadenopathy, and immunodeficiency have been reported in BIV-infected cattle, the detailed pathogenesis of BIV-infected cattle remains unclear (Burkala et al., 1999; Carpenter et al., 1992; Cyrcoats et al., 1994; Esmaeili et al., 2011; Evermann et al., 1997; Gonda et al., 1994). There is evidence that BIV can cause immunosuppression with increased incidence of secondary bacterial infections and encephalitis with high seroprevalences (Gonda et al., 1994). Following experimental infections, cattle may have transient increases in lymphocytes, lymphoid hyperplasia, atypical lymphosarcoma, and secondary bacterial infections such as *Mycobacterium bovis* (Yilmaz et al., 2008; Rola et al., 2011). Even though the virus has not been linked to any specific disease condition in cattle, it certainly can aggravate several illnesses in the animals, including impairment of the immune system (Carpenter et al., 1992). BIV seropositivity is associated with decreased milk production in dairy cattle, but no direct link has been found to clinical disease in naturally infected cattle (Burkala et al., 1999; Carpenter et al., 1992; Cyrcoats et al., 1994; Yilmaz et al., 2008). However, Walder et al. reported evidence for a possible association between bovine paraplegic syndrome and a viral agent related to BIV (Walder et al., 1995). Snider et al. determined that a herd with high seroprevalence of BIV had a high percentage of cows with encephalitis associated with depression and stupor, alteration of the immune system associated with secondary bacterial infections, and chronic inflammation of the feet and legs (Horzinek et al., 1991; Snider et al., 1996; Orr et al., 2003). The detailed pathogenesis in infected cattle still remains unclear. BIV seropositivity has been shown to be variably associated with decrease in animal production, weight loss, secondary diseases, and diminished milk production (McNab et al., 1994; Gonzalez et al., 2001).

Despite a control program being in place for over 30 years, brucellosis remains endemic in Iran and several Mediterranean countries where it is one of the most important zoonotic diseases (Esmaeili et al., 2011). The Veterinary Organization of Iran uses test and slaughter policy and vaccination against Brucella (Esmaeili, 2014). There are cases of Brucella and tuberculosis co-infection or Brucella and

HIV co-infection. Therefore, the management of HIV and tuberculosis or any other potential risk factors may be of great clinical importance in the treatment of brucellosis infection in a brucellosis endemic country like Iran (Karsen et al, 2008; Abdollahi et al, 2010;Cadmus et al, 2008). Brucellosis incidence is influenced by management factors, herd size, population density, type of animal breed, and biological features such as herd immunity (Boukary et al., 2013). BIV infection in cattle may be associated with common bacteria such as *E. coli* and *Salmonella* spp. and may also co-infect with bovine viral diarrhea virus or infectious bovine rhinotracheitis virus or Brucella (Meas et al., 2004). Up to now, studies about HIV and Brucella co-infection have been done (Hajiabdolbaghi et al., 2011), but there aren't any available reports about the co-infection of BIV and Brucella. Systemic brucellosis is characterized by involvement of tissues rich in reticuloendothelial elements and profound activation of cell-mediated immunity. Similar to other zoonotic diseases, Iran is an endemic country for Brucella infection and symptomatic brucellosis. Among the affected populations, HIV-infected patients might be at a greater risk for Brucella infection. The dramatic decline of CD4 marker level in HIV-infected patients predisposes them to organisms that are mostly eradicated via cell-mediated immunity. Therefore, a frequent association could be anticipated within geographical areas in which both brucellosis and HIV are prevalent. In the early 1990s, the possible association between brucellosis and HIV infection was assessed only in a few endemic countries. There have been evaluations of Brucella infection prevalence in hospitalized patients, most of whom were asymptomatic HIV-positive patients with a partially preserved immune system. A few studies suggest that immune reactions are probably crucial for the development of brucellosis from Brucella infection. Hence, this immune response is phenotypically polymorphic in different cases with different immuno-logical states, and the range of clinical man-ifestations widely varies among patients, so one may assume that brucellosis features are likely correlated with the state of the patient's immune system. Therefore, variable clinical responses to Brucella infection are expected in HIV-positive patients with varying CD4+ levels. However, one may conclude that CD4+ count would be inversely correlated with the severity of brucellosis complications (Hajiab-dolbaghi et al., 2011).

The bovine immunodeficiency virus (BIV) and human immunodeficiency virus types 1 and 2 (HIV-1 and -2) are members of the len-tivirus genus of retroviruses. Although the DNA sequences of these viruses have diverged considerably, the BIV genome organization, function of structural and regulatory genes, and replication cycle are very similar to that of HIV-1 (Tobin et al., 1996). So far, no re-ports on the importance of BIV as a predispos-ing factor for Brucella have been published. However, due to the biological similarities of BIV and HIV, the present study was designed according to the reports of the co-infection of HIV and Brucella. In fact, the purpose of this study was to determine the prevalence of BIV and brucella co-infection in Iranian cattle. Our study adds to the available data on BIV and Brucella and is the first report of BIV-Brucella co-infection in Iran. However, further studies should be done to determine the predisposing effects of BIV infection to other organisms like Brucella.

Materials and Methods

Herd management, blood sampling and DNA extraction: The samples were obtained from dairy industrial and non-industrial farms in Isfahan and Chaharmahal and Bakhtiari. These two provinces are among the regions with moderate incidence of brucellosis (Esmaeili, 2014). Two dairy cattle production systems

are described in these areas. One is a system of small independent farms. The herd density is about 5-50 animal per farm with a low technol-ogy level and milk production (average milk yield about 3575 Kg/cow/year based on the reports of the local veterinary organization). The second system is the commercial industri-al herds which use more advanced technology with average milk production from about 4300 to 7900 Kg/cow/year. The cow population of the tested industrial herd was 1800. All of the cows were Holstein breed. They were housed in an intensive system and were kept in indi-vidual boxes. They fed on milk, concentrate, and alfalfa. About 95% of the herds had free-stall system. All the animals were immunized against foot and mouth disease and clostridial diseases, and all female cows were vaccinated against brucellosis. All of the herds used arti-ficial insemination. Nutrition and reproduction management of the herds were controlled us-ing computerized herd health management.

Sera were isolated from 2990 peripheral blood samples (1800 cattle from an industrial dairy province in Isfahan and 490 cattle of 84 non- industrial dairy farms, in Isfahan (n=46) and Chaharmahal and Bakhtiari (n=38) areas of Iran) from 2008 to 2009. The sera were stored at -20 °C until future use. Serum samples were analyzed to detect antibodies against BIV us-ing Lab-ELISA as described by Scobie et al (1999). For PCR assay, 45 blood samples with EDTA were obtained from seropositive and se-ronegative dairy cows and genomic DNA was extracted from PBMC using the DNA isolation kit for mammalian blood (Roche Applied Sci-ence Co., Germany C. no:11 667 327 001) ac-cording to the manufacturer's directions with-in 48 h.

Labeled Avidin-Biotin enzyme-linked immunosorbent assay (Lab- ELISA): Se-rological analysis was performed on 2290 se-rum samples using a synthetic peptide derived from the available sequence of the transmem-brane (TM) glycoprotein of BIV-FL112, produced at the Veterinary Laboratories Agency, Surrey, UK (Scobie et al., 1999). The detection of antibodies against this TM peptide was performed under the following conditions: a volume of 100 µl peptide (12 µg/ml in 0.05 M carbonate-bicarbonate buffer, pH 9.6) was added to each well of a microtitre plate (Immulon 2 HB) and the plates were incubated overnight at 4 °C. The wells were washed three times with 200 µl TBS-T (138 mM NaCl, 2.6 mM of KCl, 24.8 mM Tris-Cl, 1% Tween-20, pH 7.5) and blocked with dried milk powder (2%) and goat serum (20%) in TBS-T for 1 h at room temperature. Following three washes with TBS-T, 100 µl aliquots of bovine sera diluted 1:10 in TBS-T and were incubated for 1 h at room temperature. After three additional washes, mouse monoclonal anti- bovine immunoglobulin antibody linked to Biotin diluted 1:7000 in TBS-T with 1% of non-fat milk was added to each well and incubated 1 h at room temperature. After three washes with TBS-T, alkaline-labeled streptavidin linked to antibody diluted 1:900 with TBS-T using non-fat milk was added to each well and incubated 1 h at room temperature. After three washes with TBS-T, the phosphatase reaction was visualized with Phosphate substrate tablets (Sigma-Aldrich Chemical Co., St. Louis, MO, USA, C. no:047-8203) and the optical densities (OD) were determined at 405 nm. A ratio of sample to positive control (S/P) was calculated based on the positive and negative control sera included in each plate. Samples with S/P ratios greater than 0.1 were considered positive to BIV.

Serology tests to detect Brucella antibodies: In this study, serologic tests for Brucella were conducted by the veterinary organizations in Isfahan and Chaharmahal and Bakhtiari areas. In brief, sera were initially tested using the Rose Bengal plate test (RBPT), as described by Alton et al (Alton et al., 1988), using the antigen supplied by the Razi Institute in Tehran. Positive results were confirmed with the standard tube agglutination test (STAT) and the 2-mercaptoethanol test (2ME). The STAT and 2ME tests were performed according to the method of Alton et al. (Alton et al., 1975) using the antigen supplied by the Razi Institute (Karaj, Iran). For unvaccinated and vaccinated (RB51) animals, 2ME and STAT titers were calculated and interpreted according to the Veterinary Organization of Iran's instructions (Esmaeili et al., 2012).

Nested PCR assay: Nested PCR was performed in order to detect the BIV proviral DNA 27. The first amplification was performed using a pair of outer primers specific to the BIV pol region (p01: 50-ATGCTAATGGATTTTAGGGA-30 and p36: 50-CATTTCTTGGGTGTGAGCTC-30) to amplify a 490 bp fragment. The second amplification was performed to amplify a 176 bp fragment, using a pair of inner primers from the pol region (p02: 50-CATCCTTGTGGTAGAACATT-30 and p37: 50- CCTTAC-CCTCCAGGAATTAA-30). Briefly, PCR was performed as follows: final concentrations in the reaction mixes were 1X Taq polymerase buffer (PromegaCorp., Madison, WI, USA), 3 mM MgCl2, 200 µM dNTPs, 20 pmol of each primer, 1.25U Taq polymerase and 0.5 µg of genomic DNA, in a total volume of 50 µl. The thermal cycling conditions for the first round of amplification were 1 cycle for 2 min at 94 °C, 15 s at 51 °C and 2 min at 72 °C, then 30 cycles of 45 s at 94 °C, 15 s at 51 °C and 10 min at 72 °C, and a final extension step of 10 min at 72 °C. Two microliter of the first round reaction was used in the second reaction. The thermal cycling conditions for the second round of amplification were 1 cycle for 2 min at 94 °C, 15 s at 61 °C and 1 min at 72 °C, then 30 cycles of 45 s at 94 °C, 15 s at 61 °C and 10 min at 72 °C, with a final extension step of 10 min at 72 °C. 6 microliter of the amplified products were loaded on a 1.3% agarose gel, and visualized by staining with ethidium bromide. A BIV-DNA positive control (obtained from the Veterinary Laboratories Agency, Surrey, UK) that originated from the PBMC of a calf experimentally infected with the BIV FL-112 strain was included in each analysis. The DNA for BIV-negative control was obtained from BIV-negative animals. Additionally, a water only negative control reaction was included in each reaction.

DNA sequencing: 6 PCR products were sequenced, and for this purpose, additional specific PCR products were generated using a nested amplification of the proviral pol gene by our coworkers in VLA (UK). Reactions were carried out in 50μl volumes, containing: 200μM each dNTP, 1X Promega Taq polymerase buffer (50mM KCl, 10mM Tris-HCl pH 8.8, 2.5mM MgCl2, 0.1% Trtion X-100, 2μg/ml gelatin), 0.75pM of each primer, and 0.25u of Taq DNA polymerase (Promega). The first round cycling conditions were: 94°C 2 min, 53°C for 20 s, 72°C for 2 min, followed by 36 cycles of 94°C for 45 s, 53°C for 20 s, and 72°C for 1 min and a final extension step of 72°C for 10 min. The outer primer pair sequences were: P3: 5'-GAA-CGG-GAA-GAT-GGA-GGA-TGT-3', and P38: 5'-GTT-AAG-GGG-TAT-AGA-GGG-ATT-TTT-3'. The nested reaction was carried out in 50μl volumes, using 1μl of the first round product as template, and with 200μM each dNTP, 1X Promega Taq polymerase buffer (50mM KCl, 10mM Tris-HCl pH 8.8, 3mM MgCl2, 0.1% Triton X-100, 2μg/ml gelatin), 1pM of each primer, and 0.25u of Taq DNA polymerase (Promega). The second round cycling conditions were: 94°C 2 min, 51°C 20 s, 72°C 2 min, followed by 36 cycles of 94°C 45 s, 51°C 15 s, and 72°C 1 min, with a final extension step of 72°C 10 min. The inner primer pair sequences used were: P01: 5'-ATG-CTA-ATG-GAT-TTT-AGG-GA-3', and P36: 5'-CAT-TTC-TTG-GGT-GTG-AGC-TC-3'. The specific products from the second round (491 base pairs) were then sequenced in an automated fluorescent dideoxy sequencing system using

the ABI Prism sequencing kit (ABI), with both original internal amplification primers. Sequence data were edited and analyzed with SeqMan Pro version 8.0.2 and MegAlign version 8.0.2 software (DNASTAR, Lasergene).

Statistical analysis: The results were analyzed using ANOVA, chi square, Pearson's correlation coefficient, and T-tests using SPSS software v.16.

Results

Lab- ELISA: Totally, 37 (1.61%) samples were positive for BIV antibodies. 22 / 490 (4.49%) of samples (from 84 non-industrial dairy farms) and 15 / 1800 (0.83%) of samples (from an industrial dairy farm) were BIV seropositive.

S/P ratios ranged from 0.70 to 1.86. 17 out of 84 non-industrial farms (20.2%) were BIV-positive. The age distribution of BIV seropositive animals was determined (Table 2), with 1.6% of animals less than two years of age (1-2), 7.5% of animals between 2 and 4 years of age, 5.9% of animals between 4 and 6 years, and 2.6% of animals between 6 and 8 years of age were found positive. The majority of BIV seropositive animals (77.3%) were found to be between 2 and 4 years old. For the Isfahan area, the overall seroprevalence of BIV was 1.12% (3.3% in the non- industrial farms and 0.83% in the industrial dairy farm) while for the Chaharmahal and Bakhtiari area it was 5.7 % in the non-industrial farms (see tables 3 and 4).

For the BIV S/P ratios, a 2-way analysis of variance (ANOVA) with the two factors of location and the Brucella status (negative, low, high) was performed. The Brucella status was not significant (p=0.391) but location was (p=0.034). Esfahan (SD= 1.26, SE= 0.11) was on the average slightly higher than Shahrekord (SD= 0.92, SE = 0.09).

Co-infection and statistics: Of the BIV seronegative animals (n=2253) 0.53% were sero-

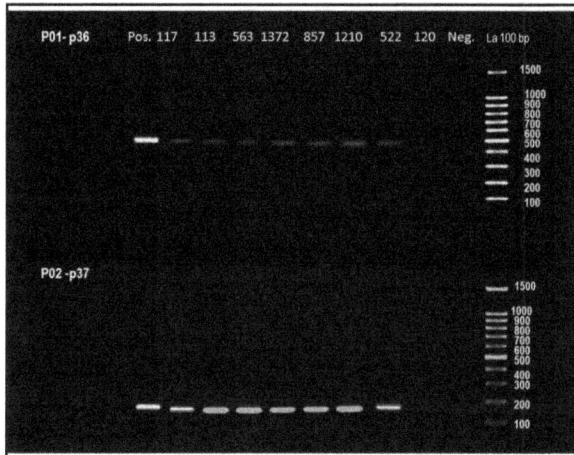

Figure 1. The picture of the agarose gel for 7 BIV-positive in nested PCR. Top row: The first amplification using a pair of outer primers specific to the BIV pol region (p01and p36) to amplify a 490 bp fragment. (Gene ruler is 100 bp). Bottom row: The second amplification to amplify a 176 bp fragment, using a pair of inner primers from the pol region (p02 and p37). (Gene ruler is 100 bp).

positive for Brucella, while 32.43% of the BIV seropositive animals (n=37) were seropositive (see tables 3 and 4). In this study, there was a statistically significant relationship between the BIV status and the Brucella status for all of the samples (p=0.0001, r=0.24), sera from Chaharmahal and Bakhtiari (p=0.044, r=0.13) and samples from industrial farms in Isfahan (p=0.001, r=0.074) using Chi square and Pearson's correlation coefficient test. The highest co- infection rate of BIV_Brucella was 9.1%, in cattle from Chaharmahal and Bakhtiari, but it was not statistically significant. Tables 2 and 3 show the results.

Nested PCR assay: Of the blood samples from BIV seropositive animals (n=37) and BIV seronegative animals (n=8), all samples (1.61%) were positive in the nested PCR test and their PCR products were in the same size of BIV positive control (some of these results have been shown in Figure 1).

DNA sequencing: The 451 nucleotide pol gene fragments sequenced from six animals were compared to the published data for BIV isolates R29 (ac. no: NC001413.1), FL112 (ac. no: L06524.1), FL491 (ac. no: L06525.1), and to each other. The sequenc-

es from five (accession numbers: KT281111, KT281112,KT281113, KT281114, KT281115) of the Iranian animals were identical, while that from the sixth (KT281116) varied in three nucleotide positions: 4- A/T, 412- C/T, and 430- C/G. The five Iranian sequences (1, 2, 7, 8, and 9) were 100% similar to the R29 isolate, 99.3% similar to the sixth Iranian sample (6), and 91.1% similar to isolates FL112 and FL491.

The translated amino acid sequences (150 amino acids) were also analyzed. There were 2 substitutions between the sequences from sample 6 and the other five, in the following positions: 1- Phe/Leu and 143- Asp/Glu.

Discussion

Serological survey is an important method to determine the distribution of BIV on livestock, and data on BIV seropositive animals may contribute to the awareness of the worldwide prevalence of the disease.

Currently, there is no gold standard (a completely accurate test) to detect BIV infection (Orr et al., 2003; Suarez et al., 1995; Nash et al., 1995) and one of the difficulties in assessing the role of BIV in predisposing cows to bovine infections or disorders is inconsistency with the methods used to detect infected cattle. Variations in infection prevalence might be influenced by the type of assays used for BIV detection. Substantial misclassification of infection would be expected in epidemiological studies of BIV regardless of which assay was used (Orr et al., 2003).

The culture of the virus is difficult and as expected, the virus could be isolated only within a short time frame. Although the use of PCR for the detection of BIV proved to be more sensitive than either serologic testing or virus isolation, the genetic variation (7-8% nucleotide divergence in the conserved pol segment) of field isolates probably plays a negative role in the results of these diagnostic tests (Meas et

Table 1. BIV seropositive cattle in Isfahan and Chaharmahal and Bakhtiari farms using Lab- ELISA.

	Non-industrial farms		Industrial farms		Total	
	No.	BIV seropositive	No.	BIV seropositive	No.	BIV seropositive
Isfahan	248	8 (3.3%)	1800	15 (0.83%)	2048	23 (1.12%)
Chaharmahal and Bakhtiari	242	14 (5.7%)	0	0(0%)	242	14 (5.7%)
Total	490	22 (4.5%)	1800	15 (0.83%)	2290	37 (1.61%)

Table 2. A) Co-infection of Brucella and BIV in cattle of different ages in non-industrial farms: (*)Brucella considered positive when serum titre ≥ 80. (**) In this study, the serum samples were randomly collected but some of them were chosen from among the dairy cattle with previous or current Brucella infection.

Age (years)	BIV+ Brucella+*	BIV+ Brucella-	BIV- Brucella+*	BIV- Brucella-	Total
1-2	0	2	54	65	121
2-4	7	2	50	61	120
4-6	5	3	57	70	135
6-8	0	3	52	59	114
Total	12	10	213 **	255	490

B) BIV infection in cattle of different ages in non-industrial farms, by area:

Age (years)	BIV Seropositive			BIV Seronegative.
	Isfahan	Chaharmahal and Bakhtiari	Total	Total
<2	0	2	2 (1.6%)	121
2-4	4	5	9 (7.5%)	120
4-6	4	4	8 (5.9%)	135
6-8	0	3	3 (2.6%)	114
Total	8	14	22 (4.5%)	490

al., 2003). It has been shown that nested PCR is 80% sensitive and 85% specific18, so we confirmed the result of PCR assay by sequencing. Earlier studies such as a study performed by Gonzalez et al. (2001) and Lew et al. (2004) indicated discordance between the serological (ID, ELISA-i, WB, PCR) and the genomic detection of BIV (Lew et al., 2004), with the genomic detection by polymerase chain reaction showing greater sensitivity and specificity. Gonzalez et al. (2001) have provided evidence that their nested PCR has a greater sensitivity than other published methods. In this study, we found a relative descriptive consistency between the serological and the genomic detection of BIV results. However, with only 37 seropositive and 8 seronegative PCR tests, it is not possible to prove any coordination between serological and molecular results definitively and more analysis is needed.

ELISA tests are, in general, relatively accurate and have been considered highly sensitive and specific in detecting specific antibodies. Therefore, Lab-ELISA based on BIV-TM peptide should also be presented as a confirmatory test for BIV because of the high sensitivity of streptavidin to biotin. We propose here that the Lab-ELISA based on recombinant viral antigen or synthetic peptides, as used in this work, should decrease the number of false positive reactions which occur when the serum reacts with non-relevant proteins and could be recommended as a diagnosis test to detect BIV seropositive animals.

BIV Proviral DNA is detectable in PBMC during the early stage of infection (from 4-60 days with peak titers 20 dpi). There is a transient viraemia from 4 to 14 dpi. An antibody

Table 3.Co-infection of Brucella and BIV in Isfahan and Chaharmahal and Bakhtiari areas of Iran. [*] - Brucella seropositive titre defined as >80.

	BIV seronegtive		BIV seropositive		Total	
	.No	Brucella* seropositive	.No	*Brucella seropositive	.No	*Brucella seropositive
Isfahan	2025	113 (5.58%)	23	2(8.7%)	2048	115 (5.61%)
Chaharmahal and Bakhtiari	228	100 (43.85%)	14	10(71.42%)	242	110 (45.45%)
Total	2253	213 (9.45%)	37	12(32.43%)	2290	225 (9.82%)

Table 4. Co-infection of Brucella and BIV in Isfahan industrial and non-industrial farms. [*] - Brucella seropositive titre defined as >80.

	BIV seronegtive samples		BIV seropositive samples		Total	
	No.	Brucella seropositive*	No.	Brucella seropositive*	No.	Brucella seropositive*
(Non-industrial farms)	240	(47.08%) 113	8	(% 25) 2	248	(46.37%) 115
(Industrial farms)	1785	(0%) 0	15	(0%)0	1800	(0%) 0
Total	2025	(5.58%) 113	23	(8.7%) 2	2048	(5.61%) 115

response to the TM glycoprotein commences 12 dpi with peak titers 10-30 wpi, and its response is detectable until 50 weeks post infection. Thus, it is suitable for the long term monitoring of the infection. An antibody response to the CA protein is detected not until 34 dpi. So a CA-based serological assay would not identify the majority of infected cattle (McNab et al., 2010).

Due to the persistent nature of the anti-TM antibody response in BIV infections (Scobie et al., 1999), the TM glycoprotein may also be a promising linear antigenic target and may, therefore, yield a potential antigen for inclusion in a differential serological assay. The inconsistency between previous serological and molecular assays may be because of the nature of antigen or antibody included in each serological assay or the time that blood sampling and tests have been done. In this study, we detected BIV-positive cows by Lab-Elisa and nested PCR within one month. Therefore, the consistency between the results of these two tests isn't unlikely. Of course, according to just 45 PCR results for 37 seropositive samples and 8 seronegative samples, it cannot definitively be concluded that both serological and molecular tests have consistency.

If there are PCR results for seronegative

samples, they should be clarified. Previously, the presence of BIV infection in the dairy cattle of industrial farms in Iran was reported by Nikbakht Borujeni et al. (Nikbakht Borujeniet al., 2010) and Tajbakhsh et al. (Tajbakhsh et al., 2010) and the BIV prevalence in these studies was 20.3% and 60% respectively, which are far larger than the world average (4-6%), but their BIV prevalence results are in the range. Sero-prevalence rates of BIV which have been reported worldwide are between 1.4% and 64%, but mostly in the range of 4% to 6%. In total, BIV prevalence varies widely worldwide (Belloc et al. 1996; Kurth et al. 2010). As described, BIV Proviral DNA is detectable in a short time during the infection, so it isn't possible to detect such a high prevalence with using only PCR. The prevalence rate varied in different dairy herds and the higher prevalence in some dairy cattle may be the result of herd management practices and of the extended productive life. In the previous studies on the BIV prevalence in Iran, the state of farms has not been well described. Therefore, large-scale serological and molecular studies with detailed long-term epidemiological observation of BIV incidences will be necessary to confirm these findings (McNab et al., 2010).

In this study, the serum samples were randomly collected, but some of them were chosen from among the dairy cattle with previous or current Brucella infection. The overall prevalence of BIV in west-central Iran in this survey was 1.61%. Out of 490 animals from 84 non-industrial dairy farms, 22 were positive (4.5%). The difference between BIV prevalence in these types of farms is mainly due to the herd management and flock density.

The results presented here give an accurate new estimate of BIV prevalence in west-central Iran. In the present study, a seroepidemiological survey of BIV and Brucellosis was performed to determine a correlation between BIV and Brucellosis infections. It has been hypothesized that infection with BIV, and potential consequent immunosuppression, might predispose cattle to infection by other agents such as Brucella or might affect their response to vaccination (Tajbakhsh et al., 2010). For example, immunosuppression with a delayed IgG response to B. abortus has been described for the closely related Jembrana disease virus in Bali cattle34. The p value for chi square and the Pearson's correlation coefficient test (p=0.0001, r=0.24) provide evidence of association between BIV and Brucellosis. Thus, in this study, statistically significant evidence has been found for the correlation of BIV and Brucella infection rates. However, the probability that BIV infection predispose the animals to infection with Brucellosis needs to be confirmed with further tests such as analysis and monitoring of brucellosis development in experimentally BIV-infected cows and comparing the findings with the results of the same test in an equal BIV-negative control group. Co-infection may simply represent prior exposure to both microorganisms and not in itself indicate any biological association and/or probable synergisms.

Seroepidemiological studies of BIV infections in cattle have been reported in many countries (Nikbakht Borujeniet al., 2010). Despite the worldwide distribution of BIV in-

fection, whether the presence of BIV in a host leads to primarily pathologic changes or can cause secondary bacterial and/or viral infections as a predisposition factor has not been fully elucidated. In the natural infection with BIV, the host is affected differently compared to what has been observed in experimental infection. The presence of BIV combined with the stresses associated with parturition and a modern dairy production system was considered causal for the development of secondary diseases in immunocompromised cattle. In the previous studies, in BIV-infected animals the secondary disease processes and their incidence were reported (Yilmaz et al., 2008).

In conclusion, the seroprevalence of BIV in industrial and non-industrial dairy cattle herds in Iran was 0.83% and 4.5%, respectively. In this study, the overall BIV seroprevalence in Iran was 1.61% and we found that there is a relatively significant relationship between BIV and Brucellosis. Further studies should be designed to investigate the pathogenic and biological properties of local field isolate strains of the virus, and these strains should be included in the assays chosen to detect BIV antibodies.

Studies such as the present work have some limitations. First, it is difficult to know whether the disorders observed were due to BIV infection alone, because of the fact that BIV-positive cattle were not further analyzed for other infectious agents like viruses or bacteria that may play a role in that kind of clinical disorder. Second, it is difficult to select uniform patient and control populations in animal studies. Therefore, control animals were selected from among BIV-serone B) BIV infection in cattle of different ages in non-industrial farms, by area: gative cattle from the same herds including BIV-positive animals, because of the fact that some factors, i.e. climate, magnitude of farm, and management, are well known to affect the health status of dairy cattle. Third, the number of lactations could have been recorded in the present study. The fact that there was no significant difference in age between the groups may have minimized the effects of lactation on differences between them (Yilmaz et al., 2008; Nikbakht Borujeniet al., 2010; Tajbakhsh et al., 2010). These findings suggest that the presence of BIV infections should be considered a health risk for cattle populations, and may have a role in predisposing cattle to infections with other pathogenic microorganisms. Further studies in a larger patient population are required to verify these observations.

Our study adds to the available data on BIV in Iran. Further studies are needed to determine the epidemiology of infections in Iran, and local farmers need to be informed of the health risks these infections pose to their animals. In addition, it cannot be said that the prevalence of Brucella infection is only due to BIV, because there are certainly numerous risk factors of Brucellosis, and our study has proposed BIV as a potential new risk factor of Brucella infection.

Acknowledgements

The authors wish to thank R. Sayers (Veterinary Laboratories Agency, UK) for statistical advice and F. Steinbach (Veterinary Laboratories Agency, UK) for assistance with the manuscript.

References

1. Abdollahi, A., Morteza, A., Khalilzadeh, O., Rasoulinejad, M. (2010) Brucellosis serology in HIV-infected patients. Int J Infect Dis. 14: 904- 946.

2. Alton, G.G., Jones, L.M., Angus, R.D., Verger, J.M. (1988) Techniques for the Brucellosis Laboratory. (3rd ed.) Institut National de la Recherche Agronomique (INRA), Paris, France.

3. Alton, G.G., Jones, L.M., Pietz, D.E. (1975) Laboratory techniques in brucellosis. WHO monograph series. Geneva: WHO. 55:1-163.

4. Amborski, G.F., Lo, J.J., Seger, C.L. (1989) Serological detection of multiple retroviral infections in cattle: bovine leukemia virus, bovine syncytial virus and bovine visna virus. Vet Microbiol. 20: 247-253.

5. Baron, T., Betemps, F., Mallet, F., Cheynet, V., Levy, D., Belli, P. (1998) Detection of bovine immunodeficiency-like virus infection in experimentally infected calves. Arch Virol. 143: 181-189.

6. Belloc, C., Polack, B., Schwartz, I., Brownlie, J., Levy D. (1996) Bovine immunodeficiency virus: facts and questions. Vet Res. 27: 395-402.

7. Boukary, A.R., Saegerman, C., Abatih, E., Fretin, D., Alambédji Bada, R., De Deken, R., Harouna, H.A., Yenikoye, A., Thys, E. (2013) Seroprevalence and potential risk factors for Brucella Spp. infection in traditional cattle, sheep and goats reared in urban, periurban and rural areas of niger. PLoS One. 8: e83175.

8. Burkala, E.J., Ellis, T.M., Voigt, V., Wilcox, G.E. (1999) Serological evidence of an Australian bovine lentivirus. Vet Microbiol. 199: 171-177.

9. Cadmus, S.I., Adesokan, H.K., Stack, J.A. (2008) Co-infection of brucellosis and tuberculosis in slaughtered cattle in Ibadan, Nigeria: a case report. Vet Ital. 44: 557-8.

10. Carpenter, S., Miller, L.D., Alexardensen, S., Whetstone, C.A., Van Der Maaten, M.J., Viuff, B., Wannermuehler, Y., Miller, J.M., Roth, J.A. (1992) Characterization of early pathogenic effects after experimental infection of calves with bovine immunodeficiency-like virus. J Virol. 66: 1074-1083.

11. Cyrcoats, K.S., Pruett, S.B., Nash, J.W., Cooper, C.R. (1994) Bovine immunodeficiency virus: incidence of infection in Mississippi dairy cattle. Vet Microbiol. 42: 181-189.

12. Esmaeili, H. (2014) Brucellosis in Islamic republic of Iran, J Med Bacteriol. 3: 47-57.

13. Esmaeili, H., Ekhtiarzadeh, H., Ebrahimzadeh, H., Partovi, R., Marhamati Khameneh, B., Hamedi, M., Khalaji, L. (2011) Evaluation of National program for control of Brucellosis

in Iran. J Arak Med Uni. 6: 9-20.

14. Esmaeili, H., Tajik, P., Ekhtiyarzadeh, H., Bolourchi, M., Hamedi, M., Khalij, M., Amiri, K. (2012) Control and eradication program for bovine brucellosis in Iran: An epidemiological survey. J Vet Res. 67: 211-221.

15. Evermann, J., Jackson, M.K. (1997) Laboratory diagnostic tests for retroviral infections in dairy and beef cattle. Vet Clin North Am Food Anim Pract. 13: 87-106.

16. Gradil, C.M., Watson, R.E., Renxhaw, R.W., Gilbert, R.O., Dubovi, E.J. (1999) Detection of bovine immunodeficiency virus DNA in the blood and semen of experimentally infected bulls. Vet Microbiol. 70: 21-31.

17. Gonda, M.A., Braun, M.J., Carte, S.J., Kost, T.A., Bess, J.W., Arthur, T.A., Van Der Maaten, M.J. (1987) Characterization and molecular cloning of a bovine lentivirus related to human immunodeficiency virus. Nature 330: 388-391.

18. Gonda, M.A., Gene Luther, D., Fong, S.E., Tobin, G.J. (1994) Bovine immunodeficiency virus: molecular biology and virus-host interactions. Virus Res. 32: 155-181.

19. Gonzalez, E.T., Oliva, G.A., Valera, A., Bonzo, E., Licursi, M., Etcheverrigaray, M.E. (2001) Leucosis enzoo´ tica bovina: Evaluacio´n de te´cnicas diagno´ sticas (ID, ELISA-i, WB, PCR) en bovine's experimentalmente inoculados. Analecta Vet J. 21: 8-15.

20. Hajiabdolbaghi, M., Rasoulinejad, M., Abdollahi, A., Paydary, K., Valiollahi, P., SeyedAlinaghi, S., Parsa, M., Jafari, S. (2011) Brucella Infection in HIV Infected Patients. Acta Med Iran. 49: 801-5.

21. Horzinek, M., Keldermans, L., Stuurman, T., Black, J., Herrewegh, A., Silliken, S.P., Koolen, M. (1991) Bovine immunodeficiency virus: immunochemical characterization and serological survey. J Gen Virol. 72: 2923-2928.

22. Karsen, H., Karahocagil, M.K., Irmak, H., Demiröz, A.P. (2008) A meningitis case of Brucella and tuberculosis co-infection. Mikrobiyol Bul. 42: 689-94.

23. Kurth, R., Bannert, N. (2010) Retroviruses: Molecular Biology, Genomics and Pathogenesis. Reinhard, K., Norbert, B. (eds.). Caister Academic Press, Norfolk, UK.

24. Lew, A.E., Bock, R.E., Miles, J., Cuttell, L.B., Steer, P., Nadin-Davis, S. (2004) Sensitive and specific detection of bovine immunodeficiency virus and bovine syncytial virus by 5´taqnuclease assays with fluorescent 3´ minor groove binder-DNA probes. J Virol Methods. 116: 1-9.

25. McNab, T.J. (2010) An Analysis of Bovine immunodeficiency virus and Jembrana disease virus Infections in Bos javanicus, thesis for the degree of Doctor of Philosophy. p. 75-89.

26. McNab, W.B., Jacobs, R.M., Smith, H.E. (1994) A survey for bovine immunodeficiency-like virus in Ontario dairy cattle and associations between test results production records and management practices. Can J Vet Res. 58: 36-41.

27. Meas, S., Kabeya, H., Yoshihara, S., Ohashi, K., Matsuki, S., Mikami, Y., Sugimoto, C., Onuma, M. (1998) Seroprevalence and field isolation of bovine immunodeficiency virus. J Vet Med Sci. 60: 1195-1202.

28. Meas, S., Nakayama, M., Usui, T., Nakazato, Y., Yasuda, J., Ohashi, K., Onuma, M. (2004) Evidence for bovine immunodeficiency virus infection in cattle in Zambia. Jpn J Vet Res. 52: 3-8.

29. Meas, S., Yilmaz, Z., Usui, T., Torun, S., Yesilbag, K., Ihashi, K., Onuma, M. (2003) Evidence of bovine immunodeficiency virus in cattle in Turkey. Jap J Vet Res. 51: 3-8.

30. Nash, J.W., Hanson, L.A., St Syr Coats, K. (1995) Detection of bovine immunodeficiency virus in blood and milk derived leukocytes by use of polymerase chain reaction. Am J Vet Res. 56: 445-449.

31. Nikbakht Borujeni, G., Taghi Poorbazargani, T., Nadin-Davis, S., Tolooie, M., Barjesteh, N. (2010) Bovine immunodeficiency virus and bovine leukemia virus and their mixed infection in Iranian Holstein cattle. J Infect Dev

Ctries. 9: 576-579.

32. Orr, K.A., O´ Reilly, K.L., Scholl, D.T. (2003) Estimation of sensitivity and specificity of two diagnostics test for bovine immunodeficiency virus using Bayesian techniques. Prev Vet Med. 61: 79-89.

33. Polack, B., Schwartz, L., Berthelemy, M., Belloc, C., Manet, G., Vuillaume, A., Baron, T., Gonda, M.A., Levy, D. (1996) Serologic evidence for bovine immunodeficiency virus infection in France. Vet Microbiol. 48: 165-173.

34. Scobie, L., Venables, C., Hughes, K., Dawson, M., Jarret, O. (1999) The antibody response of cattle infected with Bovine Immunodeficiency Virus to peptides of the viral transmembrane protein. J Gen Virol. 80: 237-243.

35. Snider, T.G., Hoyt, P.G., Coats, K.S., Graves, K.F., Cooper, R.R., Stors, R.W., Luther, D.G., Jenny, B.F. (2002) Natural bovine lentiviral type 1 infection in Holstein dairy cattle. I. Clinical serological and pathological observations. Comp Immunol Microbiol Infect Dis. 26: 89-101.

36. Snider, T.G., Luther, D.G., Jenny, B.F., Hoyt, P.G., Battles, J.K., Ennis, W.H., Balady, J., BLAS-Machado, U., Lemarchand, T.X., Gonda, M.A. (1996) Encephalitis, Lymphoid tissue depletion and secondary diseases associated with bovine immunodeficiency virus in a dairy herd. Comp Immunol Microbiol Infect Dis. 19: 117-131.

37. Suarez, D.L., Van Der Maaten, J., Whettone, C.A. (1995) Improved early and long-term detection of bovine lentivirus by a nested polymerase chain reaction test in experimentally infected calves. Am J Vet Res. 56: 579-586.

38. Suarez, D.L., Van Der Maaten, M.J., Wood, C., Whetstone, C.A. (1993) Isolation and characterization of new wild-type isolates of bovine lentivirus. J Virol. 67: 5051-5055.

39. Tajbakhsh, E., Nikbakht Borujeni, G., Momtazan, H., Amirmozafari, N. (2010) Molecular prevalence for bovine immunodeficiency virus infection in Iranian cattle population. Afr J Microbiol Res. 12: 1199-1202.

40. Tobin, G.J., Ennis, W.H., Clanton, D.J., Gonda, M.A. (1996) Inhibition of bovine immunodeficiency virus by anti-HIV-1 compounds in a cell culture-based assay. Antiviral Res. 33: 21-31.

41. Usui, T., Meas, S., Konnai, S., Ohashi, K., Onuma, M. (2003) Seroprevalence of bovine immunodeficiency virus and bovine leukemia virus in dairy and beef cattle in Hokkaido. J Vet Med Sci. 65: 287-289.

42. Van Der Maaten, M.J., Boothe, A.D., Seger, C.L. (1972) Isolation of a virus from cattle with persistent lymphocytosis. J Natl Med Assoc. 49: 1649-1657.

14

Molecular characterization of recent Iranian infectious bronchitis virus isolates based on S2 protein gene

Nazemi, K.[1], Ghalyanchi Langeroudi, A.[1*], Hashemzadeh, M.[2], Karimi, V.[3], Seger, W.[1,4], Ehsan, M.R.[1]

[1]Department of Microbiology and Immunology, Faculty of Veterinary Medicine, University of Tehran, Tehran, Iran

[2]Department of Research and Production of Poultry Viral Vaccine, Razi Vaccine and Serum Research Institute, Karaj, Iran

[3]Department of Avian Medicine, Faculty of Veterinary Medicine, University of Tehran, Tehran, Iran

[4]Department of Pathology and Poultry Diseases, Faculty of Veterinary Medicine, University of Basra, Basra, Iraq

Key words:

characterization, infectious bronchitis virus, genotyping, phylogenetic study, spike

Correspondence

Ghalyanchilangeroudi, A. Department of Microbiology and Immunology, Faculty of Veterinary Medicine, University of Tehran, Tehran, Iran

Email: ghalyana@ut.ac.ir

Abstract:

BACKGROUND: Avian infectious bronchitis (IB), with avian infectious bronchitis virus (IBV) as the causing agent, is a ubiquitous endemic disease of the chicken with devastating effects on its industry. A viral membrane surface protein called S not only induces neutralizing antibodies but also plays an important role in virus binding and entry to host cells. Technically, S1 protein gene sequencing also helps greatly in IBV genotyping. **OBJECTIVES:** The aim of this study was to characterize Iranian IBV based on S2 gene. **METHODS:** After RT-PCR amplification, the S2 gene of nine Iranian IBV isolates were sequenced and then compared with reference strains. **RESULTS:** The isolates were classified into genotype I as Massachusetts like IB Vs, genotype VII which clustered into two branches, VIIa (IS-1494 like IB viruses), and VIIb, and was related to QX- like viruses and Genotype VIII as 793/B like IBVs. **CONCLUSIONS:** As far as we know, this is the first S2-based classification study on Iranian IBV isolates providing a firm experimental basis to correlate with genotypic characterization.

Introduction

Infectious bronchitis (IB) is a ubiquitous and highly contagious disease of chickens caused by Infectious Bronchitis Virus (IBV). IBV is a member of genus Gammacoronavirus, subfamily Coronavirinae, family Coronaviridae, order Nidovirales with a single-stranded positive sense RNA genome, 27.6 kb (Jackwood, 2012). By infecting the respiratory tract, kidneys and oviduct, the virus results in reduced performance and egg quality and quantity while predisposing the chickens to other pathogens (Mo, et al., 2013). The viral genome encodes proteins including the viral RNA-dependent RNA-polymerase (RdRp), envelope (E), membrane (M), nucleocapsid (N) and structural proteins spike (S) (Jackwood, 2012). The latter, also called surface glycoprotein (S), is located on the surface of the viral membrane and is a major inducer of neutralizing antibodies while playing a vital role in virus binding and entry to host cells. It is cleaved into two subunits, amino-terminal S1 (92 kDa, ~535 amino acids) and the carboxyl-terminal S2 (84 kDa, ~627 amino acids) post-translationally. The S1 subunit forms the distal and bulbous part of the spike whereas the S2 sub unit anchors S1 to the viral membrane. The antigenic region of the S2 subunit has been proposed to play a role in protection (Mo, et al., 2013). This subunit also has a fusion peptide-like region and two heptade regions, approximately 100 to 130 Å in length (771-879 amino acid in IBV), involved in oligomerization of the protein and entry into susceptible host cells (Abro, 2012). More studies should be performed on this subunit though the S1 subunit has been examined extensively. Apparently based on the highly conservative nature of the S2 subunit among different members of the Coronavirus genus and different strains of IBV, it plays a little or no role in inducing a host immune response. Mostly, the molecular studies aimed to detect IBV genotypes were based on S1 glycoprotein. On the other hand, the S2 subunit possibly induces serotype-specific neutralizing antibodies while it is conserved within a serotype but not between serotypes (Ammayappan & Vakharia, 2009; Scott Andrew Callison, Mark W Jackwood, & Deborah Ann Hilt, 1999).

The first report of IBV isolation from Iranian chicken flocks goes back to 1994 (Seyfi Abad Shapouri, Mayahi, Assasi, & Charkhkar, 2004). Based on analyzing mainly hypervariable regions of the S1 glycoprotein gene, Genotyping of IBV strains isolated in Iran were classified into seven distinct phylogenetic groups as Mass, 793/B like, IS/1494 like, IS/720-like, QX-like, IR-1, and IR-2 (Hosseini, Bozorgmehri Fard, Charkhkar, & Morshed, 2015; Najafi, et al.,2015). At present, different vaccines for Massachusetts and 793/B types are administered in Iranian poultry industry. Nevertheless, IB outbreaks are still present. However, genotyping of Iranian IBV isolates based on sequence analysis of the S2 protein gene have not been performed, hence, the aim of this study was to understand genotype identification of the S2 gene of IBVs isolated in Iran by sequencing and phylogenetic analysis.

Materials and Methods

Samples: Nine Iranian IBV isolates with different genotypes were studied in this paper. The isolates information including the type of flock, specimens, and S1 gene-based genotypes were indicated in Table 1; the broiler chickens have shown respiratory manifestations, nephritis and mortalities .The surveillance was done from 2014 to 2015.

RNA extraction and cDNA synthesis: The total RNA of viruses was extracted using Cinna Pure RNA extraction kit (Sinaclon, Iran) and then stored at -70°C until further use. The extracted RNA was used in reverse transcription (RT) reaction to generate cDNA using Revert Aid Reverse Transcriptase (Thermo Scientific, Canada), Ribolock Rnase inhibitor (Thermo Scientific, Canada), dNTP mix (Sinaclon , Iran), and DEPC-treated water (Sinaclon, Iran). For cDNA synthesis, 5 μL of the extracted RNA was mixed with 1 μL of random hexamer primer and incubated at 65°C for 5 min, followed by addition of 14 μL of master mix (7.25 μL distilled water, 4 μL buffer 5X, 2 μL dNTP mix, and 0.5 μL RT enzyme) to make the final volume 20 μL. Then, the mixture was incubated at 25°C for 5 min, 42°C for 60 min, 95°C for 5 min, and 4°C

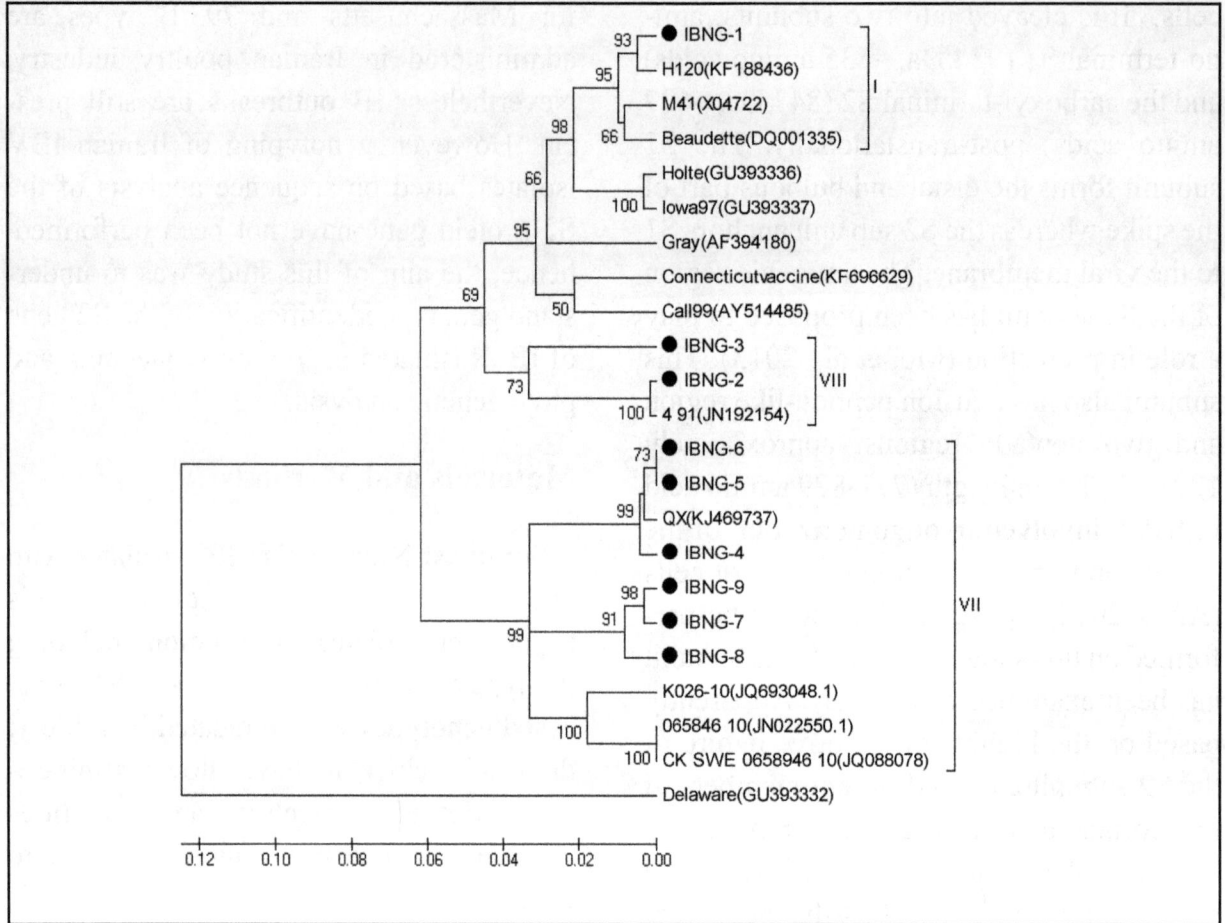

Figure 1. Phylogenetic tree based on amino acid of S2 gene of IBVs, black circles: nine Iranian strains among other reference strains; The phylogenetic tree was constructed with the MEGA version 5.0 using the neighbor-joining method with bootstrap replicates (bootstrap 1,000 values as shown on the tree). The branch number represents the percentage of the branch showing up in the tree. Bootstrap values greater than 50% are shown.

Table 1. IBV strains used in this study.

Name	Chicken species	Organ	Genotypes based on S1 gene
IBNG-1	Broiler	Trachea	Massachusetts
IBNG-2	Broiler	Trachea	793/B
IBNG-3	Broiler	Kidney	793/B
IBNG-4	Broiler	Trachea	QX
IBNG-5	Broiler	Kidney	QX
IBNG-6	Broiler	Trachea	QX
IBNG-7	Broiler	Kidney	IS-1494 like (Var-2)
IBNG-8	Broiler	Trachea	IS-1494 like (Var-2)
IBNG-9	Broiler	Kidney	IS-1494 like (Var-2)

for 1 min.

PCR for amplification of partial segment of S2 gene: PCR was performed to amplify the S2 gene using the primer pairs as forward primer S2F2, 5" GCTG-CGTCRTTTAATAAGGCCAT 3" (22756-

22778 according to Beaudette CK strain) and reverse primer S2R2, 5" CTAGGCTG-CCACAACAATAAC 3" (23752 - 23732) (PCR length : 997 pb). The reaction mix was prepared in a volume of 20μL with 3μL of cDNA, 13μL of master mix (Sinaclon, Iran),

1μl of each primer. The PCR reaction was carried out under the following conditions in a thermal cycler (Eppendorf, Germany): 35 cycles of 95°C for 3 min, denaturation 95 °C for 30 Sec, Annealing at 58°C for 30 Sec. Extension 72 °C for 60 Sec. The expected amplified fragment of PCR product is one Kb. The RT-PCR products were visualized by electrophoresis of 5 μl of each product in a 1% agarose gel, containing red safe stain, followed by UV trans illumination.

Phylogenetic analysis: The AccuPrep® PCR Purification Kit (Bioneer Co., Korea) was used for purification of the PCR products. Sequencing was performed with the same primers used in the PCR (Bioneer Co., Korea). Then, chromatograms were evaluated with CromasPro (CromasPro Version 1.5) and the multiple alignments of S2 nucleotide was achieved using Clustal W using the MEGA 5.1 software. The phylogenetic tree was constructed by using the same software with the neighbor-joining method and each tree was produced using a consensus of 1000 bootstrap replicates (Tamura, et al., 2011). The amino acid sequences of the S2 gene were compared with several S2 sequences from Gene bank including H120(KF188436), 4/91(JN19215.4) ,M41(X04722), Beaudette (DQ001335), Iowa97 (GU 393337), Holte (Gu39336), Gray (AF394180), Call99 (AY514485), QX (KJ469737) and Delaware (GU393332).

Results

Obtained Amino acid sequences of S2 gene of nine IBV isolates were aligned and compared with the reference strains from GenBank and available from the national center for biotechnology information (NCBI). Phylogenetic analysis based on the S2 gene showed that the Iranian IBV isolates were grouped into three distinct clusters I, VII & VIII. Group I (IBNG-1) closely related to Massachusetts viruses, Group VII, related to QX IBV isolate, clustered into two sub-clusters including VIIa containing IBNG-4, IBNG-5 and IBNG-6 (Variant 2 like virus) and second sub cluster VII b containing IBNG-7, IBNG- 8 and IBNG-5, and finally group VIII (IBNG-2 & IBNG-3) which were in the same cluster with 793/B viruses (Fig. 1). The amino acid identity within groups VIII and VII was 90.21% and 93.81%-100%, respectively. On the other hand, the amino acid identity between group I and group VIII was 88.19% while it was 85% between group VII and group VIII. In the case of vaccine strains, the identity level of group I with H120, M41, and Beaudette was 99.35%, 98.58%, and 98.36% respectively. Meanwhile, sequence identity between group VIII and 4/91(JN192154) and between group VII and QX (KJ1469737) was also 99.39%-99.89 % and approximately 99%, respectively.

Discussion

The infectious bronchitis virus (IBV) causes huge losses in the poultry industry. In the S2 subunit, regions of sequence variation were found interspaced with regions of high conservation causing the overall diversity of the S gene. Genotyping is often the preferred serotyping method due to its convenience and time-saving aspects compared with virus neutralization (VN) or other traditional serotyping tests (Lee, Hilt, & Jackwood, 2003). Playing a role in many biofunctions such as cell receptor's attachment and tissue tropism together with inducing IBV neutralizing antibodies makes

S1 gene the principal method to study the genetic diversity of infectious bronchitis virus. Meanwhile, S2 gene does not have any major antigenic sites. However, it was considered to be associated with antigenicity, which is affected by its conformation. This makes the analysis of the S2 gene critical to further determine the antigenicity of isolates , which might be diverse among IBV strains because of some recombination events between the virus strains classified into different genetic groups (Callison, et al., 1999). IBV in Iranian chicken flocks was first isolated by Aghakhan et al (1994) (Aghakhan, Abshar, Fereidouni, Marunesi, & Khodashenas, 1994) and found to belong to Massachusetts serotype. Hosseini et al. isolated Iran/QX/H179/11 strain in 2011 followed by Iran/QX/H255/12, Iran/QX/ H281/12, and Iran/QX/H284/12 strains in 2012 in Iran. QX-type isolates of the current study showed more than 96% homology with these Iranian strains (Bozorgmehri-Fard, Charkhkar, & Hosseini, 2014). Also, the presence of two variant viruses (IS/1494/06 like) in Iranian commercial flocks has been demonstrated in another study (Hosseini, et al., 2015). Based on phylogenetic analysis of the S1 glycoprotein gene,   six distinct phylogenetic groups as IS/1494/06 [Var2] like, 4/91-like, IS /720-like, QX-like and IR-1 and Mass-like were described recently (Najafi, Madadgar, Jamshidi, Langeroudi, & Lemraski, 2014). In case of Phylogenetic analysis based on S2 gene, the current study's IBV strains could be classified into three genetic groups: genotypes I (Massachusetts like), VII (QX & IS 1494 like) & VIII (793/B like). The present study was partially consistent with Mase et al (2008) who developed a grouping method of IBV based on the S2 glycoprotein gene and di-

vided IBV genotypes into eight clusters. The strains belonged to the Massachusetts, Gray and Connecticut types were classified into group I, II and III, respectively while those belonging to the foreign Iowa-609 type were classified as group IV and Group V consisted of Japanese strains, including the C-78 vaccine strain, only. It is necessary to mention that Group VI also mainly consisted of Japanese strains, including the comparatively newly established vaccine strains, the Miyazaki, TM86 and GN strains. Since viruses belonging to groups VII or VIII were of strains isolated after 2000, they were not used in the previous study (Mase, Inoue, Yamaguchi, & Imada, 2009). Zulperi et al studied the phylogenetic analysis and sequencing of both S1 and S2 genes of Malaysian IBV strains concluding that even with only 77% identity, MH5365/95 and V9/04 belong to non-Massachusetts strain. The S2 gene-based phylogenetic tree analysis of the study also indicated that both MH5365/95 and V9/04 isolates grouped together in a separate sub-cluster (Zulperi, Omar, & Arshad, 2009). Though showing sequence variability among different strains of IBV, which generally differ by less than 10%, Callison et al concluded S2 gene sequence is more conserved than that of the S1 gene and in fact, the serotypes were grouped based on S2 gene sequence (Callison, Jackwood, & Hilt, 1999). The diversity of the N-terminal region of the S2 gene of IBV in Iran was revealed in this study confirming the applicability of this region for IBV strain grouping. While some studies reported Iranian IBV genotyping based on S1 gene, this study highlighted the first time use of S2 gene-based IBV genotyping in Iran as far as we know. There are different reports around Iranian IBV genotyping based S1 gene. Our findings have highlighted for the first time IBV genotyping based on the S2 gene in Iran. More studies should be performed with a full-length sequence of S2 gene while genotyping the S2 gene on more IBV isolates.

Acknowledgments

This study was conducted under grant of the research council, University of Tehran (No. 28692/6/4). In addition, Iranian veterinary organization under grant (No. 22/39007) financially supported this project. The authors gratefully acknowledge Dr. Hamideh Najafi, Mr.Behrooz Asadi and Mr. Ahmad Vahedi for their extensive technical supports.

References

1. Abro, S.H. (2012) Molecular characterization and detection of infectious bronchitis virus.Vet Microbiol. 155: 237-246.

2. Aghakhan, S., Abshar, N., Fereidouni, S.R.N., Marunesi, C., Khodashenas, M. (1994) Studies on avian viral infections in Iran. Arch Inst Razi. 44: 1-10.

3. Ammayappan, A., Vakharia, V.N. (2009) Complete nucleotide analysis of the structural genome of the infectious bronchitis virus strain md27 reveals its mosaic nature. Viruses. 1: 1166-1177.

4. Bozorgmehri-Fard, M., Charkhkar, S., Hosseini, H. (2014) Detection of the chinese genotype of infectious bronchitis virus (QX-type) in Iran. Iran J Virol. 7: 21-24.

5. Callison, S.A., Jackwood, M.W., Hilt, D.A. (1999) Infectious bronchitis virus S2 gene sequence variability may affect S1 subunit specific antibody binding. Virus Genes. 19: 143-151.

6. Callison, S.A., Jackwood, M.W., Hilt, D.A. (1999) Infectious bronchitis virus S2 gene sequence variability may affect S1 subunit specific antibody binding. Virus Genes. 19: 143-151.

7. Hosseini, H., Bozorgmehri Fard, M.H., Charkhkar, S., Morshed, R. (2015) Epidemiology of avian infectious bronchitis virus genotypes in Iran (2010-2014). Avi Dis. 59: 431-5.

8. Jackwood, M. W. (2012) Review of infectious bronchitis virus around the world. Avian Dis. 56: 634-641.

9. Lee, C.-W., Hilt, D. A., Jackwood, M.W. (2003) Typing of field isolates of infectious bronchitis virus based on the sequence of the hypervariable region in the S1 gene. J Vet Diagn Invest. 15: 344-348.

10. Mase, M., Inoue, T., Yamaguchi, S., Imada, T. (2009) Genetic diversity of avian infectious bronchitis viruses in Japan based on analysis of s2 glycoprotein gene. J Vet Med Sci. 71: 287-291.

11. Mo, M.-L., Hong, S.-M., Kwon, H.-J., Kim, I.-H., Song, C.-S., Kim, J.-H. (2013) Genetic diversity of spike, 3a, 3b and e genes of infectious bronchitis viruses and emergence of new recombinants in Korea. Viruses, 5, 550-567.

12. Najafi, H., Langeroudi, A.G., Hashemzadeh, M., Karimi, V., Madadgar, O., Ghafouri, S.A., Maghsoudlo, H., Farahani, R.K. Molecular characterization of infectious bronchitis viruses isolated from broiler chicken farms in Iran, 2014-2015. Arch Virol. 161: 1-10.

13. Najafi, H., Madadgar, O., Jamshidi, S., Langeroudi, A.G., Lemraski, M.D. (2014) Molecular and clinical study on prevalence of feline herpesvirus type 1 and calicivirus in correlation with feline leukemia and immunodeficiency viruses. In: Vet Res Forum (Vol. 5, pp. 255): Faculty of Veterinary Med-

icine, Urmia University, Urmia, Iran.

14. Seyfi Abad Shapouri, M., Mayahi, M., Assasi, K., Charkhkar, S. (2004) A survey of the prevalence of infectious bronchitis virus type 4/91 in Iran. Acta Vet Hung. 52: 163-166.

15. Tamura, K., Peterson, D., Peterson, N., Stecher, G., Nei, M., Kumar, S. (2011) MEGA5: molecular evolutionary genetics analysis using maximum likelihood, evolutionary distance, and maximum parsimony methods. Mol Biol Evol. 28: 2731-2739.

16. Zulperi, Z.M., Omar, A.R., Arshad, S.S. (2009) Sequence and phylogenetic analysis of S1, S2, M, and N genes of infectious bronchitis virus isolates from Malaysia. Virus Genes. 38: 383-391.

15

Detection of chlamydial infection in Iranian turkey flocks

Tatari, Z., Peighamabri, S.M.*, Madani, S.A.

Department of Avian Diseases, Faculty of Veterinary Medicine, University of Tehran, Tehran, Iran

Key words:

Chlamydia psittaci, nested PCR, real-time PCR, turkey

Correspondence

Peighamabri, S.M.
Department of Avian Diseases,
Faculty of Veterinary Medicine,
University of Tehran, Tehran,
Iran

Email: mpeigham@ut.ac.ir

Abstract:

BACKGROUND: Avian chlamydiosis is a zoonotic disease of birds caused by the intracellular bacterium *Chlamydia psittaci*. Avian chlamydiosis leads to severe respiratory disease in young turkeys and egg production losses in layers. **OBJECTIVES:** Due to paucity of information about the prevalence of chlamydial infection in the turkey population in Iran, this study was conducted to detect chlamydial infection in some Iranian turkey flocks in different provinces. **METHODS:** A total of 177 samples were taken from turkeys and first verified as *Chlamydiaceae* by *Chlamydiaceae*-specific real-time polymerase chain reaction (real-time PCR) by detection of the 23S RNA gene of *Chlamydiaceae* (Ct values ranging from 34 to 38) and then positive samples were investigated for the presence of *C. psittaci* by a nested PCR. **RESULTS:** Seventeen of 177 samples (9.6%), corresponding to 13 farms of 48 examined farms were positive for *Chlamydiaceae* by real-time PCR. None of the positive samples were found to be *C. psittaci* in the nested PCR. **CONCLUSIONS:** This study showed no *C. psittaci* infection in the turkey population in Iran. We recommend investigation on other farm animals and wild populations for possible chlamydial infection and for better understanding of the source and epidemiology of this agent. Due to the challenges that exist for sampling and the relevant impact on reducing positive samples, investigation by parallel and complementary techniques may be useful in showing the true prevalence of infection in the target populations.

Introduction

Chlamydial infections leading to outbreaks of avian chlamydiosis in domestic, companion and wild birds are regularly reported from all parts of the world (Gade et al., 2008; Laroucau et al., 2009a; Sachse et al., 2012; Zocevic et al., 2012, Madani and Peighambari, 2013). The general importance of avian chlamydiosis includes both economic losses to the bird owners and potential zoonotic transmission to humans (Vanrompay et al., 2007; Laroucau et al., 2009a). The family *Chlamydiaceae* currently includes only the genus Chlamydia,

from which nine species including *abortus*, *caviae*, *felis*, *muridarum*, *pecorum*, *pneumoniae*, *psittaci*, *suis* and *trachomatis* have been identified (Kuo et al., 2010).

Recent investigations have provided evidence of the occurrence of chlamydial species other than *Chlamydia psittaci* (*C. psittaci*) in birds (Herrmann et al., 2000; Chahota et al., 2006; Pantchev et al., 2009; Lemus et al., 2010; Sachse et al., 2012). Moreover, atypical strains of *Chlamydiaceae* were recently detected in chickens (Gaede et al., 2008; Laroucau et al., 2009a; Zocevic et al., 2012), pigeons (Gasparini et al., 2011; Sachse et al.,

2012), gulls (Christerson et al., 2010) and wild birds (Madani and Peighambari, 2013).

The clinical feature depends on the chlamydial strains and avian host (Andersen and Vanrompay, 2000). Transmission of *C. psittaci* predominantly occurs through inhalation of contaminated material and sometimes through ingestion, from an infected bird to a susceptible bird. Humans can become infected by inhaling an organism shed by infected birds, mouth-to-beak contact or by handling the plumage and tissues of infected birds. Human infections are common following handling or processing of infected turkeys or ducks (Laroucau et al., 2009b). The disease in humans contracted from turkeys is often more severe than that contracted from psittacine birds (Andersen and Vanrompay, 2000).

Diagnosis of chlamydial infection in birds is still a considerable challenge. Clinical changes are not pathognomonical and persistent infections can also occur. The infection can therefore only be confirmed by direct identification of the agent or indirectly by detection of specific antibodies. PCR is currently the method of choice for diagnosis of chlamydial infection. Specific and sensitive PCR methods targeting the 23S rRNA gene that allows the detection of *Chlamydiaceae* and identification of Chlamydia species have been developed (Everett et al., 1999; DeGraves et al., 2003; Ehricht et al., 2006). Analysis of the gene encoding outer membrane protein A (ompA) is most often used to study avian *C. psittaci* strains into genotypes (Sachse et al., 2008). Nine genotypes of *C. psittaci* are currently accepted (A-F, E/B, WC and M56) (Geens et al., 2005a; Geens et al., 2005b; Sachse et al., 2008).

Previous research in Iran avian/poultry population showed 12.6% *Chlamydia psittaci* infection in companion and wild birds (Madani et al., 2011) and 14.3% in Pigeons (Doosti and Arshi, 2011). At present, little is known about the prevalence of chlamydial infection in the turkey population, especially in Iran. This study was, therefore, conducted to detect chlamydial infection in Iranian turkey population by real-time PCR. Samples were first verified as *Chlamydiaceae* and then were investigated for the presence of *C. psittaci*.

Materials and Methods

Samples: During 2013-2014, a total of 177 samples were collected from turkey flocks located in the provinces of Ardabil, Ghazvin, Ghom, Gilan, Golestan, Hamedan, Isfahan, Lorestan, Mazandaran and Tehran. In total, 48 farms were sampled, from which 11 farms showed clinical signs including nasal discharge, sinusitis, conjunctivitis and diarrhea. Thirty samples were also collected from free range turkeys in Golestan province and cases referred to a private poultry clinic in Tehran (Table 1).

A single sterile cotton-tipped swab was used to take triple samples from the conjunctiva, choanal cleft and cloaca of each individual randomly selected turkey in the flock. Twenty triple sample swabs were collected from each flock, then each five swabs from the same flock were pooled to form a single sample. Tissue samples including air sac exudates, lungs, spleens and livers were collected in Najafabad abattoir (Isfahan province) and from cases referred to a poultry clinic in Tehran. Tissue samples from each bird were considered as a single sample. Swab samples were placed in plastic bags or in SPG (Sucrose Phosphate Glutamate) transport media (Madani and Peighambari, 2013) and transported to the laboratory in cold condition and preserved at -20° C until further use.

DNA extraction and Real-time PCR assay for Chlamydiceae: Template DNA was extracted and prepared using the High Pure PCR Preparation kit (Roche Applied Science, Mannheim, Germany) as instructed by the manufacturer.

A *Chlamydiaceae* family-specific real-time

PCR based on partial replication of the 23S gene and yielding a 111 base pairs (bp) fragment was used (Ehricht et al., 2006). The forward Ch23S-F (5′-CTGAAACCAGTAGCT-TATAAGCGGT-3′) and reverse Ch23S-R (5′-ACCTCGCCGTTTAACTTAACTCC-3′) primers, and the probe Ch23S-p (FAMCT-CATCATGCAAAAGGCACGCCG-TAMRA) used for the amplification process were synthetized by Metabion International AG (Martinsried, Germany). Real-time PCR reactions were run in a Rotor-Gene Q (QIAGEN Marseille S.A.) instrument. Each reaction mixture contained 2 µl sample DNA template, 10 µl of qPCR Probes MasterMix 2X (Jena Bioscience GmbH, Germany), 0.5 µl of each primer (25 mM), 2 µl of the probe (1 mM), and 5 µl deionized water. The cycling profile was included and initial denaturation at 95°C for 10 min followed by 45 cycles of denaturation at 94°C for 15s and 60°C for 60s. A cycle threshold (Ct value) of <38.00 was considered as positive. The positive control DNA templates were provided from previous works in our laboratory (Madani and Peighambari, 2013). Sterile dH2O was also used as negative control. All samples were tested at least in duplicate.

OmpA nested PCR: All specimens that were positive in real-time PCR and positive control DNA were subjected to ompA nested PCR amplification for the detection of *C. psittaci* as described by Sachse and Hotzel (2003). The degenerate nested primers 191CHOMP (5′-GCIYTITGGGARTGYGGITGYGCI AC-3′) and CHOMP371 (5′-TTAGAAICK-GAATTGIGCRTTIAYGTGIGCIGC-3′) for the identification of the genus *Chlamydia* spp. were synthesized by Metabion International AG (Martinsried, Germany). A 50 µl reaction mixture was prepared with 1 µl dNTP (10 mM), 1 µl of each primer (20 pmol/µl), 1.5 µl MgCl2 (50 mM), 5 µl 10X PCR Buffer, 0.2 µl SmarTaq™ DNA Polymerase, 5 µl DNA and 35.3 µl dH2O. Amplification was programmed in a thermocycler (Gradient Mastercycler, Ep-

pendorff, Germany) as follows: an initial denaturation at 95°C for 30 s, followed by 35 cycles of denaturation (95°C for 30 s), alignment (50°C for 30 s), extension (72°C for 30 s), and a final extension at 72°C for 2 min. PCR products were visualized by agarose gel electrophoresis (1%) in TBE (Tris Base, boric acid, EDTA, pH8, 0.5 M), stained with RedSafe™ (iNtRON, South Korea). GeneRULER™ 100 bp Plus DNA Ladder (Fermentas, Germany) was used as marker on each gel running. This step provided amplicon with weights 576-597 bp. All amplification products were subjected to a second PCR to identify *C. psittaci* using the primers 218PSITT (5′-GTA-ATTTCIAGCCCAGCACAATTYGTG-3′) and CHOMP336s (5′-CCRCAAGMTTTTC-TRGAYTTCAWYTTGTTRAT-3′) in a reaction with proportions of reactants as described above but varying the amounts of $MgCl_2$ (2 µl), distilled water (38.8 µl) and DNA (1 µl). Amplification conditions, programmed in Gradient Mastercycler (Eppendorff) were as follows: 95°C for 30 s followed by 20 cycles of 95°C for 30 s, 60°C for 30 s, 72°C for 30 s, and 72°C for 2 min. The second PCR products were visualized by agarose gel electrophoresis as described above. Samples that showed bands with weights 389-404 bp were considered positive. DNA of *C. psittaci* which was extracted from the liver of a Chlamydia positive African grey parrot, taken at the Dutch Research Institute for Birds and Exotic Animals in the Netherlands (NOIVBD), was used as positive control; water was used as negative control. All PCR materials including SmarTaq™ DNA polymerase, $MgCl_2$, PCR buffer and dNTPs were purchased from Cinnagen (Tehran, Iran).

Results

Seventeen of 177 samples (9.6%), corresponding to 13 farms of 48 examined farms (Table 2) were positive for *Chlamydiaceae* by real-time PCR, i.e. the 23S RNA gene of

Table 1. The total number of examined birds and type of samples.

Sample type	No. of pooled samples/Farms	No. of samples used for pooling
Triple swab transported in dry condition	61/15	5
Triple swab in SPG transport medium	44/11	5
Tissue samples	72/22	1
Total	177/48	

Table 2. Detailed results obtained in real-time PCR assay.

Sample type (no.)	Age (Day)	Farm	Real-Time PCR		No. of positive samples in nested PCR total
			No. of positive samples in total tested	Ø Ct value	
Tissue samples (7)	56	A	7/72	36	0/7
	112	B			
	45	C			
	72	D			
	72	D			
	32	E			
	18	F			
Triple swab transported in dry condition (3)	100	G	3/61	37.44	0/3
	82	H			
	40	I			
Triple swab in SPG transport medium (7)	50	J	7/44	35.50	0/7
	50	J			
	60	K			
	160	L			
	160	L			
	65	M			
	160	Z			

Chlamydiaceae was detected (Ct values ranging from 34 to 38) (Fig. 1). None of the positive samples were found to be *C. psittaci* in the nested PCR (Fig. 2). Samples from free range turkeys in Golestan province were also negative.

Discussion

Chlamydia psittaci is a very important bacterial pathogen in veterinary and human medicine (Andersen and Vanrompay, 2000). In turkeys, *C. psittaci* causes infections of the respiratory tract followed by septicemia and localization in epithelial cells and macrophages in various organs (Vanrompay et al., 1995a). Nowadays, the increase in confinement-rearing of turkeys and the prevention of wild birds flying in and out the turkey houses seems to contribute to a decrease of severe outbreaks (van Loock et al., 2005). Since little is known about the prevalence of chlamydial infection in the turkey population of Iran, this study was designed to detect chlamydial infection in some Iranian turkey farms, for the first time in Iran, by molecular methods.

In this study, 177 sample were sampled in order to detect chlamydial infections by real-time PCR assay. Triple sample swabs were taken from each bird, as infected birds can

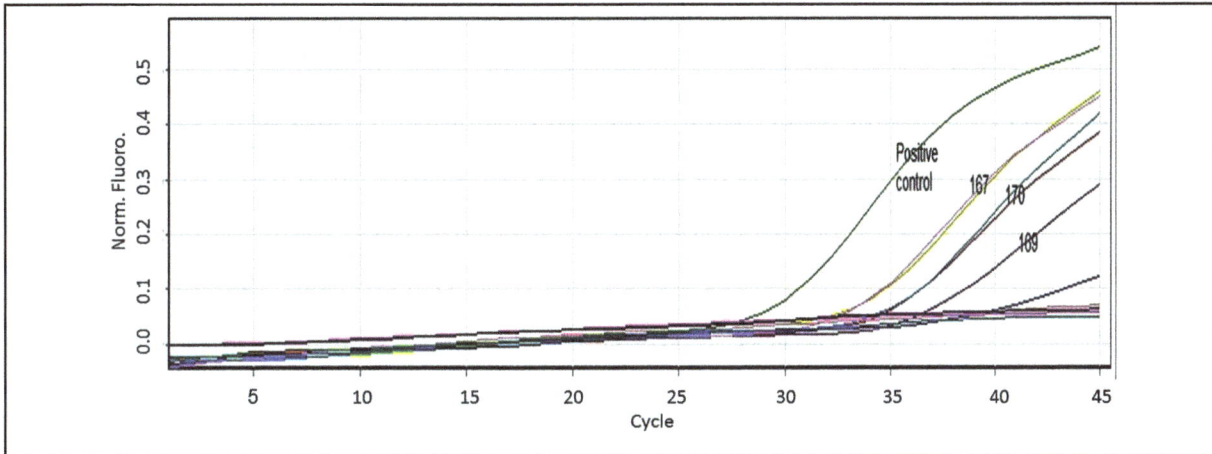

Figure 1. Curve of three positive samples in real-time PCR for 23S gene of *Chlamydiaceae*.

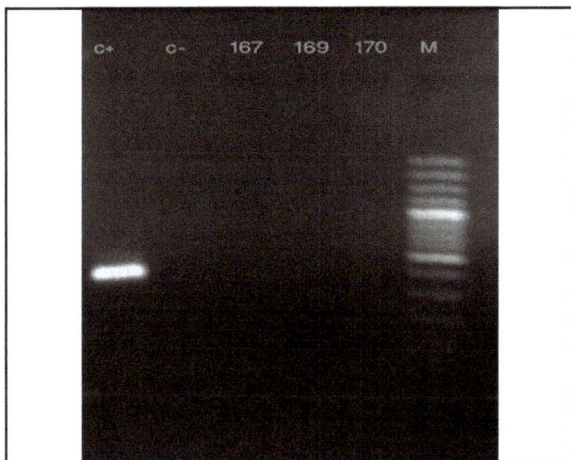

Figure 2. Gel electrophoresis of three nested-PCR amplified products previously. found as positive in real-time PCR for 23S gene of *Chlamydiaceae*. M = Molecular. weight marker (GeneRULERTM 100 bp Plus DNA Ladder, Fermentas, Germany), C+ = Positive control, C-= Negative control.

shed Chlamydiae through respiratory tract excretions and in feces (Andersen and Vanrompay, 2000; Harkinezhad et al., 2009). Seventeen out of 177 samples (9.6%), corresponding to 13 out of 48 sampled farms were positive for *Chlamydiaceae* by real-time PCR. Among the farms that were sampled in our study, 11 out of 48 (22%) farms showed clinical signs, while the others were apparently healthy.

There was considerable difference between our findings and those of others on prevalence of *C. psittaci* infection in turkey. There may be some reasons that have influenced our results. Sampling may have occurred at the times that birds had stopped shedding, as the shedding of *C. psittaci* occurs intermittently and healthy

carrier birds might not excrete bacteria for extended periods (Vanrompay et al., 1995b). Most of the sampled turkeys were clinically healthy birds; therefore, the amount of chlamydial DNA in the swabs was probably lower than required for the test. Antibacterial agents can stop shedding of Chlamydiae and Chlamydia availability (Billington, 2005). Antibiotics such as tetracyclines, macrolides, fluoroquinolones and chloramphenicol may interfere with diagnostic tests by reducing antibody production, antigen shedding, and Chlamydia viability (Krieg et al., 2010). In Iran, because of imprudent use of antibacterial agents in farms, it is really difficult to find and sample turkey flocks without previous background of antibacterial usage.

Surprisingly, none of the positive samples in real-time PCR were positive in the nested PCR. One reason for this may be that the amount of investigated DNA of *C. psittaci* was under the detection limit of our nested PCR method. Real-time PCR is one of the favored methods for the detection of DNA of *Chlamydiaceae* (Geens et al., 2005a; Ehricht et al., 2006; Pantchev et al., 2009). Nested PCR is usually a bit more sensitive, but vulnerable to DNA cross-contamination (Sachse and Hotzel, 2003). The second reason may be due to failures in ompA gene fragment amplification. This may occur because this gene is represented by a single copy per genome, unlike ribosomal RNA genes such as 23S gene that was amplified in real-time PCR (Arraiz et al., 2012). The third reason that can be speculated is the possible infection of our *Chlamydiaceae*-positive samples found in real-time PCR with a non-classified strain of *C. psittaci*. Non-classified strains that belong to another member of the Chlamydia genus are not amplified by the ompA nested PCR used in the present work. Based on systematic investigation on poultry samples submitted to laboratories for avian chlamydiosis diagnosis, Zocevic et al. (2012) confirmed that *C. psittaci* was not the predominant chlamydial species among chickens and suggested that the new chlamydial agents could putatively be widespread in poultry flocks in countries such as France, Greece, Croatia, Slovenia and China. However, Zocevic et al. (2013) suggested a limited dissemination of atypical strains compared to the usually higher prevalence of *C. psittaci* that is the main species associated with avian chlamydiosis in Parisian pigeon populations.

In conclusion, this study showed no *C. psittaci* infection in the turkey population in Iran. We recommend investigation on other farm animals and wild populations for possible chlamydial infection and for better understanding of the source and epidemiology of this agent. Due to the challenges that exist for sampling and the relevant impacts on reducing positive samples, investigation by parallel and complementary techniques such as cell culturing, serology and micro-array may be useful in showing the true prevalence of infection in the target population.

Acknowledgements

This study was funded by a research grant (no. 7508007/6/21) from the Research Council of the University of Tehran. We sincerely thank Dr. Kamyab, Dr. Yazdkhasti and Dr. Rezaeifar for their help in providing and collecting samples.

References

1. Andersen, A.A., Vanrompay, D. (2000) Avian chlamydiosis. In: Diseases of Poultry. Saif, Y.M., Barnes, H.J., Fadly, A.M., Glisson, J.R., McDougald, L.R., Swayne, D.E., (eds.). (11th ed.) Iowa State University Press. Ames, Iowa, USA. p. 863-879.

2. Arraiz, N., Bermudez, V., Urdaneta, B., Mujica, E., Sanchez, M.P., Mejía, R., Prieto, C., Escalona, C., Mujica, A. (2012) Evidence of zoonotic *Chlamydophila psittaci* transmission in a population at risk in Zulia state, Venezuela, Rev Salud Pública. 14: 305-314.

3. Billington, S. (2005) Clinical and zoonotic aspects of psittacosis. In Pract. 27: 256-263.

4. Chahota, R., Ogawa, H., Mitsuhashi, Y., Ohya, K., Yamaguchi, T., Fukushi, H. (2006) Genetic diversity and epizootiology of Chlamydophila prevalent among the captive and feral avian species based on VD2 region of ompA gene. Microbiol Immunol. 50: 663-678.

5. Christerson, L., Blomqvist, M., Grannas, K., Thollesson, M., Laroucau, K. Waldenstrom, J., Eliasson, I., Olsen, B., Herrmann, B. (2010) A novel *Chlamydiaceae*-like bacterium found in faecal specimens from sea birds from the Bering Sea. Environ Microbiol Rep. 2: 605-610.

6. DeGraves, F.J., Gao, D., Hehnen, H.R., Schlapp, T., Kaltenboeck, B. (2003) Quantitative detection of *Chlamydia psittaci* and *C. pecorum* by high-sensitivity real-time PCR reveals high prevalence of vaginal infection in cattle. J Clin Microbiol. 41: 1726-1729.

7. Doosti, A., Arshi, A. (2011) Determination of the Prevalence of *Chlamydia psittaci* by PCR in Iranian pigeons. Int J Biol. 3: 79-82.

8. Ehricht, R., Slickers, P., Goellner, S., Hotzel, H., Sachse, K. (2006) Optimized DNA microarray assay allows detection and genotyping of single PCR-amplifiable target copies. Mol Cell Prob. 20: 60-63.

9. Everett, K.D.E., Hornung, L.J., Andersen, A.A. (1999) Rapid detection of the *Chlamydiaceae* and other families in the order Chlamydiales: Three PCR tests. J Clin Microbiol. 37: 575-580.

10. Gaede, W., Reckling, K.F., Dresenkamp, B., Kenklies, S., Schubert, E., Noack, U., Irmscher, H.M., Ludwig, C., Hotzel, H., Sachse, K. (2008) *Chlamydophila psittaci* infections in humans during an outbreak of psittacosis from poultry in Germany. Zoonoses Pub Health. 55: 184-188.

11. Gasparini, J., Erin, N., Bertin, C., Jacquin, L., Vorimore, F., Frantz, A., Lenouvel, P., Laroucau, K. (2011) Impact of urban environment and host phenotype on the epidemiology of *Chlamydiaceae* in feral pigeons (Columbia livia). Environ Microbiol. 13: 3186-3193.

12. Geens, T., Desplanques, A., van Loock, M., Bönner, B.M., Kaleta, E.F. , Magnino, S., Andersen, A.A., Everett, K.D.E., Vanrompay, D. (2005a) Sequencing of the *Chlamydophila psittaci* ompA gene reveals a new genotype, E/B, and the need for a rapid discriminatory genotyping method. J Clin Microbiol. 43: 2456-2461.

13. Geens, T., Dewitte, A., Boon, N., Vanrompay, D. (2005b) Development of a *Chlamydophila psittaci* species specific and genotype-specific real-time PCR. Vet Res. 36: 787-97.

14. Harkinezhad, T., Geens, T., Vanrompay, D. (2009) *Chlamydophila psittaci* infections in birds: a review with emphasis on zoonotic consequences. Vet Microbiol. 135: 68-77.

15. Herrmann, B., Rubaiyat, R., Bergström, S., Bonnedahl, J., Olsen, B. (2000) Chlamydophila abortus in a brown skua (Catharacta antarctica lonnbergi) from a subantarctic island. Appl Environ Microbiol. 66: 3654-3656.

16. Krieg, N.R., Parte, A., Ludwig, W., Whitman, W.B., Hedlund, B.P., Paster, B.J., Staley, J.T., Ward, N., Brown, D. (2010) Bergey's Manual of Systematic Bacteriology. (2nd ed.) Vol. 4. Springer Verlag. New York, USA. p. 846.

17. Kuo, C., Stephens, R.S., Bavoil, P.M., Kaltenboeck, B. (2010) Chlamydia. In: Bergey's Manual Systematic Bacteriology. (2nd ed.) Vol. 4. Springer Verlag. New York, USA. p. 846.

18. Laroucau, K., Vorimore, F., Aaziz, R., Berndt, A., Schubert, E., Sachse, K. (2009a) Isolation of a new chlamydial agent from infected domestic poultry coincided with cases of atypical pneumonia among slaughterhouse workers in France. Infect Gen Evol. 9: 1240-1247.

19. Laroucau, K., de Barbeyrac, B., Vorimore, F., Clerc, M., Bertin, C., Harkinezhad, T., Verminnen, K., Obeniche, F., Capek, I., Bébéar, C., Vanrompay, D., Garin-Bastuji, B., Sachse, K. (2009b) Chlamydial infections in duck farms associated with human cases of psittacosis in France. Vet. Microbiol. 135: 82-89.

20. Lemus, J.A., Fargallo, J.A., Vergara, P., Parejo, D., Banda, E. (2010) Natural cross chlamydial infection between livestock and free-living bird species. PLoS ONE. 5: e13512.

21. Madani, S.A., Peighambari, S.M., Barin, A. (2011) Isolation of *Chlamydophila psittaci* from pet birds in Iran. Int J Vet Res. 5: 95-98.

22. Madani, S.A., Peighambari, S.M. (2013) PCR-based diagnosis, molecular characterization and detection of atypical strains of avian *Chlamydia psittaci* in companion and wild birds, Avian Pathol. 42: 38-44.

23. Pantchev, A., Sting, R., Bauerfeind, R., Tyczka, J., Sachse, K. (2009) New real-time PCR tests for species-specific detection of *Chlamydophila psittaci* and Chlamydophila abortus from tissue samples. Vet J. 181: 145-150.

24. Sachse, K., Hotzel, H. (2003) Detection and differentiation of Chlamydiae by Nested-PCR. In: PCR Detection of Microbial Pathogens (Methods in Molecular Biology). Sachse, K., Frey, J. (eds.) Totowa: Humana Press. p. 123-136.

25. Sachse, K., Kuehlewind, S., Ruettger, A., Schubert, E., Rohde, G. (2012) More than classical *Chlamydia psittaci* in urban pigeons. Vet Microbiol. 157: 476-480.

26. Sachse, K., Laroucau, K., Hotzel, H., Schubert, E., Ehricht, R., Slickers, P. (2008) Genotyping of *Chlamydophila psittaci* using a new DNA microarray assay based on sequence analysis of ompA genes. BMC Microbiol. 8: e63.

27. Vanrompay, D., Ducatelle, R., Haesebrouck, F. (1995a) *Chlamydia psittaci* infections: a review

with emphasis on avian chlamydiosis. Vet Microbiol. 45: 93-119.

28. Vanrompay, D., Harkinezhad, T., Van De Walle, M., Beeckman, D., van Droogenbroeck, C., Verminnen, K., Leten, R., Martel, A., Cauwerts, K. (2007) *Chlamydophila psittaci* transmission from pet birds to humans. Emerg Infect Dis. 13: 1108-1110.

29. Vanrompay, D., Mast, J., Ducatelle, R., Haesebrouck, F., Goddeeris, B. M. (1995b) *Chlamydia psittaci* infections in turkeys: pathogenesis of infections in avian serovar A, B and D. Vet Microbiol. 47: 245-256.

30. van Loock, M., Geens, T., De Smit, L., Nauwynck, H., van Empe, P., Naylor, C., Hafez, H.M., Goddeeris, B.M., Vanrompay, D. (2005) Key role of *Chlamydophila psittaci* on Belgian turkey farms in association with other respiratory pathogens. Vet Microbiol. 107: 91-101.

31. Zocevic, A., Vorimore, F., Marhold, C., Horvatek, D., Wang, D., Slavec, B., Prentza, Z., Stavianis, G., Prukner-Radovcic, E., Dovc, A., Siarkou, V.I., Laroucau, K. (2012) Molecular characterization of atypical Chlamydia and evidence of their dissemination in different European and Asian chicken flocks by specific real-time PCR. Environ Microbiol. 8: 2212-2222.

32. Zocevic, A., Vorimore, F., Vicari, N., Gasparini, J., Jacquin, L., Sachse, K., Magnino, S., Laroucau, K. (2013) A real-time PCR assay for the detection of atypical strains of *Chlamydiaceae* from pigeons. PLoS ONE. 8: e58741.

16

Heavy metal bioaccumulation and its potential relation with incidence of canine parvovirus infection in golden jackals, North Iran

Namroodi, S.[*]**, Rezaie, H., Milanlou, D.**

Department of Environmental Sciences, Faculty of Fisheries and Environmental Sciences, Gorgan University of Agricultural Sciences & Natural Resources, Gorgan, Iran

Key words:

bioaccumulation, heavy metal, jackals, parvovirus, road-killed

Correspondence

Namroodi, S.

Department of Environmental Sciences, Faculty of Fisheries and Environmental Sciences, Gorgan University of Agricultural Sciences & Natural Resources, Gorgan, Iran

Email: snamroodi2000@yahoo.com

Abstract:

BACKGROUND: Heavy metal toxicity has been confirmed to be a critical threat to animals' health. It has been proved that heavy metals can cause immunosuppression. Although, it is said that damage of immune function plays a contributing role in the increasing incidence of infectious diseases. The increasing use of rural habitats by jackals makes them suitable to monitor the anthropogenic activities impact on the health status of the animals. **OBJECTIVES:** We examined whether exposure to immunosuppressive heavy metals is associated with infectious disease in golden jackals (as representative of wild canids). So mercury and lead concentrations, frequency of CPV-2 infection and the relation between heavy metal concentrations and CPV-2 infection incidence were analyzed in golden jackals. **METHODS:** 30 Road-killed golden jackals were necropsied. Concentrations of Pb and Hg were measured by AAS in kidney and liver samples. VP2 gene of the CPV genomic DNA was applied to detect CPV-2 infection in fecal samples by PCR. **RESULTS:** Mean concentrations (mg/kg wet weight) of Hg and Pb were 0.15 ± 0.11 and 0.25 ± 0.18 in kidneys, and 2.8 ± 0.91 and 4.7 ± 1.03 in livers. CPV-2 was detected in 8 (24%) samples. Mean concentrations of Hg and Pb were meaningfully higher in the jackals that were CPV-2 infected compared to non- CPV-2 infected jackals. **CONCLUSIONS:** This pilot study has linked heavy metals bioaccumulation to viral infection. Further work is required to estimate the exact role of heavy metals in susceptibility of jackals to CPV-2 infection.

Introduction

Environmental contamination by heavy metals is one of the most dangerous anthropogenic influences on living organisms worldwide. This is due to both the occurrence of high numbers of metals' sources inside the earth's crust and human activities (Langner et al., 2011; Markert et al., 2011). Some of them (Hg and Pb) are very toxic for organisms even in low concentration and have a wide range of toxic effects on humans and animals (Lehmann, et al., 2011). Toxic effects of heavy metals frequently linked to chronic exposure include mutagenicity, carcinogenicity, teratogenicity, immunosuppression, poor body condition and impaired reproduction (Beyioersmann and Hartwig, 2008; Garcia-Leston et al., 2012; Lehmann et al., 2011).

The data related to adverse effects of heavy metals contaminations in the wild carnivores is rare. However, Hg and Pb are known to bioaccumulate and to magnify in some carnivores such as marine mammals, and have been introduced as a cause of great concern in terms of their general health (Larbi, et al., 2014). Moreover, adverse effects of non-essential heavy metals on the immune system of animals have often been stated (Jaishankar et al., 2014).

Moreover, it has been accepted that impairment of immune function plays a contributing role in the increasing incidence of infectious diseases in animals. Accordingly, nowadays pollution and pathogens represent a serious threat to the health of animals (Morley, 2010).

Golestan Province located in the north Iran is a very important region for conservation of biodiversity in Iran. More than 50% of the total Iranian mammals' species is found in Golestan Province (Majnoonian et al., 1999). Golestan's geographical situation and climate make it suitable for agricultural and industrial activities (Sharbati, 2012). Hence, it suffers from a large extent, large scale human activities and pollution.

Despite the fact that many kinds of environmental changes, such as heavy metal contamination threaten the survival of wild species in Golestan Province, heavy metals contamination and their effects on occurrence of infectious diseases in wild animals have not been surveyed by researchers in Iran.

Canine parvovirus (CPV-2) is widely circulating in the global canine population and one of the important causes of morbidity and mortality in wild and domestic canids (Goddard and Leisewitz, 2010). For example, it has been documented that CPV-2 infection was one of the major factors in decline of the Isle Royale wolf population (Peterson and Krumenaker, 1989).

Golden jackal (*Canis aureus*) is the biggest and the only jackal species outside Africa. It is the most extensively dispersed canid species, occurring in Northern and Eastern Africa, Asia Minor, the Middle East, Central and Southern Asia, and South-eastern Europe (Jhala and Moehlman, 2004). Golden jackal is supposed to be adaptable species due to its omnivorous diet which mainly consists of small mammals, livestock remains and carcasses, and human refuse (Lanszki et al. 2010; Ćirović et al. 2014; Markov and Lanszki 2012; Jaeger et al. 2007). Due to theirs opportunistic scavenging behavior, jackals are able to live in different ecosystems, with high local densities (Jhala and Moehlman, 2004; Šálek et al. 2014).

Jackals' population, being in close contact with human made pollutant, can act as a suitable reservoir for pathogens (Ćirovi et al., 2015). In addition, they may play a role in the risk of infection disease spillover from unvaccinated rural dogs to wild canids.

Golden Jackal has been introduced as one of the most abundant species of wild canids in Golestan Province (Ziae, 2008). Consequently, it can be used as a sentinel of its ecosystem for scientific studies in North Iran.

Animals respond in a different way to environmental pollution, and the presence of toxic materials in the environment and their increase in animal tissues need to be studied for a better understanding of the effects of contaminants on each of the organisms of the ecosystem.

The main objective of this study was to survey the impact of anthropogenic activities on golden jackals through heavy metal contamination and frequency of CPV-2 infection in golden jackals. So, Hg and Pb concentrations and CPV infection incidence were analyzed in road killed golden jackals to survey the relation between heavy metals concentrations and the susceptibility of golden jackals to CPV-2 infection incidence.

Materials and Methods

Sampling: Fecal samples and liver & kidney tissues were collected from 30 road-killed jackals from the main traffic road of Golestan Province which is located near numerous villages. Samples were used only from carcasses for which the close time of death could be evaluated as less than 12-24 h.

CPV-2 detection: Fecal samples were obtained in the form of a rectal swab, using sterilized swabs, and directly transferred to labeled sterile vials containing PBS. The samples were centrifuged at 10,000 rpm for 5 minutes and supernatant was used in the PCR. Total DNA were extracted from the supernatant by use of Bioneer extraction kit. The custom manufactured forward (5' GAAGAGTGGTTGTAAATAATA 3') and reverse (5' CCTATATCACCAAAGTTAG-TAG 3') primers specific for the VP2 gene of the CPV-2 genomic DNA were applied to amplify the DNA of 681 bp in length having the following cyclic conditions. Initial denaturing temperature of 94 °C for 5 min for one cycle, 30 cycles of denaturation at

94 °C for 30 sec, primer annealing at 55 °C for 2 min, 72 °C for 2 min, 30 cycles and final extension of 5 min at 72 °C (Pereira et al., 2000). The amplified products were electrophoresed on 1% agarose gel, stained with ethidium bromide and then visualized under the UV transilluminator against the 100 bp DNA ladder.CPV-2 Vaccine strain and ultra-water were used as positive and negative control, respectively.

Heavy metal analysis: To measure Hg and Pb concentrations in kidney and liver tissue samples, wet tissue weight was recorded. Then samples were digested with concentrated nitric and perchloric acid (1:1). After heating on a hot plate for 1 h, the digested samples were examined two times for measuring Hg and Pb concentrations with an atomic absorption spectrophotometer using an air/acetylene flame (GBc I, Australia) (FAO, 1993).

Statistical analysis: SPSS 18 and Excel 2010 software were used for statistical analyses. Mean concentrations of Pb and Hg were represented in mean WW ± standard deviation. Differences in trace elements concentrations of different tissues and incidence of CPV-2 infection were calculated by T-test.

Results

Frequency of CPV-2 infection: There was no apparent clinical sign of CPV-2 infection in road-killed jackals. VP2 partial gene was detected in 8 of 30 (24%) fecal samples (Fig. 1). There was no difference between female and male jackals in frequency of CPV-2 infection.

Tissues Hg and Pb concentrations: Mean Hg concentrations in livers and kidneys of sampled golden jackals were 0.25

Table 1. Group Statistics. 1= Kidney, 2= Liver.

	Salembimar	N	Mean	Std. Deviation	Std. Error Mean
Hg K[1]	1.00	22	.1101	.08563	.01826
	2.00	8	.2913	.05718	.02022
Hg L[2]	1.00	22	.1809	.09851	.02100
	2.00	8	.4463	.21804	.07709
Pb K	1.00	22	2.4436	.66175	.14109
	2.00	8	3.9637	.46325	.16378
Pb L	1.00	22	4.3155	.83583	.17820
	2.00	8	5.8238	.68930	.24371

Table 2. Results of Independent Samples T-test between heavy metals concentration and CPV2 incidence. 1= Kidney, 2= Liver

		Levene's Test for Equality of Variances		t-test for Equality of Means					95% Confidence Interval of the Difference	
		F	Sig.	t	df	Sig. (2-tailed)	Mean Difference	Std. Error Difference	Lower	Upper
Hg K1	Equal variances assumed	.683	.415	-5.519	28	.000	-.18111	.03281	-.24833	-.11390
	Equal variances not assumed			-6.649	18.886	.000	-.18111	.02724	-.23815	-.12408
Hg L2	Equal variances assumed	5.810	.023	-4.643	28	.000	-.26534	.05715	-.38241	-.14827
	Equal variances not assumed			-3.321	8.063	.010	-.26534	.07990	-.44934	-.08135
Pb K	Equal variances assumed	.292	.593	-5.956	28	.000	-1.52011	.25520	-2.04287	-.99735
	Equal variances not assumed			-7.032	17.949	.000	-1.52011	.21617	-1.97437	-1.06586
Pb L	Equal variances assumed	.002	.964	-4.557	28	.000	-1.50830	.33100	-2.18631	-.83028
	Equal variances not assumed			-4.996	15.052	.000	-1.50830	.30191	-2.15160	-.86499

± 0.18 and 0.15 ± 0.11 mg/kg, respectively. Although Pb concentrations in livers and kidneys of sampled golden jackals were 4.7 ± 1.03 and 2.8 ± 0.91 mg/kg, respectively, no significant difference was observed between levels of Hg and Pb concentration in male and female jackals. Livers Hg and Pb concentrations were higher than kidneys.

Correlation between levels of heavy metals concentrations and incidence of CPV-2 infection: There was a positive correlation between CPV-2 infection incidence and levels of Hg & Pb concentrations in sampled golden jackals. Results of T-test revealed that mean concentration of the Hg and Pb was higher in CPV-2 infected jackals than CPV-2 negative jackals (Table 1 and 2).

Discussion

There is limited data regarding heavy metals contamination, frequency of CPV-2 infection and potential relationship between

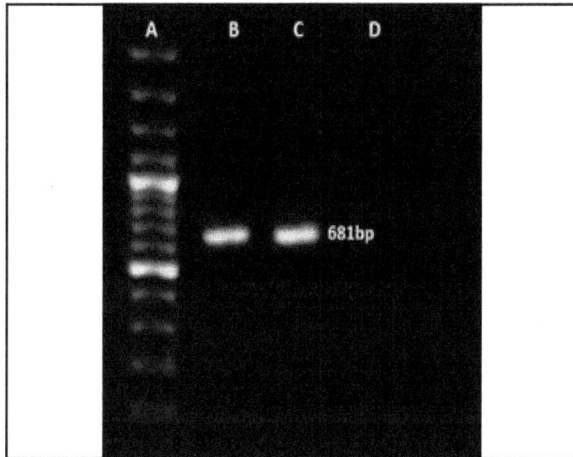

Figure 1. PCR results: A= DNA Ladder, B= Positive control, C= Positive sample, D= Negative control.

heavy metals contamination and incidence of viral diseases in golden jackals. For this study, as for other surveys explained in the scientific papers, the obtained results were step by step compared to linked results reported in the peer-reviewed scientific literature.

Frequency of Canine parvovirus infection incidence: Infectious diseases have been documented as important threats to wildlife population throughout the world and have been introduced in some areas where populations of some species such as Africa wild dogs have been declining (Prager et al., 2012).

CPV-2 was detected in 8 out of 30 (24%) fecal samples by PCR which seems a high value. CPV-2 can persist in the environment for a long period of time, and can also be spread not only by direct contact but also through vectors such as flies (Greene and Apple 2011). Therefore, this information together with the suitable climate situation of Golestan Province for CPV persisting in environment can also be part of the explanation for high CPV-2 infection of sampled golden jackals.

Measurement of serum antibody titer can be a useful method to reveal the history of animals CPV-2 exposures. But it is not valid for determination of CPV-2 infection incidence in canids (Greene and Apple 2011). Hence, in this study CPV-2 infection was surveyed in golden jackals to measure the actual CPV-2 contamination risk that golden jackals are facing in Golestan Province.

With regard to CPV, detection of antibody titer to CPV-2 has been frequently used to analyze canids' population.

There are very limited epidemiological surveys on CPV-2 infection in wild canids. One of the first reports of CPV-2 infection of wild canids was documented by Mech and Fritts (1987). They reported CPV-2 infection led to the death of 11 wolf pups in a captive wolf colony in Minnesota (USA). Mech and Goyal (1993) explained that the small population of wolves has been significantly affected by CPV-2 mortality.

Results of serological studies which are not comparable with our study have shown high frequency of wild canids and free-living dogs' exposures to CPV-2 in some countries.

13 of 19 wolves' serum from Montana (USA) were recorded as positive for CPV-2 antibody (Johnson, 1984).

Based on data achieved in this study, it cannot be concluded exactly whether CPV-2 spill over from golden jackals to other wild canids species in Golestan Province. However, the presence of CPV-2 in sampled golden jackals suggests the possible danger of CPV-2 infection in other wild canids and the need for designing continues via monitoring plans for actively restricting this lethal disease through vaccination.

So, it seems that the government should be encouraged to vaccine rural dogs and also the golden jackals' population in north Iran, to protect endangered species   from

CPV-2 infection.

Therefore, this study must be extended to include the testing of higher numbers of golden jackals in North Iran.

Pb and Hg contamination: Assessment of environmental contamination can be indirectly surveyed by analysis of toxic elements concentration in living organisms.

To the best of our knowledge, this is the first study that surveyed the concentrations of Pb and Hg in golden jackals, which are at the top of the food web and may be very sensitive to any levels of non-essential heavy metals, in Iran.

Pb is a very toxic heavy metal that disrupts numerous physiological processes and it does not have any biological function in animals (Kalisinska et al., 2012, Najeeb et al., 2014). Lead toxicity can cause anemia, impaired nervous system and kidney function, delayed healing of fractures and immunosuppression (Liu, 2003). There are many natural and anthropogenic sources of Pb in the environment. The chief causes of lead contamination are industrial activities, coal combustion, automotive industry, agricultural activities (Najeeb et al., 2014).

Pb concentrations in livers and kidneys of sampled golden jackals were 4.7 ± 1.03 and 2.8 ± 0.91 mg/kg, respectively. Toxic threshold of Pb concentration in golden jackals has not been surveyed. However, based on laboratory tests on rodents from the order Rodentia, it was found that Pb bone concentration near the level of 50 mg/kg dw, could lead to adverse effects of this metal on skeletal formations (Andrews, et al., 1989).

As there was no data about the health status of sampled road killed jackals, the toxic effect of Pb on sampled jackals cannot be concluded. Nevertheless this metal can be toxic for animals even at very low levels.

There are just two similar studies on golden jackals in the world and most of the related surveys have been done on foxes.

Ćirović1 and his colleagues (2014) surveyed concentrations of seven trace elements (Pb, Cd, Zn, Cu, Fe, Mn, and Ni) in livers of 129 golden jackals from Serbia. The highest and lowest Pb concentration were recorded 23.00 mg/kg ww and 3.46 mg/kg ww, respectively, with average range of 9.59 mg/kg.

Markov and his colleagues (2016) detected Pb concentration of 6.88 ± 1.67 mg/kg dw and 4.03 ± 1.32 mg/kg dw in livers and kidneys of golden jackals from Bulgaria, respectively, which seems lower than results of the current study.

Pb skin concentration in red foxes from Spain, Croatia and Poland has been documented 0.053 mg/kg, 0.043 mg/kg and 1.445 mg/kg, respectively (Milla´n et al., 2008, Bilandzic et al., 2010).

Hg is a well-known environmental toxicant and pollutant which causes severe changes in the body tissues and causes a wide range of adverse health effects such Gastro-intestinal disorders, respiratory tract irritation, renal failure, neurotoxicity and immunosuppression (Scheuhammer et al. 2008).

The chief sources of Hg contamination include anthropogenic activities such as agriculture, municipal wastewater discharges, mining, incineration, metallurgy, burning coal and discharges of industrial wastewater (Liao et al., 2006).

Mean Hg concentrations in livers and kidneys of sampled golden jackals were 0.25 ± 0.18 and 0.15 ± 0.11 mg/kg, respectively. To the best of our knowledge, there is not any report on golden jackals Hg contamination. So, we compared our results with other canids' species such as foxes.

Hg poisoning in wild canids has been rarely documented. One known case was documented in a Swedish wild fox with Hg poisoning signs: running around, staggering, apparently blind without olfactory sense. A mixed sample from the liver and kidney from that individual contained 30 mg Hg/kg ww (Borg et al., 1969).

Although there were a few previous reports on Hg contamination in foxes as representative of wild canids, the Hg threshold value for wild canids (above which adverse effects happen) was not reported. Such data is accessible for the domestic dogs (*Canis lupus*) which also belong to the family Canidae. The laboratory tests performed on the dogs revealed that the typical concentration of Hg in the liver and kidney is <0.1 mg/kg wet weight, ww (~0.3 mg/kg dw), while 2.8 and 3.3 mg/kg ww are introduced as lethal (9.3 and 11 mg/kg dw) (Farrar et al., 1994).

Generally, the effects of Hg contamination on sampled golden jackals in this study are not clear. However, as it can be toxic to cells in low concentration, the toxic effect of Hg on sampled jackals seems possible (Borg et al., 1969).

From the results of similar studies, starting from the 1980s, red foxes and Arctic foxes were found to have kidney and liver Hg levels not higher than 10 mg/kg dw, which is equal to ~2.5 mg/kg ww (Kalisinska et al., 2012).

In recent years, the highest Hg concentrations in the liver and kidney of the red fox ranged from about 4.2 to 5.4 mgHg/kg dw and were observed only in single individuals in Poland and Spain. In both cases, the considerable Hg concentrations were due to unusual environmental conditions and diet

(Cybulski et al., 2009, Millan et al., 2008).

Kalisinska and her colleagues (2012) determined the concentrations of total Hg in samples of liver, kidney and skeletal muscle of 27 red foxes from northwestern Poland.

The median concentrations of Hg in the liver, kidney and skeletal muscle were 0.22, 0.11 and 0.05 mg/kg dw, respectively. As it can be concluded, the results of this study are lower than the results of current study. Although when compared with the kidney and liver Hg levels reported by Cybulski et al. (2009) for the farmed silver fox (0.056 and 0.082 mg/kg dw, respectively), golden jackals in this study had higher levels of Hg in the kidneys and livers.

Observed differences in noted results originate from many factors, including difference in diet of each species, habitat condition, type of biological samples, and biological characteristics of each species of animals (Millan, et al., 2008).

Sources of Hg and Pb have not been diagnosed in this study. However, that consumption of contaminated foods has been introduced as one of the major means of heavy metal contamination (Millan, et al., 2008). Golden jackals usually feed on small mammals which can absorb trace elements from soil, water, plant, air and have been introduced as a potential source of contamination for predatory animals inhabiting natural and agricultural ecosystems (Fritsch, et al., 2010).

So, Hg and Pb contaminations in sampled road -killed jackals are strongly correlated with rural and wild regions condition of Golestan Province and indirectly show heavy metal contamination of rural and wild ecosystems in this province.

In this study like most of the studies which have been done on tissues heavy metals contaminations of animals, higher concentration of heavy metals was observed in livers than kidneys (Kalisinska et al., 2012, Markov et al., 2016).

One main part of the explanation is liver tissue activities in detoxification of blood in the body of the animals. Conversely, Lopez et.al, detected a higher concentration of Hg in kidneys (0.053 mg/kg ww) than livers (0.032 mg/kg ww) in free living dogs.

There are conflicting results regarding the effects of gender on heavy metals contamination in animals. Gender effect on heavy metals accumulation is assumed to be related to the biology of the species. The extent of golden jackal`s home range can be influenced by food resource distribution, extent of human pressure, type of habitat, and is estimated to be in the range from 1.1 to 20 km2 (Jhala and Moehlman, 2004).

Generally, male jackals have wider home ranges than females (Giannatos, 2004). Furthermore, the removal rate of foreign compounds per unit body weight in mammals decreases as body weight increases (Prater, 1980).

Thus, males being heavier and more mobile are more prone to collecting contaminants, including heavy metals although the difference in level of metals between genders occurs, no significant sex-related differences in heavy metals accumulation were found in this study. Similar results were reported by Cirovicl et al. (2014) in golden jackals and Kalisinska et al., (2012) in red foxes.

Conversely, in the survey of Millán et al., (2008) on levels of heavy metals and metalloids contamination in critically endangered Iberian lynx and other wild carnivores from southern Spain, liver concentrations of Se, Cd, Pb and Hg were higher in females than in males.

Totally, results of the current study revealed potential risk of heavy metal contamination for wild carnivores and rural habitats in Golestan Province regions and also showed that golden jackals can be a good indicator for environmental pollution.

Relation between Hg and Pb contamination levels and CPV-2 incidence: Presence of heavy metals in biological tissues reflects the chronic intake of heavy metals. Since there is no useful procedure for the removal of trace elements accumulation in various tissues, low levels of chronic intake can lead to harmful effects on long living organisms (Bilandzic et al., 2010).

The presence of Pb and Hg has been detected in most tissues of mammals, and it has been proved that even minimum concentrations of them can cause metabolic disturbances, reducing physical efficiency, weakening immune and enzymatic processes, and leading to many diseases and sometimes death (Rittschof et al., 2005). For example, the interactions between infectious diseases and pollutants in aquatic communities have become an increasing area of concern (Morley, 2010). In combination, these two types of stressors may potentially be synergistically harmful to affected population. Interestingly, a noteworthy positive connection between CPV-2 infection incidence and levels of Hg & Pb contaminations was detected in our study. Jackals with high levels of Hg and Pb tissues concentration were also positive for CPV-2 infection.

To the best of our knowledge, this survey is one of the principal epidemiological studies that provides evidence for a relationship between heavy metals contamination and incidence of viral disease in wild canids. The consequent immunomodulation by Pb and Hg contamination may increase sampled golden jackals susceptibility to CPV-2.

There are some studies with similar results which showed interactions between heavy metals contaminations and infectious and non- infectious diseases in humans and animals.

Nguyen and his colleagues (2016) reported a positive relationship between aerial heavy metals and itchy eyes and coughing in chronic cough patients.

Heavy traffic exposure, one source of heavy metals, has been associated with growth in the incidence and prevalence of childhood asthma and wheeze as well as allergic sensitization, bronchial hyper responsiveness and respiratory symptoms in children (Janssen, et al., 2003).

Bennett and his colleagues showed that long-term exposure to heavy metals, including immunosuppressive metals, like mercury (Hg), is associated with infectious disease in wild cetacean.

Like the results of this study, they found that mean liver concentration of Hg was significantly higher in the porpoises that died of infectious disease compared to healthy porpoises that died from physical trauma.

It has been documented that pretreatment of mice with Hg compounds enhances susceptibility to experimental infections with murine leishmaniasis or sporozoites.

Chou et al.(1998) used host-virus system to examine the effects of heavy metals (cadmium, copper, zinc, mercury) on clam susceptibility to viral infection. Introduction to virus followed by metals resulted in increased clam mortalities compared to controls of up to 52% after 5 weeks.

Liao et al. (2006) and Liao and Yeh (2007) showed that the immunomodulating effects of metal pollution is a significant factor in-

fluencing population dynamics of disease transmission, increasing susceptibility of molluscs to infection. However, size of host population, life stage or density and the way of stress exposure (virus +metal or metal + virus) are critical factors in disease dynamics.

Nevertheless, a number of mammalian studies have demonstrated that chemical exposure can cause reactivation of latent viral infections or that viruses may modify the detoxification of other pollutants (Sattar et al., 2007).

It has been supposed that survival and transmission of free-living viral stages in polluted conditions are influenced by the specific contaminants present (Sattar et al., 2007).

These studies, in line with the present study, suggest that heavy metal contamination can affect susceptibility rate of animals to diseases. However, the correlation found between CPV-2 infection and levels of heavy metals concentrations in the present study does not necessarily reveal a causal relationship between these two factors. Indeed, other factors associated to habitat geographical conditions could have been involved in occurrence of such a correlation. It is very likely that this correlation might also be enhanced by the habitat (sanitation, temperature, diet) of the golden jackals and further studies are needed to monitor long-term concentrations of heavy metals with long-term effect on immune system of golden jackals and also frequency of CPV-2 infection.

Moreover, the survey points to the necessity of extra investigation using golden jackals as bioindicators of environmental capacity, and not only with respect to heavy metals. It shows the importance and necessity of assessment of the potential risk associated with environmental pollution.

Acknowledgements

The authors thank all the local minibus drivers that helped us access the road-killed jackals Mr. poorghaz, Dr. kheirabad (employee of Golestan Province Environmental Department) and also students who helped us in collection of the samples.

References

Andrews, S.M., Johnson, M.S., Cooke, J.A. (1989) Distribution of trace elements pollutants in a contaminated grassland ecosystem established on metalliferous fluorspar tailings. Lead. Environ Pollut. 58: 73-85.

Bennett, P.M., Jepson, P.D., Law, R.J., Jones, B.R., Kuiken, T., Baker, J.R. (2001) Exposure to heavy metals and infectious disease mortality in harbour porpoises from England and Wales. Environ Pollut. 112: 33-40.

Bilandzic, N., Dezdek, D., Sedak, M., Dokic, M., Solomun, B., Varenina, I., Knezevic, Z., Slavica, A. (2010) Concentrations of trace elements in tissues of red fox (*Vulpes vulpes*) and stone marten (*Martes foina*) from suburban and rural areas in Croatia. Bull Environ Contam Toxicol. 85: 486-491.

Borg, K., Wanntorp, H., Erne, K., Hanko, E. (1969) Alkyl mercury poisoning in terrestrial Swedish wildlife. Viltrevy. 6: 301-379.

Ćirović, D.A., Penezić, M., Milenković, M.P. (2014) Winter diet composition of the golden jackal (*Canis aureus*) in Serbia. Mamma Biol. 79: 132-137.

Cybulski, W., Chalabis-Mazurek, A., Jakubczak, A., Jarosz, L., Kostro, K., Kursa, K. (2009) Content of lead, cadmium, and mercury in the liver and kidneys of silver foxes (*Vulpes vulpes*) in relation to age and reproduction

disorders. Bull Vet Inst Pulawy. 53: 65-69.

FAO/ SIDA (1993) Manual of Methods in Aquatic Environmental Research, part9, Analysis of metals and organochlorines in fish. FAO Fisheries Technical Paper No.212.

Farrar, W.P., Edwards, J.F., Willard, M.D. (1994) Pathology in a dog associated with elevated tissue mercury concentrations. J Vet Diagn Invest. 6: 511-514.

Fritsch, C.R.P., Cosson, M., Coeurdassier, F., Raoul, P., Giraudoux, N., Crini, A. (2010) de Vaufl eury and R. Scheifl er. Responses of wild small mammals to a pollution gradient: Host factors influence metal and metallothionein levels. Environ Pollut. 158: 827-840.

García-Lestón, J., Roma-Torres, J., Vilares, M., Pinto, R., Prista, J., Teixeira, J.P., Mayan, O., Conde, J., Pingarilho, M., Gaspar, J.F., Pásaro. E., Méndez. J., Laffon. B. (2012) Genotoxic effects of occupational exposure to lead and influence of polymorphisms in genes involved in lead toxicokinetics and in DNA repair. Environ Int. 43: 29-36.

Giannatos, G. (2004) Conservation Action Plan for the golden jackal Canis aureus in Greece. WWF Greece.

Greene, C.E., Apple, M.J.G. (2011) Canine viral enteric pathogens. In Infectious Diseases of the Dog and Cat. W.B Saunders Elsevier. St.Louis. Mo., USA. 8: 75-76.

Goddard, A., Leisewitz, A.L. (2010) Canine Parvovirus. Vet Clin Small Anim Pract. 40: 1041-1053.

Janssen, N.A.H., Brunekreef, B., Van Vliet, P., Aarts, F., Meliefste, K., Harssema, H., Fischer, P. (2003) The relationship between air pollution from heavy traffic and allergic sensitization, bronchial hyperresponsiveness, and respiratory symptoms in Dutch schoolchildren. Environ Health Perspect. 111: 1512-1518.

Jaeger, M.M.E., Haque, P., Sultana, R.L., Bruggers. (2007) Daytime cover, diet and space-use of golden jackals (*Canis aureus*) in agro-ecosystems of Bangladesh. Mammalia. 71: 1-10.

Jaishankar, M., Tenzin, T., Anbalagan, N., Blessy, B., Krishnamurthy, N.B. (2014) Toxicity, mechanism and health effects of some heavy metals. Interdiscip Toxicol. 7: 60-72.

Jhala, Y.U., Moehlman, P.D., Jackal, G., Sillero-Zubiri, C.M., Hoffmann, D.W. (2004) Canids, Foxes, Wolves, Jackals and dogs. International Union for Conservation of Nature and Natural Resources. p. 156-161.

Johnson, P.T. (1984) Viral diseases of marine invertebrates. Helgolander Meer. 37: 65-98.

Kalisinska, E., Lisowski, P., Izabela, D. (2012) Kosik-Bogacka. Red fox *Vulpes vulpes* (L., 1758) as a bioindicator of mercury contamination in terrestrial ecosystems of North-Western Poland. Biol Trace Elem Res. 145: 172-180.

Langner, A.N., Manu, A., Tabatabai, M.A. (2011). Heavy metals distribution in an Iowa suburban landscape. J Environ Qual. 40: 83-89.

Lanszki, J.G., Giannatos, A., Dolev, G., Bino, M.H. (2010) Late autumn trophic flexibility of golden jackal *Canis aureus*. Acta Theriologica. 55: 361-370.

Larbi, D.K, Bouslah, Y., Bouderbala, M., Boutiba, Z. (2014) Heavy metals in soft tissues of short-beaked common dolphins (*Delphinus delphis*) stranded along the Algerian West coast. Sci Res. 4 (2).

Lehmann, I., Sack, U., Lehmann, J. (2011) Metal ions affecting the immune system. Met Ions Life Sci. 8: 157-185.

Liao, C.M., Chang, C.F., Yeh, C.H., Chen, S.C., Chiang, K.C., Chio, C.P., Chou, B.Y.H., Jou, L.J., Lien, G.W., Lin, C.M., Shen, H.H., Wu, G.D. (2006) Metal stresses affect the population dynamics of disease transmission in aquaculture species. Aquaculture. 257: 321-332.

Liao, C.M., Yeh, C.H. (2007) Hard clam Meretrix lusoria to Hg-stressed birnavirus susceptibility revealed through stage-structured disease transmission dynamics. Aquaculture. 264: 101-118.

Liu, Z.P. (2003) Lead poisoning combined with cadmium in sheep and horses in the vicinity of non-ferrous metal smelters. Sci Total Environ. 309: 117-126.

Lopez-Alonso, M., Miranda, M., García-Partida, P., Cantero, F., Hernandez, J., Benedito, J.L. (2007) Use of dogs as indicators of metal exposure in rural and urban habitats in NW Spain. Sci Total Environ. 372: 668-675.

Majnoonian, H., Zehzad, B., Dareshouri, F.B., Meigouni, H. (1999) Golestan National Park. Department of Environment of Islamic Republic of Iran, Tehran, Iran. p. 450- 463.

Markert, B., Wuenschmann, S., Fraenzle, S., Graciana Figueiredo, A.M., Ribeiro, A.P., Wang, M. (2011) Bioindication of atmospheric trace metals with special references to megacities. Environ Pollut. 159: 1991-1995.

Markov, G., Kocheva, M., Gospodinova, M. (2016) Assessment of Heavy Metal Accumulation in the Golden Jackal (*Canis aureus*) as a Possible Bioindicator in an Agricultural Environment in Bulgaria. Bull Environ Contam Toxicol. 96: 458-64.

Mechand, S.H., Frui, I.S. (1987) Parvovirus and heartworm found in Minnesota wolves. Endangered Species Technical Bulletin Number 12, U.S. Fish and Wildlife Service, Washington D.C. p. 5-6.

Mechand, S. M., Goyal. (1993) Canine parvovirus effect on wolf population change and pup survival. J Wildlife Dis. 29: 330-333.

Millan, J., Mateo, R., Taggart, M.A., Lopez-Bao, J.V., Viota, M., Monsalve, L., Camarero, P.R.,

Blazquez, E., Jimenez, B. (2008) Levels of heavy metals and metalloids critically endangered Iberfian lynx and other wild carnivores from Southern Spain. Sci Total Environ. 399: 193- 201.

Morley, N.J. (2010) Interactive effects of infectious diseases and pollution in aquatic molluscs. Aquat Toxicol. 96: 27-36.

Najeeb, U., Ahmad, W., Zia, M.H., Malik, Z., Zhou, W. (2014) Enhancing the lead phytostabilization in wetland plant Juncus eff usus L. through somaclonal manipulation and EDTA enrichment. Arab J Chem. 5: 27-33.

Nguyen, T.T.T., Higashi, T., Kambayashi, Y., Anyenda, E.O., Michigami, Y., Hara, Y. (2016) A longitudinal study of association between heavy metals and itchy eyes, coughing in chronic cough patients: related with non-immunoglobulin E mediated mechanism. Int Environ Res Public Health. 13: 110-21.

Pereira, C.A., Monezi, T.A., Mehnert, D.U.D 'Angelo, M., Durigon, E.L. (2000) Molecular characterization of canine parvovirus in Brazil by PCR. Vet Microbiol. 75: 127-133.

Peterson, E., Krumenaker, H. (1989) Wolf approach extinction on Isle Royale: Abiologucal and policy conundrum. George Wright Forum. 6: 10-15.

Prager, K.C., Mazet, J.A.K., Munson, L., Cleaveland, S., Donnelly, C.A., Dubovi, E.J. (2012) 'The effect of protected areas on pathogen exposure in endangered African wild dog (Lycaon pictus) populations',. Biol Conserv. 150: 1-15.

Prater, S.H. (1980). The Book of Indian Animals. Bombay Natural History Society, Bombay, India.

Rittschof, D., and McClellan-Green, P. (2005) Molluscs as multidisciplinary models in environmental toxicology. Mar Pollut Bull. 5: 369-373.

Šálek, M.J., Červinka, B.C., Ovidiu, M., Krofel, D., Ćirović, I., Selenec, A., Penezić, S., Grill, J., Reigert. (2014) Population densities and habitat use of the golden jackal (Canis aureus) in farmlands across the Balkan Peninsula. Europ J Wildlife Res. 60: 193-200.

Scheuhammer, A.M., Basu, N., Burgess, N.M., Elliott, J.E., Campbell, G.D., Wayland, M., Champoux, L., Rodrigue, J. (2008) Relationships among mercury, selenium, and neurochemical parameters in common loons (Gavia immer) and bald eagles (Haliaeetus leucocephalus). Ecotoxicology. 17: 93-101.

Sharbati, A. (2012) The Ecotourism Potentials of Golestan Province. J Basic Appl Sci Res. 2: 564-570.

Ziaee, H. (2008) Field handbook of Iran's mammals. Introduction wildlife center institute publication, Tehran, Iran.

17

A molecular survey of *Chlamydial* infection in pet and zoo captive reptiles

Rostami, A.[1], Shahabi, M.[1*], Madani, A.[2]

[1]*Department of Internal Medicine, Faculty of Veterinary Medicine, University of Tehran, Tehran, Iran*
[2]*Department of Poultry Diseases, Faculty of Veterinary Medicine, University of Tehran, Tehran, Iran*

Key words:

chlamydia, reptiles, real time PCR, zoonotic disease

Correspondence

Shahabi, M.
Department of Internal Medicine, Faculty of Veterinary Medicine, University of Tehran, Tehran, Iran

Email: majidshahabi@ut.ac.ir

Abstract:

BACKGROUND: Chlamydiosis is a worldwide zoonotic disease caused by different microorganisms in the order Chlamydiales. **OBJECTIVES:** The aim of this study was to detect and determine the prevalence of Chlamydia infection in pet and zoo reptiles in Tehran, Iran. **METHODS:** In a period of 10 months from April 2015 to February 2016, swab samples were collected from cloaca and conjunctiva of 130 pet or zoo reptiles (18 snakes, 81 turtles, and 31 iguanas). A Real Time-PCR assay targeting 23s rRNA of chlamydial organisms was performed to detect chlamydial infection in clinical specimens. **RESULTS:** No positive sample could be detected in the investigated clinical specimens in the present study. **CONCLUSIONS:** Regarding the negative results which were achieved in this study, reptiles could not be important hosts of chlamydial organisms at least in the region of the present study, Tehran, Iran. Despite the present findings in reptiles, pet and aviary birds were previously shown to be remarkable hosts of *Chlamydia* spp. in Iran. Further studies particularly serologic surveys and other PCR methods are needed to thoroughly evaluate the significance of the chlamydial infection in reptiles. A rapid, accurate and cost-effective method was applied for Chlamydiaceae spp detection and discrimination of the most significant *Chlamydia* spp., causing disease complications in reptiles. The results indicated low zoonotic risk of *Chlamydia* spp in Iranian reptiles.

Introduction

Chlamydiosis is a worldwide zoonotic disease caused by microorganisms called Chlamydia. These bacteria are obligate intracellular parasites that belong to the family Chlamydiaceae (Suchland et al., 2003).

Several animal species can become infected by chlamydial organisms. According to a previous study by Krauss et al., 2003 the chlamydiosis was recognized in 32 species of mammals. Sheep, cats and goats are the most probable affected (Matsui et al., 2008, Stuen et al., 2011). Many infected animals do not show any clinical signs. The infection with *Chlamydia psittaci* in reptiles has broad spectrum clinical signs such as distress, purulent nasal discharge, diarrhea, frequent urination, lethargy, sinusitis and disorders of the central nervous system (Soldati et al., 2004, Yucesan et al., 2001). Commonly, reptiles such as chameleon and snakes sporadically develop Chlamydiosis with diverse clinical signs (granulomatous inflammation and erythema), iguanas and giant turtles (inflammatory changes on various organic systems) and crocodiles (conjunctivitis) (Frutos et al.,2015, Gaydos et al., 1992). The severity of clinical sign depends on the species of *Chlamydia*, species of reptiles and age (Ebani and Fratini, 2005).

Human can occasionally get infected from animal contact (Andersen and Vanrompay., 2003). Meyers in 2009 indicated no transition of *C. pneumonia* from animal to humans (Myers et al., 2009). Immunodeficient and immunosuppressed human beings, pediatrics and geriatrics, are included as high risk population to chlamydiosis, which is transferred by reptiles (Pospisil et al., 2004, Mendall et al., 1995).

Identification of the infected reptile with bacterial agents is critical to control the disease in high risk people who are exposed to the mentioned animals (Jacobson et al.,2004). In general, the diagnosis of chlamydial infections by conventional methods is difficult and has a highly variable response (Black, 1997). Gold standardized methods (observing inclusion body by light or electron microscopy) for most Chlamydia spp. are not widely available (Bodetti et al., 2002). In order to speed up the analysis, the usage of PCR methods has been introduced to identify Chlamydia spp. in human and reptiles samples (Boman et al., 1999). Increasing demand for a quantitative, more sensitive and specific and rapid procedures are prompting the development of real-time quantitative PCR methods.

People who raise reptiles as pets have increased recently but microbiological information is limited. The purpose of the present study was to evaluate the presence of clinical and subclinical chlamydial infection in some pet and zoo captive reptiles in Tehran.

Material and Method

Clinical samples: All parts of sampling and DNA extraction were coordinated based on previous studies (Taylor-Brown et al., 2015, Madani and Peighambari, 2013, Di Ianni et al., 2015). For this purpose a single swab was used to take the samples from conjunctiva and cloaca, respectively. In a period of ten months from April 2015 to February 2016, 130 swab samples were collected from cloaca and upper respiratory tract or conjunctiva of different reptile species. The investigated animals were either admitted to Tehran small animal research and teaching hospital or were housed in Tehran zoo (24 zoo animals and 106 pet animals). The swabs were placed in sucrose-phosphate glutamine medium (SPG) and frozen for the future investigation. SPG contain 75 g of sucrose, 0.52 g of KH2PO4, 1.22 g of Na2HPO4 and 0.72 g of glutamic acid, distilled water to 1 liter (pH 7.4) (Merck Co., Germany), with 10% fetal calf serum (FCS) supplement, 500 mg vancomycin, 500 mg streptomycin, 200 mg of gentamicin and amphotericin 50 mg.

Real-time PCR assay: Total genomic DNA was extracted using High Pure PCR Template Preparation Kit (Roche, Germany) as instructed by the manufacturer. Extracted DNA samples were stored at −20 °C. All clinical samples were amplified on the Rotor Q machine (QIAGEN co., Germany) using the 23s rRNA-based Chlamydiaceae family-specific real-time PCR as described previously (Ehricht et al., 2006). The spe-

Table1. The scientific names and the number of pet and zoo reptiles which were sampled in the present study for molecular survey of chlamydia infection.

Common name	Scientific sample Name	Number
Python	*Pythonidae family*	5
Boa	*Boidae family*	6
Blind snakes	*Typhlopidae family*	1
Streaked snakes	*Oligodon taeniolatus*	2
Javelin sand boa	*Eryx jaculus*	3
Diadem snakes	*Spalerosophis diadema schiraziana*	1
Caspian turtle	*Mauremys caspica*	28
Pond slider	*Trachemys scripta*	41
Russian tortoise	*Testudo horsfieldii*	1
European pond turtle	*Emys orbicularis*	11
green iguana	*Iguana iguana*	22
bearded dragons	*Pogona*	4
Egyptian mastigure	*Uromastyx aegyptia*	1
desert iguana	*Dipsosaurus dorsalis*	4

cific primers were used for amplification of Chlamydia spp., including: Ch23S-F (5′-CTGAAACCAGTAGCTTATAAG-CGGT-3′), Ch23S-R (5′-ACCTCGC-CGTTTAA CTTAACTCC-3′), and probe Ch23S-p (FAM-CTCATCATGCAAAAG-GCACGCCG-TAMRA) (Ehricht et al.,2006). The primers targeted an amplicon in 23s rRNA gene with the size of 111 bp. In each reaction, 2.5 µl of extracted DNA was added to a mixture of reagents containing 12.5 µl of 2×TaqMan® Fast Universal PCR Master Mix (Jena Bioscience, Germany, Jena), with final concentration of 5 pmol/µl of each primer and the probe (Macrogen, South Korea) to yield a final volume of 25 µl. The cycling profile included an initial denaturation (95 °C, 10 min) followed by 45 cycles of denaturation at 94 °C for 15 s and 60 °C for 60 s. A cycle threshold (Ct value) of <38.00 was considered as positive, and all samples were tested at least in duplicate also all samples were compared to UT-NOIVBD (Veldhoven, the Netherland) as positive control and deionized water as negative control (Madani and Peighambari, 2013).

Results

A total 130 clinical samples were obtained from 16 snakes, 81 turtles, 33 iguanas. Ages vary from 1 month to 12 years. The frequency of conjunctivitis and respiratory lesions was 21% and 11%, respectively. According to positive control test, the results were interpreted as questionably positive if one threshold cycle (Ct) value was less than 38 while the other showed no Ct value. If one Ct value was above 38 and the other showed no Ct value, the result was interpreted as questionably negative. Thus, our results indicated no amplification products from 130 clinical samples by real time PCR. There were no positive samples with different strains of Chlamydia sp.

Discussion

Chlamydia spp. are a widespread group of obligatory intracellular bacteria in both warm-blooded and cold-blooded animals. Their infection was reported in different

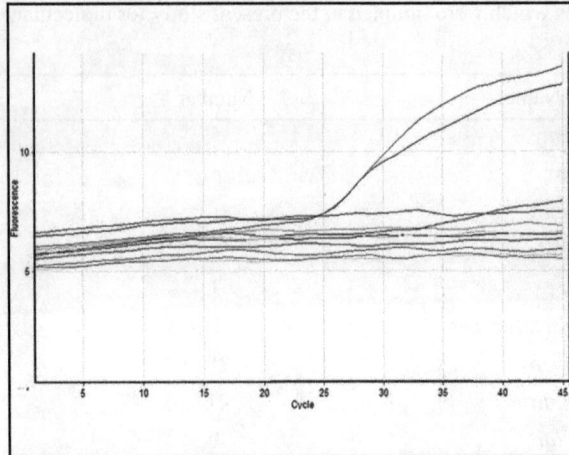

Figure1. As the graph illustrates, all of our samples were plateau, while control positive samples peaked in the 25ᵗʰ cycle and prove real time PCR efficiency.

hosts including human, cats, birds, sheep, dogs, pigs, koalas, and cattle (Suchland et al, 2003). Chlamydiosis was also described in various species of reptiles including turtles, chameleons, crocodiles, iguanas and snakes (Andreoletti et al., 2007, Corsaro and Venditti, 2004). In the present study 130 clinical specimens from 14 reptile species were subjected to Chlamydiaceae specific real-time PCR. None of them were positive for Chlamydia spp. 23s rRNA DNA using the highly sensitive molecular method.

Although it was relatively scarce in the literature, chlamydial infection was previously reported in reptiles. Using the conventional PCR, Jacobson et al., (1989) detected the bacterial DNA in a group of turtles with myocarditis, pneumonia, hepatitis, and splenomegaly. Kabeya et al., (2015) reported 8.1% of Chlamydia infection in reptiles. The incidence of *Chlamydia pneumoniae* DNA was significantly higher in reptiles (5.8%) than in mammals (0.3%) and birds (0.3%). Taylor-Brown et al., (2015) illustrated the variable occurrence of Chlamydia from 5% to 33% in captive snakes. In another report from Argentina, *C. pneumoniae*

infection was diagnosed in a single collection of captive reptiles (Frutos et al., 2014). Hotzel et al., (2005) reported Chlamydia spp infection in 16 out of 155 (10.3%) nasal lavage specimens from tortoises. Di Ianni et al., (2015) found *Chlamydia* spp in a single animal with severe conjunctivitis using a PCR diagnosis. The Chlamydia sp. was isolated from the respiratory lesions of a Burmese python and also a *Corallus hortulanus* suffered from a chronic pulmonary thromboembolism, respectively in 2001 and 2002 (Jacobson et al., 2001, Bodetti et al., 2002). Soldati et al., (2004) detected *C. pneumonia*e DNA in nine out of 90 (10%) reptile samples. To the best of the authors' knowledge it was the first attempt in the molecular detection of chlamydiosis in captive and zoo reptiles in Iran.

The isolation of Chlamydia sp. is very time consuming and relatively difficult considering the obligatory intracellular nature of these organisms. Molecular methods are superior to the traditional isolation regarding the test sensitivity and the rapid one day results (Gaydos et al., 1992, Sachse et al., 2005). In the previous studies real time PCR was used for chlamydia sp. detection in birds and a koala (Madani and Peighambari, 2013, Krawiec et al., 2015, Mackie et al., 2016) and in reptiles Jacobson et al., (2004) used it in an emerald tree boa. The real-time PCR which was applied in the present study was very sensitive and a robust diagnostic method which has been repetitively employed in different studies since its invention by Ehricht et al., (2006).

Chlamydiosis is a zoonotic infection and it can cause a severe clinical condition in human (Andersen and Vanrompay, 2003, Bodetti et al., 2002, Jacobson et al., 2004, Huchzermeyer et al., 2008, Homer et al.,

1994). It was previously indicated that *C. pneumoniae* infection might be correlated with different pathologies such as atherosclerosis, coronary heart disease and Alzheimer in human (Roulis et al., 2013). The population of pet reptiles is growing in Iran (Darvish and Rastegar-Pouyani, 2012, Esmaeili et al., 2008). The captive reptiles can be a potential reservoir of different zoonotic organisms like Chlamydia infection. Their role in this specific infection could not be demonstrated in the present study. According to this survey, it can be concluded that the investigated captive reptiles were not a major threat for their owner regarding the chlamydial infections. The significance of chlamydial infection in farm animals (Esmaeili et al.,2015, Ebadi et al., 2014), birds (Madani et al., 2013, Ghorbanpoor et al., 2015, Tatari et al., 2016) and human (Hashemi et al., 2009, Ghazvini et al., 2012) have been previously shown in Iran.

Di Ianni et al., (2015) were unable to prove a cause-effect correlation between the presence of chlamydia and the disease situation in reptiles. Furthermore, the clinical manifestations of Chlamydia infection in the investigated cases were low. The necropsy was not performed in the current survey and consequently internal organs were not submitted for thorough investigation. While real time PCR has a promising sensitivity and specificity for the detection of bacterial infectious agents, Kabeya et al., (2015) indicated some limitations in the application of these molecular methods. It is recommended for future studies to apply two or more concurrent PCR methods to get a more reliable result.

A review on previous studies in which a high number of infections were reported revealed that almost all specimens in those studies were collected from a limited captive population or even a single population in a unique location. In contrast, the samples of the current study were mostly collected from pet reptiles which were owned by different owners and also were kept individually at home. The higher infection rate in other studies might be correlated with those specific captive populations. It is a common practice in pet markets of Iran to treat the animals with different antibiotics. Previous treatment with different antibiotics could decrease the infection rate. Unfortunately, there was no recorded history of antibiotic administration in our cases. However, larger sample size, different sampling methods especially collecting internal organs during necropsy, and applying various detection tests can increase our understanding about reptile chlamydiosis in Iran.

Acknowledgments

With best regard of our colleagues and staff of laboratory.

References

Andersen, A., Vanrompay, D. (2003) Avian chlamydiosis (psittacosis, ornithosis). Poult Dis J. 61: 863-79.

Andreoletti, O., Budka, H., Buncic, S., Colin, P., Collins, J.D., De Koeijer, A. (2007) Public health risks involved in the human consumption of reptile meat scientific opinion of the panel on biological hazards. EFSA J. 583: 1-64.

Black, C.M. (1997) Current methods of laboratory diagnosis of *Chlamydia trachomatis* infections. Clin Microbiol Rev. 10: 160-84.

Bodetti, T.J., Jacobson, E., Wan, C., Hafner, L., Pospischil, A., Rose, K. (2002) Molecular evidence to support the expansion of the hostrange of *Chlamydophila pneumoniae* to include reptiles as well as humans, horses, koalas and amphibians. Syst Appl Microbiol. 25: 146-52.

Boman, J., Gaydos, C.A., Quinn, T.C. (1999) Molecular diagnosis of *Chlamydia pneumoniae* infection. J Clin Microbiol. 37: 3791-9.

Corsaro, D., Venditti, D. (2004) Emerging chlamydial infections. Crit Rev Microbiol. 30: 75-106.

Darvish, J., Rastegar-Pouyani, E. (2012) Biodiversity conservation of reptiles and mammals in the Khorasan provinces, Northeast of Iran. Prog Biol Sci. 2: 95-109.

Di Ianni, F., Dodi, P., Cabassi, C., Pelizzone, I., Sala, A., Cavirani, S., Parmigiani, E., Quintavalla, F., Taddei, S. (2015) Conjunctival flora of clinically normal and diseased turtles and tortoises. Vet Res. 11: 91.

Ebadi, A., Moosakhani, F., Jamshidian, M. (2014) Phylogenetic analysis of *Chlamydia abortus* isolated from fetus aborted ewes of Alborz Province. Bull Environ Pharmacol Life Sci. 4: 122-126.

Ebani, V., Fratini, F. (2005) Bacterial zoonoses among domestic reptiles. Ann Fac Med Vet. 58: 85-91.

Ehricht, R., Slickers, P., Goellner, S., Hotzel, H., Sachse, K. (2006) Optimized DNA microarray assay allows detection and genotyping of single PCR-amplifiable target copies. Mol Cell Probes. 20: 60-3.

Esmaeili, H.R., Teimory, A., Khosravi, A.R. (2008) A note on the biodiversity of Ghadamgah spring-stream system in Fars province, southwest Iran. Iran J Anim Biosyst. 3: 15-23.

Esmaeili, H., Bolourchi, M., Mokhber-Dezfouli, M. (2015) Seroprevalence of *Chlamydia abortus* infection in sheep and goats in Iran. Iran J Vet Res. 9: 73-77.

Frutos, M.C., Monetti, M.S., Re, V.E., Cuffini, C.G. (2014) Molecular evidence of *Chlamydophila pneumoniae* infection in reptiles in Argentina. Rev Argent Microbiol. 46: 45-48.

Frutos, M.C., Monetti, M.S., Vaulet, L.G., Cadario, M.E., Fermepin, M.R. (2015) Genetic diversity of Chlamydia among captive birds from central Argentina. Avian Pathol. 44: 50-6.

Gaydos, C.A., Quinn, T.C., Eiden, J.J. (1992) Identification of *Chlamydia pneumoniae* by DNA amplification of the 16S rRNA gene. J Clin Microbiol. 30: 796-800.

Ghazvini, K., Ahmadnia, H., Ghanaat, J. (2012) Frequency of *Chlamydia trachomatis* among male patients with urethritis in northeast of Iran detected by polymerase chain reaction. Saudi J Kidney Dis Transpl. 23: 316-320.

Ghorbanpoor, M., Bakhtiari, N., Mayahi, M., Moridveisi, H. (2015) Detection of *Chlamydophila psittaci* from pigeons by polymerase chain reaction in Ahvaz. Iran J Vet. 7: 18-22.

Hashemi, F.B., Pourakbari, B., Yazdi, J.Z. (2009) Frequency of *Chlamydia trachomatis* in women with cervicitis in Tehran, Iran, Infect Dis Obstet Gynecol. 4: 67014.

Hotzel, H., Blahak, S., Diller, R., Sachse, K. (2005) Evidence of infection in tortoises by Chlamydia-like organisms that are genetically distinct from known Chlamydiaceae species. Vet Res Commun. 29: 71-80.

Homer, B., Jacobson, E., Schumacher, J., Scherba, G. (1994) Chlamydiosis in mariculture-reared green sea turtles (*Chelonia mydas*). Vet Pathol. 31: 1-7.

Huchzermeyer, F., Langelet, E., Putterill, J. (2008) An outbreak of chlamydiosis in farmed Indopacific crocodiles (*Crocodylus porosus*). J S Afr Vet Ass. 79: 99-100.

Jacobson, E.R., Heard, D., Andersen, A. (2004) Identification of *Chlamydophila pneumoniae* in an emerald tree boa, Corallus caninus. J Vet Diagn Invest. 16: 153-4.

Jacobson, E.R., Gaskin, J.M., Mansell, J. (1989)

Chlamydial infection in puff adders (Bitis arietans). J Zool Wild Med. 20: 364-9.

Jacobson, G.F., Autry, A.M., Kirby, R.S., Liverman, E.M., Motley, R.U. (2001) A randomized controlled trial comparing amoxicillin and azithromycin for the treatment of *Chlamydia trachomatis* in pregnancy. Am J Obstet Gynecol. 184: 1352-6.

Jones, K. E., N. G., Patel, M. A., Levy, A., Storeygard, D., Balk, J. L., Gittleman, Daszak, P. (2008) Global trends in emerging infectious diseases. Nature. 451: 990-993

Kabeya, H., Sato, S., Maruyama, S. (2015) Prevalence and characterization of Chlamydia DNA in zoo animals in Japan. Microbiol Immunol. 59: 507-15.

Krawiec, M., Piasecki, T., Wieliczko, A. (2015) Prevalence of *Chlamydia psittaci* and other *Chlamydia* Species in wild birds in Poland. Vector Borne Zoonotic Dis. 15: 652-5.

Mendall, M., Carrington, D., Strachan, D., Patel, P., Molineaux, N., Levi, J. (1995) *Chlamydia pneumoniae*: risk factors for seropositivity and association with coronary heart disease. J Infec. 30: 121-8.

Madani, A., Peighambari, M. (2013) PCR-based diagnosis, molecular characterization and detection of atypical strains of avian *Chlamydia psittaci* in companion and wild birds. Avian Pathol. 42: 38-44.

Matsui, T., Nakashima, K., Ohyama, T., Kobayashi, J., Arima, Y., Kishimoto, T. (2008) An outbreak of psittacosis in a bird park in Japan. Epidemiol Infect. 136: 492-5.

Mackie, J., Gillett, A. K., Palmieri , C., Feng, T., Higgins, D.P. (2016) Pneumonia due to *Chlamydia pecorum* in a Koala (Phascolarctos cinereus). J Comp Pathol. S0021-9975(16) 30101-3.

Myers, G.S., Mathews, S.A., Eppinger, M., Mitchell, C., O'Brien, K.K., White, O.R., Benahmed, F., Brunham, R.C., Read, T.D.,

Ravel, J., Bavoil, P.M., Timms, P. (2009) Evidence that human *Chlamydia pneumoniae* was zoonotically acquired. J Bacteriol. 191: 7225-33.

Pospisil, L., Canderle, J. (2004) *Chlamydia* (Chlamydophila) *pneumoniae* in animals: a review. Vet Med. 49: 129-34.

Roulis, E., Polkinghorne, A., Timms, P. (2013) *Chlamydia pneumoniae*: modern insights into an ancient pathogen. Trends Microbiol. 2: 120-128.

Sachse, K., Hotzel, H,. Slickers, P., Ellinger, T., Ehricht, R. (2005) DNA microarray-based detection and identification of Chlamydia and Chlamydophila spp. Mol Cell Probes. 19: 41-50.

Soldati, G., Lu, Z., Vaughan, L., Polkinghorne, A., Zimmermann, D., Huder, J. (2004) Detection of mycobacteria and chlamydiae in granulomatous inflammation of reptiles: a retrospective study. Vet Pathol. 41: 388-97.

Stuen, S., Longbottom, D. (2011) Treatment and control of chlamydial and rickettsial infections in sheep and goats. Vet Clin North Am Food Anim Prac. 27: 213-33.

Suchland, R., Geisler, W., Stamm, W.E. (2003) Methodologies and cell lines used for antimicrobial susceptibility testing of *Chlamydia* spp. Antimicrob Agents Chemother. 47: 636-42.

Tatari, Z., Peighamabri, S.M., Madani, S.A. (2016) Detection of Chlamydial infection in Iranian turkey flocks. Iran J Vet Med. 10: 83-90.

Taylor-Brown, A., Rüegg, S., Polkinghorne, A., Borel, N. (2015) Characterisation of *Chlamydia pneumoniae* and other novel chlamydial infections in captive snakes. Vet microbiol. 178: 88-93.

Yucesan, C., Sriram, S. (2001) *Chlamydia pneumoniae* infection of the central nervous system. Curr Opin Neurol. 14: 355-9.

18

Evaluate *Toxocara canis* excretory-secretory antigens in experimental allergic encephalomyelitis (EAE)

Borhani Zarandi, M.[1], Hoseini, S.H.[1*], Jalousion, F.[1], Etebar, F.[1], Vojgani, M.[2]

[1]Department of Parasitology, Faculty of Veterinary Medicine, Tehran University, Tehran, Iran

[2]Department of Immunology and Biology, School of Medicine, Tehran University of Medical Sciences, Tehran, Iran

Key words:

disability score, EAE gene expression, experimental allergic encephalomyelitis, immune system in EAE *Toxocara canis* excretory-secretory antigens

Correspondence

Hoseini, S.H.

Department of Parasitology,

Faculty of Veterinary Medicine,

Tehran University, Tehran, Iran

Email: hhoseini@ut.ac.ir

Abstract:

BACKGROUND: *Toxocara canis* is the most prevalent intestinal roundworm of canid species. **OBJECTIVES:** This study aims to evaluate the effects of *Toxocara canis* excretory-secretory antigens (TcES Ag) on modulating the immune system in Experimental Allergic Encephalomyelitis (EAE) model. **METHODS:** Adult worms of *T.canis* were collected from dogs to obtain excretory-secretory antigens. Female C57BL/6 mice were divided to four groups (5 mice in each) including: group 1 (MOG +TcES Ag), 2 (MOG), 3 (normal) and 4 (TcES Ag). EAE was induced in groups 1 and 2 using myelin oligodendrocyte glycoprotein peptide. Before EAE induction, TcES Ag was injected in group 1. Twenty-nine after EAE induction, mice spleens were removed. Mononuclear cells were cultured and used for RNA extraction.Real Time PCR was performed to evaluate RNA expression levels of T-bet (Th1 lineage-specific transcription factor), GATA-3 (Th2 transcription factor), and FOXP3 (Treg transcription factor). **RESULTS:** Our results indicated the clinical signs (disability score) of mice in group 1 were decreased significantly as compared to the control group. Gene expression of T-bet in the TcES Ag treatment group were noticeably diminished compared to MOG and normal group. The expression of GATA-3 gene in group 1 was lower than that in group 2. **CONCLUSIONS:** It seems that the TcES Ag may reduce disability score in multiple sclerosis EAE model, and other recombinant antigens should be examined.

Introduction

According to the "hygiene hypothesis", lack of serious infection in children leads to defects in the immune system. It has been indicated that exposure to infectious agents such as bacteria, viruses, and parasites, especially in childhood, can reduce the risk of autoimmune diseases (Osada and Kanazawa 2010). A number of previous investigations support the hygiene hypothesis, assuming that infections can have a protective role rather than inducing or accelerating autoimmune diseases such as MS (Bach 2002). Worms are known as the most important factors in modulation of the immune response (Maizels, et al., 2004). In vitro models have shown that worms and their products interfere with the proliferation of lymphocytes and decreases in B lymphocytes, resulting in IgE production and activation of macrophages type 2 modulators.

Chronic infection of worms can modulate the immune response to the Th2, T reg, and Th2-related cytokine, including IL4, IL5, and IL13. Moreover, safety regulation in response to chronic infection is caused by worms and leads to reduction of the incidence of autoimmune diseases and allergies (Chow et al., 2000; Harnett 2006; Smits et al., 2010; Daniłowicz-Luebert, O'Regan et al., 2011; Cooke 2012; Elliott Weinstock 2012). Based on the theory, it has been demonstrated that worms' products have potential therapeutic effects for treatment of allergies as well as inflammatory and autoimmune diseases (Van Riet et al., 2007).

The prevalence of allergic diseases and autoimmune diseases such as multiple sclerosis is rising in developed and developing countries. Multiple sclerosis is an inflammatory disease of the central nervous system (a related-myelin membrane destruction) (Goldenberg 2012; Hafler 2012). In mouse models of autoimmune diseases, the presence of helminthes infections has been reported to be associated with disease resistance, and the infection by eggs and adult worm of *Schistosoma mansoni* has been indicated to inhibit the development of type 1 diabetes(Cooke, et al., 1999; El-Wakil, et al., 2002; Zaccone, et al., 2003).

Moreover, the previous studies have shown therapeutic effects of parasitic worms including nematodes (*Heligmosomoides polygyrus* and *Trichinella spiralis*), trematodes (*Schistosoma mansoni*, *Schistosoma japonicom*, and *Fasciola hepatica*), and cestodes (*Taenia crassiceps*) in the Experimental Allergic Encephalomyelitis Mod-

el (Sewell et al., 2003; Zheng et al., 2008; Walsh et al., 2009; Gruden-Movsesijan et al., 2010; Wilson et al., 2010; Kuijk et al., 2012; Zhu et al., 2012).

In developed and developing countries allergic and autoimmune diseases like multiple sclerosis are increasing due to reduced exposure of infectious agents.

Recently, it has been shown that some products of parasites can be effective in modulating immune response. Therefore, evidence reveals that helminthes infections are associated with reduced severity of autoimmune disease in animal models. It has been suggested that helminthes infection or products play an effective role in the course of autoimmune pathology in both spontaneous and induced models of human autoimmune diseases (Khan et al., 2002;La Flamme et al., 2003;Walsh, Brady et al., 2009;Wilson, Taylor et al., 2010). In the present study, the effects of TcES Ag on experimental models of autoimmune diseases are evaluated to understand the therapeutic effects of this antigen.

Materials and Methods

Sample collection and antigen preparation: *T.canis* adult worms were collected from dogs, rinsed with salt, and cultured in RPMI-1640 which contained 100u/ml penicillin, 100u/ml streptomycin, and 0.25μg amphotericin B (Page et al., 1991).

T.canis was kept in the medium for 5 days at 30°C and 5% CO_2, and the culture medium was collected every 24 hours as a source of excretory-secretory antigens.

Protein measurement and concentration

TcES Ag were concentrated using dialysis bags (cut off 12) and were measured by Bradford method (Bradford 1976).

Injection of the antigen to rabbits: TcES Ag (500 µl RPMI-1640 containing 30 µg Ag) were subcutaneously injected with complete adjuvant (1:1) to the rabbit (10 weeks-old and male). Two boosters (250 µl RPMI-1640 containing 10 µg Ag) with incomplete adjuvant were also injected (1:1) 10 and 20 days after the first injection. Furthermore, the sera were separated 2 days after the third injection. Western blot was performed to determine immunogenicity of antigens.

TcES Ag injection into C57BL/6 mice: The female C57Bl/6 mice (10 weeks old) were classified into four groups as follows (5 mice in each group).

In the first group, excretory-secretory antigens of *T.canis* with adjuvants were subcutaneously injected (6µg antigen) to mice, and booster injection with incomplete adjuvant was performed after 7 days (3µg antigen). In the second group, the distilled water was injected to mice. In the third group, mice were used without injection of TcES Ag, but distilled water was injected (normal group). Seven days later, injection with distilled water was repeated. In the fourth group, mice were assigned as the control group and 250 ml of excretory-secretory antigens of *T.canis* with complete adjuvant (6µg antigen) were subcutaneously injected, and 125 ml antigen incomplete adjuvant was used for injection after 7 days (3µg antigen).

EAE induction and scoring: In the first and second groups, mice were injected subcutaneously with 300µg myelin oligodendrocyte glycoprotein peptide35-55 (MOG35-55). Two hours later, 100 ng of Pertussis Toxin were intra-peritoneally injected, which was repeated 24 hours later according to the manufacturer's protocol.

All animals were checked daily for clinical signs, and the weighting and scoring were as follows: grade 0, no abnormality; grade 0.5, tip of tail is limp; grade 1, limp tail; grade 1.5, limp tail and hind leg inhibition; grade 2.0, limp tail and weakness of hind legs; grade 2.5, limp tail and dragging of hind legs; grade 3.0, limp tail and complete paralysis of hind legs; grade 3.5, limp tail and complete paralysis of hind legs and mouse is moving around the cage, but when placed on its side, is unable to right itself; grade 4.0, limp tail, complete hind leg and partial front leg paralysis; grade 4.5, complete hind and partial front leg paralysis, no movement around the cage; grade 5.0, the mouse is spontaneously rolling in the cage or death (scoring was performed according to the manufacturer's protocol).

Cell culture: Twenty-nine days after induction of EAE, mice spleens were removed.

Mononuclear cells in culture medium RPMI-1640 (containing 10%FBS, 100 units of penicillin, streptomycin, 2ml Glutamine, and 25 ml Hepes) to 3×10^6 cells/ml were cultured in each well. 25µg of antigens of *T.canis* were added to the medium, and the culture was collected after 72 hours of incubation at 37°C and 5% CO_2 and subsequently centrifuged at 10,000rpm. Furthermore, and the precipitate was separated and stored at -70°C until use.

Real Time PCR: RNA was extracted from cultured mononuclear cells by the DNA binding column, and 8µl of RNA was used for reverse transcriptase. Eva green jumpstart Taq Ready mix (5 X HOT FIRE-Pol®EvaGreen®qPCR Mix Plus) in a final volume of 20µl each sample was submitted to 36 cycles in a real time thermal cycler (ABI) according to the manufacturer's protocol.

Sequences for our target genes were βActin (Forward: ATGCTCCCCGGGCT-GTAT Reverse: CATAGGAGTCCTTCT-GACCCATTC), T-bet (Forward: GC-CAGGGAACCGCTTATATG Reverse: AACTTCCTGGCGCATCCA), GATA-3 (Forward: CAGAACCGGCCCCTTAT-CA Reverse: CATTAGGAGAGGTGT-GAAAGC), and FOXP3 (Forward: GCAG-GGCAGCTAGGTATCTGTAG Reverse: TCGGGAGATCCCCTTTGTCTATC). Gene expression was normalized to the expression of the constitutively expressed gene βActin.

Results

Western blot is a rapid sensitive technique that uses antibody for the specific detection of proteins. This method showed that our T.cES antigen extracted from adult worm had high quality.

Western blot of TcES antigens with anti-TcES rabbit: The western blot using anti-TcES rabbit serum is shown in Fig. 1. The recognized immunogenic bands of the T.c ES antigen were 57, 35, 80, 60, and 180 KDa.

Scoring in EAE: Our results indicated that the clinical signs (disability score) in the treatment group (MOG +TcES) of female C57BL/6 mice significantly decreased when compared with the control group (Fig. 2). In addition, the average weight was lower in the control group (MOG) as compared with TcES Ag treatment group(MOG +TcES) (Fig. 3).

Immune response results: Real time PCR results showed that the gene expression T-bet in the treatment group 1 noticeably decreased compared to MOG and nor-

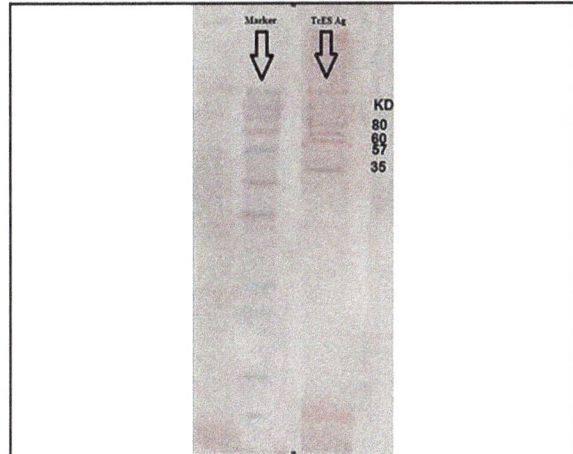

Figure 1. Western blot analysis of TcES antigens with anti-TcES rabbit.

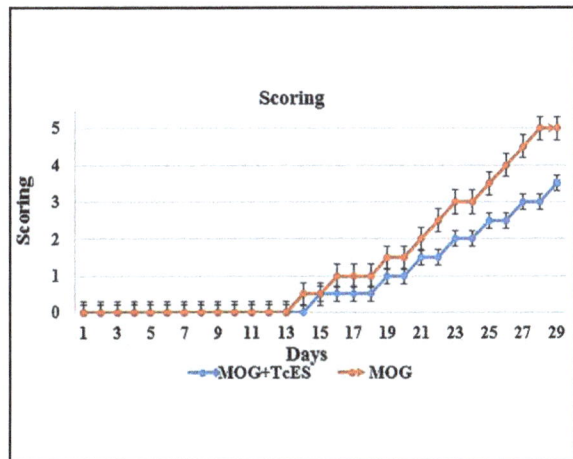

Figure 2. Average score disability of group1 (MOG +TcES Ag) and group2 (MOG) in EAE model: disability score of treatment group (MOG +TcES Ag) markedly decreased when compared with the MOG group.

mal groups.

The gene expression of FOXP3 and GATA-3 in TcES Ag challenge group (group 1) was not significantly different from those of the other groups (Fig. 4). Furthermore, the expression of GATA-3 gene in group 1 was lower than that in group 2.

Discussion

Helminthes are known as the most crucial factor in modulating immune system (Maizels et al., 2004). It has been demonstrated that helminthes can modify the host

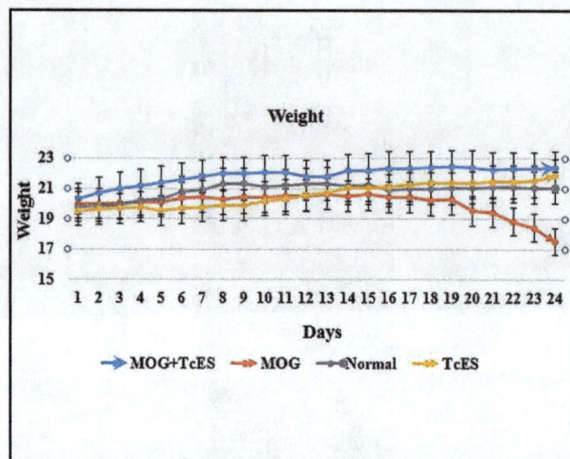

Figure 3. Clinical signs of group 1 (MOG +TcES Ag) and group 2 (MOG) in EAE model: the average weight declined in the control group (MOG) in comparison withTcES Ag treatment group (MOG +TcES Ag).

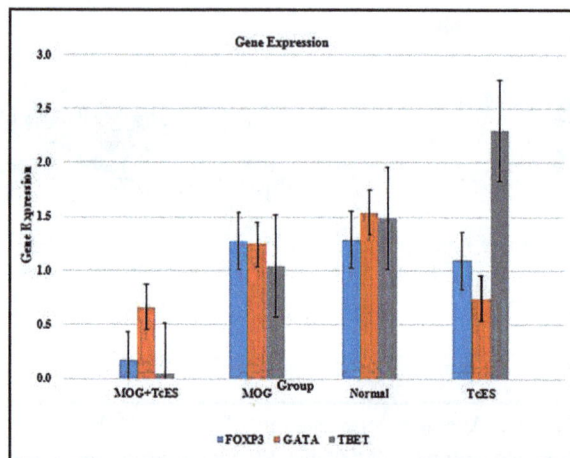

Figure 4. Real time PCR findings showed that the gene expression of TcES Ag T-bet in the treatment group 1 strongly diminished compared with MOG and normal groups.

immune system. At least 20 immune modulatory mechanisms are expressed by worms, including the production of Treg cytokine (Fleming et al., 2011).

Parasitic helminthes is considered as a potential treatment for a wide range of diseases like inflammatory bowel disease, autoimmune diseases, and asthma. Many experimental studies have shown that infection by worms has a protective effect against autoimmune diseases in animal models (colitis, arthritis, and diabetes) and allergies in human (Osada 2010).

In experimental mouse models with diabetes, it has been indicated that immunization with *Taenia crasiseps* metasestod can reduce the inflammation and lead to significant inhibition of improving clinical score. Therefore, soluble worm products (soluble egg antigen and soluble worm) followed by homogenized and live worm are used as therapeutic agents for a wide variety of diseases such as inflammatory bowel disorders, autoimmune diseases, and asthma (Kuijk et al., 2012).

Moreover, treatment with live worms is not desirable for most people. It is reported that worms' soluble products (*Schistosoma mansoni* eggs injected i.p) play an important role in regulating the immune system (Pearce 2002; Harn et al., 2009; Andersen et al., 2009; Everts et al., 2010; Van Die 2010).

Several researches have confirmed that the expression of FOXP3 gene has increased in infected mice with the gastrointestinal nematode parasite (Finney et al., 2007; Mc-Sorley et al., 2008; Rausch, et al., 2008).

Previous studies indicated that the soluble products of intestinal helminthes suppress Th1 and Th17, which are important in the pathogenesis of autoimmune and inflammatory diseases (Kuijk et al., 2012).

In vitro studies have shown that *Trichuris Suis* and *Trichinella spiralis* products can suppress the secretion of proinflammatory cytokines such as TNF (Van Vliet et al. 2007).

In the present study, TcES Ag was injected into mice and then EAE was induced.

Our study showed that the expression of T-bet gene decreased in the group 1, reducing the number of Th1 cells and the disability score.

In this study, the expression of GATA-3 gene diminished in the group 1, suggesting that the number of Th2 cells was reduced. The minimum number of parasite antigens should be used for regulation of the immunemodulatory system, because increase of Th2 cells and their cytokines led to adverse reactions (allergic disease).

Jose et al. reported that expression of T reg cells declined in EAE model (Reyes et al., 2011). In this research, expression of FOXP3 gene did not increase, suggesting that the number of T reg cells did not increase either.

Optimization of the antigen in the worm therapy is necessary and can solve the limitation of using helminthes antigens for helminthes therapy.In conclusion, it seems that the TcES Ag may reduce disability score in EAE model, and other recombinant antigens can be examined independently.

Ethics committee: The present study was confirmed by the local ethical board in Faculty of Veterinary Medicine, Tehran University.

Acknowledgements

This study was supported by grant number: 93016151 from Iran National Science Foundation. The authors would like to thank Ms. Narges Amininia for her close collaboration in this study.

References

Bach, J.F. (2002) The effect of infections on susceptibility to autoimmune and allergic diseases. N Engl J Med. 347: 911-920.

Bradford, M.M. (1976) A rapid and sensitive method for the quantitation of microgram quantities of protein utilizing the principle of protein-dye binding. Anal Biochem. 72: 248-254.

Chow, S.C., Brown, A., Pritchard, D. (2000) The human hookworm pathogen Necator amer-

icanus induces apoptosis in T lymphocytes. Parasite Immunol. 22: 29-37.

Cooke, A. (2012) Parasitic worms and inflammatory disease. Curr Opin Rheumatol. 24: 394-400.

Cooke, A., Tonks, P., Jones, F.M., O'shea, H., Hutchings, P., Fulford, A.J. (1999) Infection with Schistosoma mansoni prevents insulin dependent diabetes mellitus in non-obese diabetic mice. Parasite Immunol. 21: 169-176.

Daniłowicz-Luebert, E., Oregan, N.L., Steinfelder, S., Hartmann, S. (2011) Modulation of specific and allergy-related immune responses by helminths. J Biomed Biotechnol. 10: 155-1173.

El-Wakil, H., Aboushousha, T., El Haddad, O., Gamil, N., Mansour,T., El-Said, H. (2002) Effect of schistosoma mansoni egg deposition on multiple low doses streptozotocin induced insulin dependent diabetes. J Egypt Soc Parasitol. 32: 987-1002.

Elliott, D.E., Weinstock, J.V. (2012) Helminth-host immunological interactions: prevention and control of immune-mediated diseases. Ann N Y Acad Sci. 1247: 83-96.

Everts, B., Smits, H.H. Hokke, C.H., Yazdanbakhsh, M. (2010) Helminths and dendritic cells: sensing and regulating via pattern recognition receptors, Th2 and Treg responses. Eur J Immunol. 40: 1525-1537.

Finney, C.A., Taylor, M.D., Wilson, M.S., Maizels., R.M. (2007) Expansion and activation of CD4+ CD25+ regulatory T cells in Heligmosomoides polygyrus infection. Eur J Immunol. 37: 1874-1886.

Goldenberg, M.M. (2012) Multiple sclerosis review. P T. 37: 175.

Gruden-Movsesijan, A., Ilic, N., Mostarica-Stojkovic, M., StosiC-Grujicic, S., Milic, M., Sofronic-Milosavljevic, L. (2010) Mechanisms of modulation of experimental autoimmune encephalomyelitis by chronic Trichinella spi-

ralis infection in Dark Agouti rats. Parasite Immunol. 32: 450-459.

Harn, D.A., McDonald, J., Atochina, O., Da'dara, A.A. (2009) Modulation of host immune responses by helminth glycans. Immunol Rev. 230: 247-257.

Harnett, W., Harnett, M. (2006) Molecular basis of worm-induced immunomodulation. Parasite Immunol. 28: 535-543.

Khan, W., Blennerhasset, P., Varghese, A., Chowdhury, S., Omsted, P., Deng, Y., Collins, S. (2002) Intestinal nematode infection ameliorates experimental colitis in mice. Infect Immun 70: 5931-5937.

Kuijk, L.M., Klaver, E.G., Kooij, G., van der Pol, S.M., Heijnen, P., Bruijns, S.P., Kringel, H., Pinelli, E., Kraal, G., De Vries, H.E. (2012) Soluble helminth products suppress clinical signs in murine experimental autoimmune encephalomyelitis and differentially modulate human dendritic cell activation. Mol Immunol. 51: 210-218.

La Flamme, A.C., Ruddenklau, K., Bäckström, B.T. (2003) Schistosomiasis decreases central nervous system inflammation and alters the progression of experimental autoimmune encephalomyelitis. Infect Immun. 71: 4996-5004.

Maizels, R.M., Balic, A., Gomez-Escobar, N., Nair, M., Taylor, M.D., Allen, J.E. (2004) Helminth parasites-masters of regulation. Immunol Rev. 201: 89-116.

McSorley, H.J., Harcus, Y.M., Murray, J., Taylor, M.D., Maizels, R.M. (2008) Expansion of Foxp3+ regulatory T cells in mice infected with the filarial parasite *Brugia malayi*. J Immunol. 181: 6456-6466.

Nylander, A., Hafler, D.A. (2012) Multiple sclerosis. J Clin Invest 122: 1180-1188.

Osada, Y., Kanazawa. (2010) Parasitic helminths: new weapons against immunological disorders. J Bioed Biotechnol. 2010: 743758

Page, A., Richards, D., Lewis, J., Omar, H., Maizels, R. (1991) Comparison of isolates and species of Toxocara and Toxascaris by biosynthetic labelling of somatic and ES proteins from infective larvae. Parasitology. 103: 451-464.

Pearce, E.J., MacDonald, A.S. (2002) The immunobiology of schistosomiasis. Nat Rev Immunol. 2: 499-511.

Rausch, S., Huehn, J., Kirchhoff, D., Rzepecka, J., Schnoeller, C., Pillai, S., Loddenkemper, C., Scheffold, A., Hamann, A., Lucius, R. (2008) Functional analysis of effector and regulatory T cells in a parasitic nematode infection. Infect Immun. 76: 1908-1919.

Reyes, J.L., Espinoza-Jimenez, A.F., Gonzalez, M.I., Verdin, L., Terrazas, L.I. (2011) *Taenia crassiceps* infection abrogates experimental autoimmune encephalomyelitis. Cell Immunol. 267: 77-87.

Sewell, D., Qing, Z., Reinke, E., Elliot, D., Weinstock, J., Sandor, M., Fabry, Z. (2003) Immunomodulation of experimental autoimmune encephalomyelitis by helminth ova immunization. Int Immunol. 15: 59-69.

Smits, H.H., Everts, B., Hartgers, F.C., Yazdanbakhsh, M. (2010) Chronic helminth infections protect against allergic diseases by active regulatory processes. Curr Allergy Asthma Rep. 10: 3-12.

Steinfelder, S., Andersen, J.F., Cannons, J.L., Feng, C.G., Joshi, M., Dwyer, D., Caspar, P., Schwartzberg, P.L., Sher, A., Jankovic, D. (2009) The major component in schistosome eggs responsible for conditioning dendritic cells for Th2 polarization is a T2 ribonuclease (omega-1) J Exp Med. 206: 1681-1690.

Van Die, I., Cummings, R.D. (2010) Glycan gimmickry by parasitic helminths: a strategy for modulating the host immune response. Glycobiology. 20: 2-12.

Van Liempt, E., van Vliet, S.J., Engering, A.,

Vallejo, J.J.G., Bank, C.M., Sanchez-35. Hernandez, M., van Kooyk, Y., van Die, I. (2007) *Schistosoma mansoni* soluble egg antigens are internalized by human dendritic cells through multiple C-type lectins and suppress TLR-induced dendritic cell activation. Mol Immunol. 44: 2605-2615.

Van Riet, E., Hartgers, F.C., Yazdanbakhsh, M. (2007) Chronic helminth infections induce immunomodulation: consequences and mechanisms. Immunobiology. 212: 475-490.

Walsh, K.P., Brady, M.T., Finlay, C.M., Boon, L., Mills, K.H. (2009) Infection with a helminth parasite attenuates autoimmunity through TGF-β-mediated suppression of Th17 and Th1 responses. J Immunol. 183: 1577-1586.

Wilson, M.S., Taylor, M.D., O'Gorman, M.T., Balic, A., Barr, T.A., Filbey, K., Anderton, S.M., Maizels, R.M. (2010) Helminth-induced CD19+ CD23hi B cells modulate experimental allergic and autoimmune inflammation. Eur J Immunol. 40: 1682-1696.

Zaccone, P., Fehervari, Z., Jones, F.M., Sidobre, S., Kronenberg, M., Dunne, D.W., Cooke, A. (2003) *Schistosoma mansoni* antigens modulate the activity of the innate immune response and prevent onset of type 1 diabetes. Eur J Immunol. 33: 1439-1449.

Zheng, X., Hu, X., Zhou, G., Lu, Z., Qiu, W., Bao, J., Dai, Y. (2008) Soluble egg antigen from *Schistosoma japonicum* modulates the progression of chronic progressive experimental autoimmune encephalomyelitis via Th2-shift response. J Neuroimmunol. 194: 107-114.

Zhu, B., Trikudanathan, S. , Zozulya, A.L., Sandoval-Garcia, C., Kennedy, J.K., Atochina, O., Norberg, T., Castagner, B., Seeberger, P., Fabry, Z. (2012) Immune modulation by Lacto-N-fucopentaose III in experimental autoimmune encephalomyelitis. Clin Immunol. 142: 351-361.

19

A survey on detection of coronavirus in neonatal calf diarrhea in dairy farms of Iran

Mohebbi, M.R.[1], Lotfollahzadeh, S.[1*], Madadgar, O.[2], Mokhber Dezfouli, M.[1]

[1]*Department of Internal Medicine, Faculty of Veterinary Medicine, University of Tehran, Tehran, Iran*
[2]*Department of Microbiology, Faculty of Veterinary Medicine, University of Tehran, Tehran, Iran*

Key words:

bovine coronavirus, calf diarrhea, dairy farms, fever RT-PCR

Correspondence

Lotfollahzadeh, S.
Department of Internal Medicine, Faculty of Veterinary Medicine, University of Tehran, Tehran, Iran

Email: samdlzadeh@ut.ac.ir

Abstract:

BACKGROUND: Bovine coronavirus (BCoV) is a primary cause of neonatal calf diarrhea worldwide, and is also associated with acute diarrhea in adult cattle during the winter season, resulting in heavy economic losses to both dairy and beef industry throughout the world. **OBJECTIVES:** The objective of the present study was to screen the fecal samples for BCoV collected from diarrhea from six geographic regions of Iran, with the aim of deepening the knowledge of BCoV prevalence and epidemiology in Iran. **METHODS:** 194 fecal samples from diarrheic calves up to one-month of age, based on the geographic area were collected. Samples from all the cases were screened for the presence of BCoV by commercially available ELISA kit. Furthermore, all samples were subjected to RT-PCR for confirmation. **RESULTS:** ELISA examination revealed that 7.2 % of taken samples were positive. All positive samples in ELISA were also positive in RT-PCR. All samples from northwest, northeast, and west, were negative. The average age of positive calves was nine days. The average stool scores in positive samples and negative samples were 2.5 and 2.1 respectively. 71/4 % of positive samples had fever. **CONCLUSIONS:** The results of the present study showed that the occurrence of BCoV in stool samples of diarrheic calves in dairy farms of Iran is lower than the other reports in the world.

Introduction

Bovine coronavirus (BCoV) is an important livestock pathogen with a high prevalence worldwide. The virus causes diarrhea and respiratory disease in neonatal calves and winter dysentery in adult cattle. These diseases result in substantial economic losses and reduced animal welfare (Boileau and Kapil, 2010; Oma et al., 2016). It has been found that in beef calves, BCoV infection was more frequent among calves up to 30 days of age (Quinn et al., 2002; Afshari et al., 2012).

Serological surveys indicate that approximately 90% of the worldwide cattle population has antibodies (Abs) against BCoV (Boka et al., 2015). A number of researchers showed wild ruminants, dogs, and horses harbor similar strains of BCoV which is transmissible to cattle and vice versa (Barros et al., 2013; Saif et al., 2010).

Inter-herd transmission is possible either directly via import of live animals (Decaro et al., 2008, Fulton et al., 2011), or indirectly via contaminated personnel or equipment (Mee et al., 2012). Measures to prevent the virus spread between herds must be based upon knowledge of viral shedding, the potential for transmission to susceptible animals and the role of protective immunity (Oma et al., 2016). In two experimental studies, infected calves were not protected against reinfection with a different BCoV strain three weeks after the first challenge, but did not develop clinical signs (Cho KO et al., 2011; El-Kanawati et al., 1996). BCoV is transmitted via the fecal-oral or respiratory route. The virus infects epithelial cells of the respiratory tract (the nasal turbinates, trachea and lungs) and the intestines (the villi and crypts of the small and large intestine) (Park et al., 2007, Saif et al., 1986).

Three antigenic groups of coronaviruses have been established, and all BCoV strains belonged to the subgroup initially designated as 2a (Hasoksuz et al., 2008). The International Committee for Taxonomy Viruses (ICTV) has proposed a revision of the family Coronaviridae to create a new subfamily, Coronavirinae, that includes the Alpha, Beta and Gammacoronavirus genera. Following this new suggested taxonomy, BCoV belongs to the Betacoronavirus genus, cluster within the Coronavirinae subfamily, Coronaviridae family and the order Nidovirales (http://ictvonline.org/virusTaxonomy.asp).

The virus genome is comprised of single stranded nonsegmented positive-sense RNA (32 kb) associated to the nucleoprotein (N) and forming a nucleocapsid with helical symmetry (Clark, 1993). Viral particles are large (100-150 nm), pleomorphic and enveloped with four major structural proteins comprising a membrane (M) gly-

coprotein, an envelope (E) protein, a spike (S) glycoprotein and the hemagglutinin-esterase (HE) glycoprotein (Lai, 2001). It is interesting to note that the hemagglutinating activity of the HE from BCoVs strains is lower than the hemagglutinating activity of the S glycoprotein, which forms large spike-like projections in the viral envelope (Schultze et al., 1991).

Moreover, the S glycoprotein harbors domains responsible for receptor binding and induction of neutralizing antibodies, and is the most polymorphic viral protein among CoV species and also among strains of the same species. It is utilized for the molecular characterization of the isolates (Collins et al., 1982). The S glycoprotein consists of two subunits, S1 (N-terminal half) and S2 (C-terminal half). The S1 hypervariable region is useful to study the variability and evolution of this virus (Brandao et al., 2006; Hasoksuz et al., 2002).

BCoV has worldwide distribution and is reported from several countries (Jeong et al 2005; Khalili et al., 2006; Takiuchi et al 2006; Traven et al 2006; Gumusova et al 2007; Park et al 2007, Boileau and Kapil, 2010; Dash et al 2012; Ohlson et al., 2013; Mawatari et al., 2014; Ammar et al., 2014). However epidemiological data on BCOV in Iran is scarce.

Therefore, the aim of the present study was to screen the fecal samples for BCoV collected from clinical cases with the history of diarrhea from six geographic region of Iran covering 27 dairy farms.

Materials and Methods

Sample collection: Selected geographical regions for sampling, which were chosen based on density of dairy farms and climates, were northwest, northeast, south-west, south of Alborz Mountains, west, and central regions of Iran, (Table 1).

Totally 194 samples were collected from diarrheic neonatal calves up to one-month of age from May 2014 to June 2016. Samples were collected directly from the calves' rectum into sterile bottles and transferred to Virology laboratory of the Veterinary Faculty of University of Tehran on ice pack and stored at -18 °C. Sample's specifications such as: name of farm, province, geographic region, age, gender, stool consistency score, and rectal temperature were recorded.

BCoV antigen ELISA. An indirect antigen-capture ELISA kit employing monoclonal antibodies to BCoV was used as described by the manufacturer (IDEXX Rota-Corona-k99, USA).

Then the positive samples in ELISA were conducted on RT-PCR for confirmation.

Preparation of oligonucleotide primers. The oligonucleotide primers used in the RT-PCR were designed from the published sequence of N gene of Mebus strain (GenBank accession No.U00735). The sequences of primers are shown in Table 2, and the predicted RT-PCR product size was 407 bp (Table 2).

RNA extraction and RT-PCR. RNA from faeces was extracted using RNX-Plus solution for total RNA isolation (Sinaclon Bioscience, Iran) as instructed by the manufacturer. Then the complementary DNA (CDNA) was conducted by Maxime RT premix kit (Intron Biotechnology, Korea) as instructed by the manufacturer. The RT-PCR was conducted using the following procedure: in a tube 3 µL of CDNA sample was added to 2 µL of the Reverse and forward primers and 5.5 µL of nuclease-free water, and finally 12.5 µL master mix was

Table 1. Selected geographical regions for sampling, dairy farms and climates.

Region	Province	Sample numbers	Farms numb
northwest	Zanjan	10	1
northeast	Mashhad	30	4
northeast	Gorgan	10	2
south of Alborz	Tehran	40	6
south of Alborz	Varamin	10	1
south of Alborz	Qazvin-Alborz	20	5
Central	Qom	10	2
Central	Isfahan	30	1
Central	Saveh	12	1
west	Kermanshah	10	1
southwest	Ahvaz	12	3
Total	11	194	27

added to the solution. Then the solution waspreheated for 5 min at 94 °C, 40 cycles, including 45 seconds at 94 °C, 45 seconds at 52 °C, 1 min at 72 °C and, finally, 10 min incubation at 72 °C was applied. The PCR products were visualized on 1.5% agarose gel stained with ethidium bromide. PCR products of 407 bp were detected.

Results

ELISA examination of stool samples revealed that 14 samples (7.2%) out of 194 taken samples, which belonged to 10 dairy farms (37.03%) out of 27 farms were positive (7.2%). The positive samples were found in Tehran (three samples), Qom (two samples), Isfahan (three samples), Qazvin (two samples), Alborz (two samples), Saveh (one sample) and Ahvaz. The Zanjan, Mashhad, Gorgan, Varamin, and Kermanshah samples were negative. On the other hand, all samples from northwest, northeast, and west, were negative while samples from three other geographic regions were pos-

Table 2. The sequences of primers and the predicted RT-PCR product size.

virus	target gene	primer	sequence (5 '-3 ')	position	product length	refrence no.
BCV	Nucleocapsid	BCV-N-f	GCCGATCAGTCCGACCAATC	29475-29494	407	Tsunemitsu et al, 1999
		BCV-N-R	AGAATGTCAGCCGGGGTAT			Masaharu et al, 2012

itive. All positive samples in ELISA were positive in RT-PCR.

The average age of positive calves was nine days, and 38% were male and 62 % were female.

The average stool score in the positive samples and negative samples was 2.5 and 2.1 respectively (based on 0-3 scoring). Fecal consistency data were recorded on a scale of 0-3, with score increasing severity (0 = normal feces, 3 = severe diarrhea) (Operario et al, 2015). Degree of fecal consistency: 0 = normal, manure is normal and well formed; 1 = abnormal feces but not diarrhea, manure is pasty (softer than normal); 2 = mild diarrhea (feces are semi liquid, but still have a solid component); and 3 = liquid feces only (Mathur et al, 2001).

10 samples from the positive samples (71/4 %) had fever (rectal temperature≥40 °C).

Discussion

In the present study, Coronavirus was detected in 7.3% of diarrheic calves. Almost the same results about occurrence of BCoV were found in some other studies in Sweden (De Verdier, 2006), Japan (Kirisawa et al., 2007), Switzerland (Uhde et al 2008) and Holland (Bartels, 2010). In contrast, BCoV appeared to be of more importance with higher prevalence in some other studies in countries such as Spain (De la Fuente et al 1998; Perez et al 1998), France (Bendali et al., 1999), Brazil (Stipp et al., 2009), India (Hansa et al., 2012), Australia (Izzo et al., 2011), Korea (park et al., 2007) and Turkey

(Hasoksuz et al., 2005). A few studies also had lower prevalence, including studies in Pakistan (Alikhan, 2009, 2 %) and Argentina (Bok et al., 2015, 5 %).

In one regional study in Iran, 12.03% of diarrhetic samples were positive with both capture ELISA and RT-PCR (Khalili et al., 2006). Mayameei et al., 2010 in Tehran dairy farms showed that the prevalence of Coronavirus infection in diarrheic calves is 3.17%. In another study in Mashhad province, Coronavirus antigen was detected in 2.7% and 1.8% of diarrheic and non-diarrheic calves, respectively (Afshari et al., 2012). In the present study 28.57 % and 71.43 % of positive samples were in the age group 0-7 days and >7 days respectively. In another study, calves were divided to different age groups 1-15, 16-30, 31-45, and 46-60 days. Age group 16-30 days had most positive samples (29 %), but at least one or more positive samples were seen in other groups (Stipp et al., 2009).

In the present study, there was not any significant association between the presence of Coronavirus in feces and stool score and fever (rectal temperature >40) of calves (p> 0.05). More than 85% of positive samples had a stool score ≥2 with an average of 2.5. Also, about 71% of positive samples had a rectal temperature >40. In some studies (Busato et al 1998; Bjorkman et al 2003; Erdogan et al 2003) no significant association was found between the presence of Coronavirus in feces and clinical diarrhea but in some other studies, there was a significant association between shedding of Corona-virus in feces and diarrhea (Reynolds et al 1986, Perez et al 1998, Bendali et al 1999a, Stipp et al., 2009).

The results of the present study showed that the occurrence of coronavirus in stool samples of diarrheic calves in dairy farms of Iran is lower than the other reports in the world. The occurrence and also diagnosis of enteropathogens in the feces of diarrheic and non-diarrheic calves varies depending on the geographic location, the farm, the age and type of calves being examined and the extent to which the diagnostic laboratory is capable of isolating or demonstrating the causative pathogens. On the other hand, the role of other infectious agents in diarrhea in different countries and regions and the sensitivity and specificity of used tests in each study can explain the observed differences in prevalence of Coronavirus among a variety of studies. In addition, some of the possible reasons for low prevalence of Coronavirus in the present study are that most samples were not collected during winter, the season in which the prevalence of calf diarrhea caused by Coronavirus is higher than other seasons. Also, the sensitivity of ELISA test, used as screening test in this study, is lower than PCR, moreover, Iran has a hot, dry climate, opposed to the Coronavirus desirable stability condition.

Acknowledgments

The authors thank the staff of the microbiology department of Faculty of Veterinary Medicine, University of Tehran for providing equipment and lab. We are also grateful to all people helping us for sample collection.

References

Afshari Safavi, E.A., Mohammadi, G.R., Rad, M., Naghibi, A. (2012) A case-control study of association between diarrhea in newborn calves and infection with rotavirus and coronavirus in some industrial dairy herds of Mashhad aarea, Iran in 2008. Arch Razi Inst. 67: 35-41.

Ammar, S.S., Mokhtaria, K., Tahar, B.B., Amar, A.A., Redha, B.A., Yuva, B., Mohamed, H.S., Abdellatif, N., Laid, B. (2014) Prevalence of rotavirus (GARV) and coronavirus (BCoV) associated with neonatal diarrhea in calves in western Algeria. Asian Pac J Trop Biomed. 4: 318-322.

Bartels, C.J., Holzhauer, M., Jorritsma, R., Swart, W.A., Lam, T.J. (2010) Prevalence, prediction and risk factors of enteropathogenes in normal and non-normal faeces of yang Dutch dairy calves. Prev Vet Med. 93: 162-169.

Bendali, F., Bichet, H., Schelcher, F., Sanaa, M. (1999) Pattern of diarrhea in newborn beef calves in southwest France. Res Vet Sci. 30: 61-74.

Bjorkman, C., Svensson, C. Christensson, B., De Verdier, K. (2003) Cryptosporidium parvum and Giardia intestinalis in calf diarrhoea in Sweden. Acta Vet Scand. 44: 145-152.

Boileau, M.J., Kapil, S. (2010) Bovine coronavirus associated syndromes. Vet Clin North Am Food Anim Pract. 26: 123-146.

Boka, M., Miñoa S., Rodrigueza, D., Badaraccoa, A., Nuñesc, I., Souzac, S.P., Bilbao, G., Louge Uriarte, E., Galarza, R., Vega, C., Odeon, A., Saif, L.J., Parreño, V. (2015) Molecular and antigenic characterization of bovine Coronavirus circulating in Argentinean cattle during 1994-2010. Vet Microbiol. 181: 221-229.

Brandao, P.E., Gregori, F., Richtzenhain, L.J., Rosales, C.A., Villarreal, L.Y., Jerez, J.A., (2006) Molecular analysis of Brazilian strains of bovine coronavirus (BCoV) reveals a deletion within the hypervariable region of the S1 subunit of the spike glycoprotein also found in human coronavirus OC43. Arch Virol. 151: 1735-1748.

Busato, A., Lentze, T., Hofer, D., Burnens, A., Hentrich, B., Gaillard, C. (1998) A case control study of potential enteric pathogens for calves raised in cow-calf herds. J Vet Med B. 45: 519-528.

Cho, KO., Hasoksuz, M., Nielsen, PR., Chang, KO., Lathrop, S., Saif, LJ. (2001) Crossprotection studies between respiratory and calf diarrhea and winter dysentery coronavirus strains in calves and RT-PCR and nested PCR for their detection. Arch Virol. 146: 2401-2419.

Clark, M.A. (1993) Bovine coronavirus. Br Vet J. 149: 51-70.

Dash, S.K., Kumar, K., Goel, A., Bhatia, A.K. (2012) Detection of coronavirus antigen by ELISA from diarrhoetic cow calves in Mathura, India. Vet World. 5: 166-168.

De la Fuente, R., Garcia, A., Ruiz-Santa-Quiteria, J.A., Luzon, M., Cid, D. Garcia, S., Orden, J.A., Gomez-Bautista, M. (1998) Proportional morbidity rates of enteropathogens among diarrheic dairy calves in central Spain. Prev Vet Med. 36: 145-152.

de Verdier, K. (2006) Infektionspanoramat vid diarréer hos svenska kalvar. Svensk Veterinärtidning. 8-9: 29-32.

Decaro, N., Mari, V., Desario, C., Campolo, M., Elia, G., Martella, V., Greco, G., Cirone, F., Colaianni, M.L., Cordioli, P., Buonavoglia, C. (2008) Severe outbreak of bovine coronavirus infection in dairy cattle during the warmer season. Vet Microbiol. 126: 30-9.

El-Kanawati, Z.R., Tsunemitsu, H., Smith, D.R., Saif, L.J. (1996) Infection and cross-protection studies of winter dysentery and calf diarrhea bovine coronavirus strains in colos-

trum-deprived and gnotobiotic calves. Am J Vet Res. 57: 48-53.

Erdogan, H.M., Unver, A., Gunes, V., Citil, M. (2003) Frequency of rotavirus and coronavirus in neonatal calves in Kars district. KAFKAS ÜNİVERSİTESİ, Veteriner Fakültesi Derg. 9: 65-68.

Fulton, R.W., Step, D.L., Wahrmund, J., Burge, L.J., Payton, M.E., Cook, B.J., Burken, D., Richards, C.J., Confer, A.W. (2011) Bovine coronavirus (BCV) infections in transported commingled beef cattle and sole-source ranch calves. Can J Vet Res. 75: 191-199.

Gumusova, S.O., Yazici, Z., Albayrak, H., Meral, Y. (2007) Rotavirus and coronavirus prevalence in healthy calves and calves with diarrhea. Medycyna Weterynaryjna. 63: 62-64.

Hansa, A., Rai, R.B., Yaqoob Wani, M., Dhama, K. (2012) ELISA and RT-PPCR based detection of Bovine Coronavirus in north India. Asian J Anim Vet Adv. 7: 1120-1129.

Hasoksuz, M., Sreevatsan, S., Cho, K.O., Hoet, A.E., Saif, L.J. (2002) Molecular analysis of the S1 subunit of the spike glycoprotein of respiratory and enteric bovine coronavirus isolates. Virus Res. 84: 101-109.

Hasoksuz, M., Vlasova, A., Saif, L.J. (2008) Detection of group 2a coronaviruses with emphasis on bovine and wild ruminant strains. Virus isolation and detection of antibody antigen, and nucleic acid. Methods Mol Biol. 454: 43-59.

Izzo, M.M., Kirkland, P.D., Mohler, V.L., Perkins, N.R., Gunn, A.A., House, J.K. (2011) Prevalence of major enteric pathogens in Australian dairy calves with diarrhea. Aust Vet J. 89: 167-73.

Jeong, J.H., Kim, G.Y., Yoon, S.S., Park, S.J., Kim, Y.J., Sung, C.M., Jang, O.J., Shin, S.S., Koh, H.B., Lee, B.J., Lee, C.Y., Kang, M.I., Kim, H.J., Park, N.Y., Cho, K.O. (2005) Detection and isolation of winter dysentery bovine coronavirus circulated in korea during 2002-2004. Vet Med Sci. 67: 187-189.

Khalili, M., Morshedi, A., Keyvanfar, H., Hemmatzadeh, F. (2006) Detection of bovine coronavirus by RT-PCR in a field study. Vet Ski Arh. 76: 291-29.

Kirisawa, R., Takeyama, A., Koiwa, M., Iwai, H. (2007) Detection of bovine torovirus in fecal specimens of calves with diarrhea in Japan. J Vet Med Sci. 69: 471-476.

Lai, M.H.K.V. (2001) Coronaviridae: the viruses and their replication. In: Fields Virology. Fields, B.N., Howley, P.M., DMK (eds.). Lippincott - Raven, Philadelphia, USA. p. 1163-1186.

Masaharu, F., Kazufumi K., Ayako M., Tohru S., Keito T., Tsunehiko A., Masaji, M., Makoto, S., Hiroshi, T. (2012) Development and application of one-step multiplex reverse transcription PCR for simultaneous detection of five diarrheal viruses in adult cattle. Arch Virol. 157: 1063-1069

Mathur, S., Constable, P.D., Eppley, R.M., Waggoner, A.L., Tumbleson, M.E., Haschek, W.M. (2001) Fumonisin B1 is hepatotoxic and nephrotoxic in milk-fed calves, Toxicol Sci. 60: 385-396.

Mawatari, T., Hirano, K., Ikeda, H., Tsunemitsu, H., Suzuki, T. (2014) Surveillance of diarrhea-causing pathogens in dairy and beef cows in Yamagata prefecture, Japan from 2002 to 2011. Microbiol Immunol. 58: 530-535.

Mayameei, A., Mohammadi, Gh., Yavari, S., Afshari, E., Omidi, A. (2010) Evaluation of relationship between Rotavirus and Coronavirus infections with calf diarrhea by capture ELISA. Comp Clin Pathol. 19: 553-557.

Mee, J.F., Geraghty, T., O'Neill, R., More, S.J. (2012) Bioexclusion of diseases from dairy and beef farms: risks of introducing infectious agents and risk reduction strategies.

Vet J. 194: 143-50.

Ohlson, A., Alenius, S., Traven, M., Emanuelson, U. (2013) A longitudinal study of the dynamics of bovine corona virus and respiratory syncytial virus infections in dairy herds. Vet J. 197: 395-400.

Operario, D.J., Bristol, L.S., Liotta, J., Nydam, D.V., Houpt, E.R. (2015) Correlation between diarrhea severity and oocyst count via quantitative PCR or fluorescence microscopy in experimental cryptosporidiosis in calves. Am J Trop Med Hyg. 92 45-49.

Park S.J., Kim G.Y., Choy H.E., Hong Y.J., Saif L.J., Jeong J.H., Park, S.I., Kim, H.H., Kim, S.K., Shin, S.S., Kang, M.I., Cho, K.O. (2007) Dual enteric and respiratory tropisms of winter dysentery bovine coronavirus in calves. Arch Virol. 152: 1885-900.

Park, S.J., Lim, G.K., Park, S.I., Kim, H.H., Koh, H.B., Cho, K.O. (2007) Detection and molecular characterization of calf diarrhoea bovine corona viruses circulating in south Korea DURING 2004-2005. Zoonoses Public Health. 54: 223-30.

Perez, E., Kummeling, A., Janssen, M.M., Jimenez, C., Alvarado, R., Cabal, M., Caballero, M., Donado, P., Dwinger, R.H. (1998) Infectious agents associated with diarrhea of calves in the canton of Tilarán, Costa Rica. Prev Vet Med. 33: 195-205.

Quinn, P.J., Markey, B. K., Leonard, F. C., Hartigan, P., Fanning, S., FitzPatrick, E.S. (2002) Veterinary Microbiology and Microbial Disease. Blackwell Science Ltd. Iowa State University Press, Ames, Iowa, USA. p. 709.

Reynolds, D.J., Morgan, J.H., Chanter, N., Jones, P.W., Bridger, J.C., Debney, T.G., et al. (1986) Microbiology of calf diarrhea in southern Britain. Vet Rec. 119: 34-39.

Saif, L.J., Redman, D.R., Moorhead, P.D., Theil, K.W. (1986) experimentally induced coronavirus infections in calves: viral replication in the respiratory and intestinal tracts. Am J Vet Res. 47: 1426-1432.

Schultze, B., Gross, H.J., Brossmer, R., Herrler, G. (1991) The S protein of bovine coronavirus is a hemagglutinin recognizing 9-O-acetylated sialic acid as a receptor determinant. J. Virol. 65: 6232-6237.

Stipp, D.T., Barry, A.F., Alfieri, A.F., Takiuchi, E., Amude, A.M., Alfieri, A.A. (2009) Frequency of BCoV detection by a semi-nested PCR assay in faeces of calves from Brazilian cattle herds. Trop Anim Health Prod. 41: 1563-1567.

Takiuchi, E., Stipp, D.T., Alfieri, A.F., Alfieri, A.A. (2006) Improved detection of bovine coronavirus N gene in faeces of calves infected naturally by a semi-nested PCR assay and an internal control. J Virol Methods. 131: 148-154.

Tsunemitsu, H., Smith, D.R., Saif L.J. (1999) Experimental inoculation of adult dairy cows with bovine coronavirus and detection of coronavirus in feces by RT-PCR. Arch Virol. 144: 167-75.

Uhde, F.L., Kaufmann, T., Sager, H., Albini, S., Zanoni, R., Schelling, E., Meylan, M. (2008) Prevalence of four enteropathogens in the feces of young diarrheic dairy calves in Switzerland. Vet Rec. 163: 362-366.

Veslemøy, S.O., Madeleine, T., Stefan, A., Mette, M., Maria, S. (2016) Bovine coronavirus in naturally and experimentally exposed calves; viral shedding and the potential for transmission. Virol J. 13: 100.

20

Comparative assessment of rEPC1 antigen and copro-antigen for diagnosis of echinococcosis in dogs

Jalousian, F.[1*], Hosseini, S.H.[1], Fathi, S.[1], Shirani, D.[2], Aghaei, S.[1], Kordafshari, S.[1]

[1]*Department of Parasitology, Faculty of Veterinary Medicine, University of Tehran, Tehran, Iran*

[2]*Department of Internal Medicine, Faculty of Veterinary Medicine, University of Tehran, Tehran, Iran*

Key words:

copro-antigen, diagnosis, dog echinococcosis, Dot-ELISA, recombinant EPC1 antigen

Correspondence

Jalousian, F.

Department of Parasitology,

Faculty of Veterinary Medicine,

University of Tehran, Tehran,

Iran

Email: jalousian_f@ut.ac.ir

Abstract:

BACKGROUND: Diagnosis of *Echinococcus granulosus* in the definitive host particularly in dog is a significant complication in the endemic area. **OBJECTIVES:** The aim of this study is serological detection of *E. granulosus* in the infected dogs. **METHODS:** Dot-ELISA based on the copro-antigen and recombinant EPC1 antigen (rEPC1) for antibody detection was performed. Blood and fecal samples were collected from eleven treated puppies with 90000-100000 protoscoleces (90% viability) and four treated puppies with distilled water as controls, on day before challenge and 7, 14, 21, 28 and 35 days post challenges. Furthermore, the blood and fecal samples were collected from 35 naturally infected dogs. **RESULTS:** In terms of experimentally infected dogs, sensitivity and specificity of Dot- ELISA were close for both antigens (copro- antigen, rEPC1) that were determined to be 100%, 88% for copro-antigen, and 100 and 94% for rEPC1, respectively. In the context of naturally infected dogs, our findings showed similar sensitivity in Dot -ELISA based on the anti-body detection (using rEPC1), and antigen detection (using copro-antigen), (100%), while these methods provided different specificity, about 75% for rEPC1 and 58% for copro-antigen. **CONCLUSIONS:** Our findings indicated that both antigens are qualified. REPC1 antigen is not able to detect the infection during the first 15 days post-infection, whereas the antibody cannot be detectable. REPC1 protein may work for screening of *E. granulosus*, while copro-antigen can be useful for diagnosis of current acute infection. However, both methods are recommended for screening of sheepdog, guard dogs and police dogs.

Introduction

Echinococcus granulosus is considered as one of the most significant parasitic infections throughout the world as a causative agent of cystic hydatid disease which is transmitted between canines and numerous herbivorous livestock animals as intermediate hosts (das Neves et al. 2017). It is thought to be an important global parasitic disease of humans and animals. Cystic echinococcosis (CE) is endemic in Iran, where a variety of animals act as intermediate hosts (Eslami and Hosseini 1998; Umhang et al. 2013). Fasihi Harandi et al, (2012) estimated annual surgical incidence of CE (Cystic echinococcosis) with a rate of 1.27/100,000 population from 2000-2009 in Iran. Furthermore, average annual cost of CE in Iran was estimated at US$232.3 million, including both direct and indirect costs (Fasihi Harandi et al. 2012). The cost associated with human CE was estimated at US$93.39 million and the annual cost related to CE in livestock was estimated at US$132 million (Fasihi Harandi et al. 2012), indicating the importance of infection control. Therefore, detection of *E. granulosus* in the definitive host is an important problem in endemic areas. Control of infection in dogs is much cheaper than those in the intermediate host. The diagnosis of hydatid cyst is mainly focused on human but diagnosis and screening of infection in dogs is most important in endemic area for control programs, and also can be useful for assessing the dynamics of hydatidosis transmission (Carmena et al 2006, Allan and Craig 2006). The diagnosis of canine echinococcosis can be a challenge in surveillance of control programs, because there is no perfect gold standard test. Several diagnostic method have been employed for diagnosis of *E. granulosus*, including necropsy of dogs, examination of the small intestine, coprological examinations and purging of dogs with arecoline hydrobromide (Ibrahem, 2017). Routine stool exam cannot differentiate the eggs of echinococcus from other taenia species due to morphological similarity (Dinkel et al, 1998). These techniques are time consuming, labor intensive, hazardous and suffer from low sensitivity (Jenkins et al. 1990). The immunological methods such as ELISA and dot-blotting are highly used, although their accuracy is largely dependent on the specificity and sensitivity of antigens (Carmena et al 2006; Wachira et al

1990). Despite the development of sensitive and specific methods, the immunodiagnosis of CE and echinococcosis remains a complex task (Ortona et al 2003; Siracusano and Bruschi 2006). Majority of the available screening tests can produce a high percentage of false-negative results (up to 25 %), as well as false-positive results which occur using different assays and can be caused by co-infection with other cestodes or helminths (Carmena et al 2006). Recombinant antigens and synthetic peptides can be useful applications for human hydatidosis as specific peptides (Hernandez-Gonzalez et al 2008). Recombinant EPC1, a 8.5-kDa antigen from *E. granulosus*, has been shown to be effective for diagnosis of human hydatidosis (Li et al 2003; Cai et al 2011), without any report about the usefulness of this recombinant antigen for detection of dog echinococcosis. Dogs have an immune response against the adult parasites (Zhang et al 2003), indicating that serological tests using specific antigens may be useful. The current study was aimed to assess the efficacy of copro-antigen detection and antibody detection (based on the rEpC1) in the diagnosis and monitoring of echinococcosis.

Materials and Methods

Positive and negative reference serum samples: We performed a cross-sectional study on 15 dogs (2-3 months old). Dogs were raised from birth at the Small Animal Hospital, Faculty of Veterinary Medicine, University of Tehran. They were maintained on commercial dog food and water. Puppies were vaccinated against distemper, Rabies virus, parvoviruses and leptospirosis and treated orally with Praziquantel. Puppies were kept in separate cages with complete sanitary conditions and were divided into two groups. The first group (11 puppies) was inoculated with 90000-100000 (viability more than 90%) protoscoleces. Protoscoleces were collected from fertile hydatid cysts of ovine liver. Each dog was fed about 100000 protoscoleces. In the second group, 4 puppies were selected as a negative control group, and were kept in the same condition, but not fed any protoscolex. It is worth noting that worm infections were not found in puppies of the control group. In addition, no change in blood parameters and clinical signs were seen in experimentally infected puppies and control group.

Stool sampling was performed six times including the day before challenge, 7, 14, 21, 28 and 35 days post infection. In addition, blood was collected from dogs in these days. The blood was clotted at room temperature for 30 min and then at 4 oc for 4 h. The clot was separated from the serum by centrifugation at $3,000 \times g$ for 10 min and the serum stored at -20 oc, until use.

Other parasites infection (Naturally infected dogs): The small intestines of 35 stray dogs were opened and immersed in warm PBS. Detached worms and the intestinal contents were passed through sieves, and worms were enumerated under a bright light on a black background (WHO, 2006). The blood and fecal samples were collected from dogs with natural infection. Inspection of small intestine of these dogs showed that dogs were infected with other carnivores' intestinal worms.

***Echinococcus granulosus* copro-antigen:** trips were dipped into 1: 50, 1; 100, 1; 250, 1: 500, 1: 1000 dilution of dogs sera (5 00 µl) and placed on shaker for 1 h. The strips were then washed 3 times in PBS-T

for 5 min. Then, 100 µl of horseradish peroxidase conjugated rabbit anti-dog IgG (Sigma_Aldrich) at a 1:10000 dilution was added at 1: 2500 dilution and placed for 1 h on shaker in dark place. After rinsing, peroxidase reaction was visualized with 0.06% (w/v) diaminobenzidine tetrahydrochloride in 50 mM Tris-HCl (pH 7.6) and 0.03% (v/v) H2O2. The reaction was stopped after 2 min with distilled water.

The sensitivity, specificity and efficacy were calculated as follows:

Sensitivity=Number of true positives/ Number of true positives+Number of false negatives

Specificity=Number of true negatives/ Number of true negatives+number of false positives

Efficacy=Sensivity+specifity/2

Results

Copro-antigen Dot-Elisa in experimentally infected dog: In this method, copro-antigen showed positive reaction on days 15, 28, 35 after challenge and also control dogs showed a negative reaction.

Sensitivity and specificity of Dot -ELISA based on the copro-antigen for diagnosis of experimentally infected dogs were 100% and 88%; moreover, the efficacy of copro-antigen was 95.5% (Table 1 and Fig. 4).

Copro-antigen Dot-Elisa in naturally infected dogs: In naturally infected dogs with other carnivores' intestinal worms, copro-antigen showed sensitivity and specificity of 100% and 58% (the gold standard was necropsy of dogs). Copro antigen-based tests have a greater number of false positives which reduces the specificity of the test. Moreover, efficacy of copro- antigen was 70.5% (Table 1 and Fig. 5).

Table 1. Comparison of sensitivity, specificity, efficacy, positive and negative predictive values of Copro-Ag dot-ELISA and rEPC1 Ag dot-ELISA in detection of dog echinococcosis.

Type of Ag	Experimentally infected dogs with *Echinococcus granulosus* No.11	Healthy Puppies No.4	Sera of puppies before challenge (negative control sera) No.11	Sera of dogs with other parasites (Natural infection) No.35	True positive	False positive	True negative	False negative
Copro-Ag dot-ELISA	11 (positive sera)	0 (positive)	2 (positive sera)	34 (positive sera)	11	36	50	0
rEPC1 Ag dot-ELISA	11 (positive sera)	0 (positive)	1 (positive sera)	16 (positive sera)	11	17	50	0

REPC1 Dot-Elisa in experimentally infected dogs: Dogs with a serum dilution of 1: 50, 1; 100, 1; 250, 1: 500 and 1: 1000 were studied by Dot-ELISA. Maximum and minimum color spots were observed at a dilution of 1:50 and 1:1000. Sera of infected dogs showed positive reaction at all dilutions and also against the rEPC1. Furthermore, control group showed a negative reaction.

Furthermore, sensitivity and specificity of Dot -ELISA based on the rEpC1 for serodiagnosis of experimentally infected dogs were 100% and 94%. Moreover, the efficacy of rEpC1 Ag was calculated to be 95.5% (Table 1 and Fig. 4).

REPC1 Dot-Elisa- in naturally infected dogs: REPC1 showed a sensitivity and specificity of 100% and 75%, with naturally infected sera (other carnivores intestinal worms). The gold standard was necropsy. Furthermore, efficacy of rEPC1 was 87.5 (Table 1 and Fig. 5).

Discussion

The diagnosis of hydatid cyst is mainly focused on human, but the diagnosis of infection in dogs (adult worm) is most important in endemic areas for surveillance of control programs, also it can be useful for assessing the dynamics of hydatidosis transmission (Dinkel et al. 2011, Allan and Craig 2006). Two main immunodiagnostic approaches for diagnosis of *E. granulosus* infection in definitive hosts are antibody detection and copro-antigens detection in feces. The most common diagnostic tests in dog are based on copro-antigen detection technique. Copro-antigen ELISA by using antibodies against Echinococcus proglottid somatic antigens and or excretory/secretory (ES) antigens are the most practical approach for the diagnosis of the intestinal E. granulosus infection in dogs (Mastin et al, 2015; Deplazes et al, 1992; Jenkins et al, 2000; Dinkel et al., 2011). Moreover, copro-antigen ELISA is far more sensitive than arecoline and can be used for *E. granulosus* detection in dog populations in both laboratory and field conditions (Jenkins et al, 2000; Eckert and Deplazes, 2004). The sensitivity and specificity of copro-antigen ELISA for detection of *E. granulosus* infection in canids permits the detection of the parasite during the prepatent period (Ahmad and Nizami, 1998). As matter of fact, it can show the current status of the infection (Jenkins et al., 2000), whereas its results correlated with the worm burden in the dog intestine (Mastin et al, 2015). In the present study, none of the experimentally infected dogs had clinical sign and changes in blood parameters also were shown to be negative

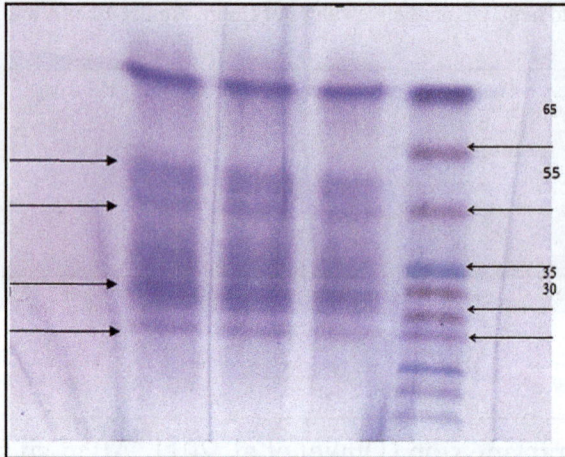

Figure 1. SDS-PAGE of Copro-antigen with 12% concentration under denatured conditions. Four bands with molecular weights of 30, 35, 55 and 60 KDa were observed.

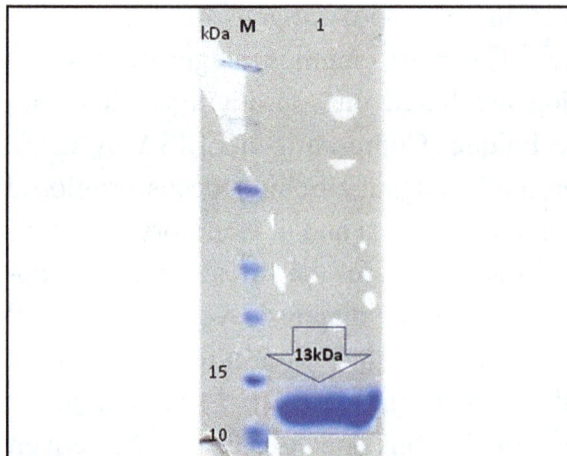

Figure 2. SDS-PAGE of rEPC1 antigen with 12% concentration under denatured conditions. A band with 13KDa molecular weight was observed.

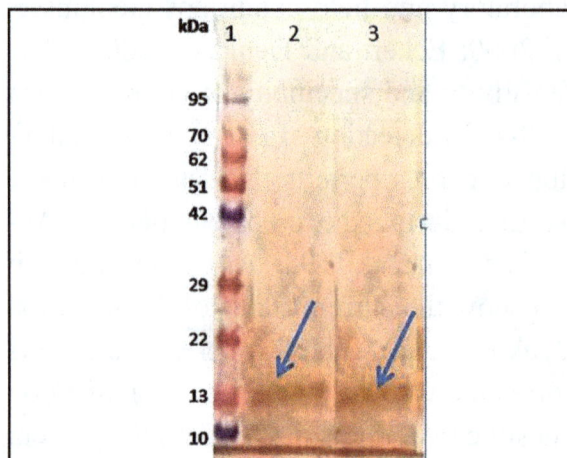

Figure 3. Reactions of rEPC1antigen (13kDa subunit) with E.granulosus positive serum samples (1:50 an 1:100, Western blotting).

after a lag phase of up to 2 weeks. This initial delay in copro-antigen production may be related to the development of the worms in intestine (Al-Jawabreh, 2015; Jenkins et al, 2000). The researchers have suggested that the amount of copro-antigen and its diagnosis is heavily dependent on burden of infection, indicating the disadvantage of method based upon copro-antigen (Deplazes et al, 1992; Jenkins, et al, 2000; Allan and Craig, 2006; Allan and Craig, 1989; Allan et al, 1992; Jenkins et al, 2000). In this study, sera from puppies infected in the laboratory were used to determine the diagnostic sensitivity of copro-antigen and simultaneously, the sera of naturally infected dogs were used to determine the diagnostic specificity of copro- antigen.The sensitivity of copro-antigen detection in this study was acceptable. Its sensitivity has been reported to be generally good with moderate to high worm burdens (>100 worms), but less in animal with low worm burdens (Pierangeli et al., 2010). The specificity of Dot -ELISA based on the copro-antigen for diagnosis of experimentally infected dogs, naturally infected dogs with other carnivores' gastrointestinal worm parasites were 88%, and 58%. Copro antigen is highly specific and can be detected by antibody in experimentally infected dogs by days 5-10 post infection, an therefore does not depend on the presence of eggs (Deplazes et al, 1992). Allan et al, (1992) reported 96% specificity for copro-antigen and good sensitivity (77-88%) based on confirmation by arecoline purge (Mastin et al, 2015; Lopera et al, 2003). The sensitivity and specificity of copro-antigen Dot-ELISA was good in experimentally infected dogs by high burden of infection (Craig, 1995; WHO, 2006). However, the specificity was relatively low in naturally infected dogs

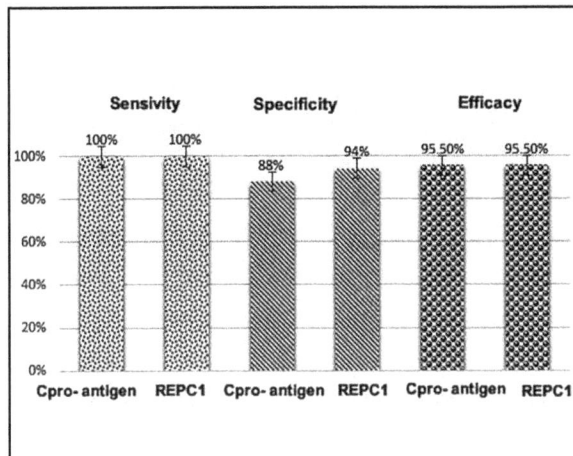

Figure 4. Comparison of sensitivity, specificity and efficacy of copro-Ag Dot-ELISA and rEPC1 Dot-ELISA for detection *E. granulosus* infection in experimentally infected dogs.

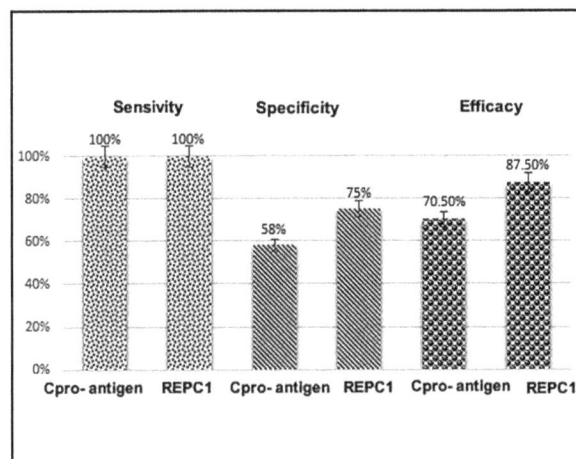

Figure 5. Comparison of sensitivity, specificity and efficacy of Copro-Ag Dot-ELISA and rEPC1 Dot-ELISA for detection of *E. granulosus* infection in naturally infected dogs.

which indicates the actual performance in naturally infected dogs is less certain than experimentally infected dogs, because of potential cross reactivity with antigens from Taenia species or other helminths and needs to be defined in fields. It should be noted that sensitivity and specificity have often been obtained in experimentally infected dogs. However, test parameters will vary with the population. We hope the method in this study will be optimized in the future with a comprehensive study which is aimed at screening of dogs. As evident from the

recent literature, recombinant antigens and fusion peptides can be useful for diagnostic applications mainly in humans as specific peptides (Zhang et al. 2003). In this study, recombinant protein (Echinococcus protoscolex gene) EPC1 was used as antigen for the detection of specific antibodies of *E. granulosus* in dogs. Therefore, the ability of recombinant protein EPC1 in dog serum samples was also analyzed by Dot-ELISA. Specific serum antibodies were shown to be detectable in the serum of dogs after experimental infection with *E. granulosus* using metacestode antigen and others confirmed the appearance of specific antibodies by using antigens derived from the oncosphere in ELISA (Barriga, 1986, Singh and Dhar, 1988; Sixl et al, 1988). Our results showed that sensitivity and specificity of Dot -ELISA based on the rEPC1 Ag for serodiagnosis of experimentally infected dogs, naturally infected dogs were 100%, 94%, 100% and 75%, respectively. This result indicated a high sensitivity compared with previous studies for detection of serum antibodies that showed variable sensitivities, ranging from 40 to 90% (Benito et al, 2001; Gasser et al, 1994; Mastin et al, 2015; Jenkins et al,1990), and also cross-reactivity with other parasite species may occur (Gasser et al, 1988), while sensitivity was reported to be high (73%) for natural canine *E. granulosus* infection using a protoscolex antigen-ELISA in south-east Australia, there was no correlation with worm burden. Gasser et al (1990) reported that a recombinant *E. granulosus* protoscolex antigen was 100% specific for *E. granulosus* antibodies in dog sera, but sensitivity was significantly low for the native protoscolex antigen that is in contrast with our study. But the specificity was relatively low in naturally infected dogs, suggesting the actual performance of antigen in naturally infected dogs is less certain than experimentally infected dogs. In our study, the relative good efficacy of rEPC1 Ag enables useful application in determination of presence or absence of Echinococcus spp. and estimating relative exposure rates in dog populations. However, antibodies persist after the elimination of the worm burden, accordingly, antibody prevalence does not correlate with the actual prevalence. Furthermore, antibody detection is not correlated with the worm burden, while copro- antigen detection is indicative of acute infection (Pierrangeli et al, 2010). However, rEPC1 antigen seems to work for screening of infected dogs. On the other hand, copro-antigen production is easy and inexpensive but the major limitations of copro-antigen are associated with the *E. granulosus* worm burden. Nonetheless, copro-antigen efficiency is important for the detection of current infection of dogs with *E. granulosus*. The specificity of copro-antigen was relatively low in naturally infected dogs than experimentally infected dogs, indicating the actual performance in naturally infected dogs can be decreased, which can also be true for rEPC1 antigen. We proposed that if the goal is screening of *E. granulosus*, rEPC1 may work for this purpose, but if the goal is detection of current infection, copro-antigen can be applicable in this matter.

Acknowledgments

This study was funded by a grant number 88000408 from Iran National Science Foundation. The authors declare that they do not have any conflicts of interest.

References

Ahmad, G., Nizami, W.A. (1998) Coproantigens: early detection and suitability of an immunodiagnostic method for echinococcosis in dogs. Vet Parasitol. 77: 237-244.

Allan, J.C., Craig, P.S (1989) Coproantigens in gut tapeworm infections: Hymenolepis diminuta in rats. Parasitol Res. 76: 68-73.

Allan, J.C., Avila G., Garcia Noval, J., Flisser, A., Craig, P.S. (1992) Immunodiagnosi of taeniasis by coproantigen detection. Parasitology. 101(Pt 3): 473-477

Allan, J.C., Craig, P.S., Garcia Noval, J., Mencos, F., Liu, D., Wang, Y., Wen, H., Zhou, P., Stringer, R., Rogan, M., Zeyhle, A. (1992) Coproantigen detection for immunodiagnosis of echinococcosis and taeniasis in dogs and humans. Parasitology. 104: 347-355.

Allan, J.C., Craig, P.S. (2006) Coproantigens in taeniasis and echinococcosis. Parasitol Int. 55: 75-80.

Al-Jawabreh, A., Dumaidi, K., Ereqat, S., Nasereddin, A., Al-Jawabreh, H., Azmi, K., Al-Laham, N., Abdeen, Z. (2015) Incidence of *Echinococcus granulosus* in Domestic Dogs in Palestine as Revealed copro-PCR. PLoS Negl Trop Dis. 9: 1-10.

Barriga, O.O., Al-Khalidi, N.W. (1986) Humoral immunity in the prepatent primary infection of dogs with *Echinococcus granulosus*. Vet Immunol Immunopathol. 11: 375-389.

Benito, A., Carmena, D., Spinelli, P., Postigo, I., Martı́nez, J., Estı́-balez, J.J., Martı́n de la Cuesta, F., Guisantes, J.A. (2001) The serological diagnosis of canine echinococcosis by an enzyme immunoassay useful for epidemiological surveys. Res Rev Parasitol. 61: 17-23.

Cai, H.X., Shen, Y.J., Han, X.M., Yuan, Z.Y., Wang, H., Xu, Y.X., Hu, Y., Lu, W.Y., Guan,Y.Y. , Cao, J.P. (2011) Cloning, expression and immunodiagnostic evaluation of antigen EPC1 from *Echinococcus granulosus*. Zhongguo ji sheng chong xue yu ji sheng chong bing za zhi. 29: 167-71.

Carmena, D., Benito, A. and Eraso, E. (2006) Antigens for the immunodiagnosis of *Echinococcus granulosus* infection. Acta Tropica. 98: 74-86.

Das Neves, L.B., Ferlini Teixeira, P.E., Silva, S., de Oliveira,F.B., Garcia, D.D., de Almeida, F.B., Rodrigues-Silva, R., Machado-Silva, J.R. (2017) First molecular identification of *Echinococcus vogeli* and *Echinococcus granulosus* (sensu stricto) G1 revealed in feces of domestic dogs (*Canis familiaris*) from Acre, Brazil. Parasit Vectors. 10: 28-33.

Deplazes, P., Gottstein, B., Eckert, J., Jenkins, DJ., Ewald, D., Jime´nezPalacios, S. (1992) Detection of *Echinococcus coproantigens* by ELISA in dogs, dingoes and foxes. Parasitol Res. 78: 303-308.

Dinkel, A., Kern, S., Brinker, A., Oehme, R., Vaniscotte, A., Giraudoux, P. (2011) A real-time multiplex-nested PCR system for coprological diagnosis of *Echinococcus multilocularis* and host species. Parasitol Res. 109: 493-8

Dinkel, A., Nickisch-Rosenegk, M., Bilger, B., merli, M., lucius, R., Romig, T. (1998) Detection of *Echinococcus multilocularis* in the definitive host: coprodiagnosis by PCR as an alternative to necropsy. J Clin Microbiol. 36: 1871-1876.

Eckert, J., Deplazes, P. (2004) Biological, epidemiological, and clinical aspects of echinococcosis, a zoonosis of increasing concern. Clin Microb Rev. 17: 107-35.

Eckert, J., Gemmel, M.A., Meslin, F.X. and Pawlowski, Z.S. (2006) Geneva: World Health Organization (WHO). Recent advances in the immunology and diagnosis of echinococcosis. FEMS Immunol Med Microbiol. 47: 24-41.

Eslami, A., Hosseini, SH. (1998) *Echinococcus granulosus* infection of farm dogs of Iran. Parasitol Res. 84: 205-207.

Fasihi Harandi, M., Budke, C.M., Rostami, S. (2012) The monetary burden of cystic echinococcosis in Iran. PLoS Negl Trop Dis. 6: 1915.

Gasser, R.B., Lightowlers, M.W., Obendorf, D.L., Jenkins, D.J., Rickard, M.D. (1988) Evaluation of a serological test system for the diagnosis of natural *Echinococcus granulosus* infection in dogs using *E. granulosus* protoscolex and oncosphere antigens. Aust Vet J. 65: 369-373.

Gasser, R.B., Lightowlers, M.W., Rickard, M.D. (1990) A recombinant antigen with potential for serodiagnosis of *Echinococcus granulosus* infection in dogs. Int J Parasitol. 20: 943-950.

Gasser, R.B., Parada, L., Acuna, A., Burges, C., Laurenson, M.K., Gulland, F.M., Reichel M.P., Paolillo, E. (1994) Immunological assessment of exposure to *Echinococcus granulosus* in a rural dog population in Uruguay. Acta Trop. 58: 179-185.

Hernandez-Gonzalez, A., Muro, A., Barrera, I., Ramos, G., Orduna, A., Siles-Lucas, M. (2008) Usefulness of four different Echinococcus granulosus recombinant antigens for serodiagnosis of unilocular hydatid disease (UHD) and postsurgical follow-up of patients treated for UHD. Clin Vaccine Immunol. 15:147-53.

Jenkins, D.J., Gasser, R.B., Zey hle, E., Roming, T., Macpherson, C.N.L. (1990) Assessment of a serological test for the detection of Echinococcus granolosus infection in dogs in Kenya. Acta Trop. 47: 245-248.

Jenkins, D.J., Fraser, A., Bradshaw, H., Craig, P.S. (2000) Detection of *Echinococcus granulosus* coproantigens in Australian canids with natural or experimental infection. J Parasitol. 86: 140-5.

Kordafshari, S., Hosseini, S.H., Jalousian, F., Rajabibazl, M., Jones, M., Etebar, F. (2015) Evaluation of dot immunogold filtration assay (DIGFA) by recombinant protein EPC1 for anti-*Echinococcus granulosus* IgG antibody. Iran J Parasitol. 10: 30-38.

Li, J., Zhang, W.B., Wilson, M., Jun, L., Zhang, W.B., Wilson, M., Ito, A., McManus, D.P. (2003) A novel recombinant antigen for immunodiagnosis of human cystic echinococcosis. J Infect Dis. 188: 1952-61.

Lopera, L., Moro, P.L., Chavez, A., Montes, G., Gonzales, A., Gilman, R.H. (2003) Field evaluation of a coproantigen enzyme-linked immunosorbent assay for diagnosis of canine echinococcosis in a rural Andean village in Peru. Vet Parasitol. 117: 37-42.

M. Ibrahem, M., M. Ibrahem,W., M. Ibrahem, K., B. Annajar, B. (2017) Incidence and the history of *Echinococcus granulosus* infection in dogs within the past few decades in Libya: A review. JVMAH. 9: 1-10.

Mastin, A., van Kesteren, F., Torgerson, P.R., Ziadinov, I., Mytynova, B., Rogan, M.T., Tursunov, T., Craig, P.S. (2015) Risk factors for Echinococcus coproantigen positivity in dogs from the Alay valley, Kyrgyzstan. J Helminthol. 89: 655-63.

Ortona., E., Rigan, O.R., Buttari, B., Delunardo, F., Ioppolo, S., Margutti, P., Profumo, E., Teggi, A., Vaccari, S., Siracusano, A. (2003) An update on immunodiagnosis of cystic echinococcosis. Acta Trop. 85: 165-171.

Pierangeli, N.B., Soriano, S.V., Roccia, I., Bergagna, H.F.J., Lazzarini, L.E., Celescinco, A., Kossman, A.V., Saiz, M.S., Basualdo, J.A. (2010) Usefulness and validation of a coproantigen test for dog echinococcosis screening in the consolidation phase of hydatid control in Neuquen, Argentina. Parasitol Int. 59: 394-399.

Singh, B.P., Dhar, D.N. (1988) Indirect fluorescent antibody test for the detection of antibodies to *Echinococcus granulosus* in experimentally infected pups. Vet Parasitol. 28: 185-190.

Siracusano, A., Bruschi, F. (2006) Cystic echinococcosis: progress and limits in epidemiology and immunodiagnosis. Parasitologia. 48: 65-66.

Sixl, W., Wisidagama, E., Stunzner, D., Withalm, H., Sixl-Voigt, B. (1988) Serological examinations of dogs (*Canis familiaris*) in Colombo/Sri Lanka. Geogr Med. Suppl. 1: 89-92.

Umhang, G., Richomme, C., Boucher, J.M., Hormaz, V., Boue, F. (2013) Prevalence survey and first molecular characterization of *Echinococcus granulosus* in France. Parasitol Res. 112: 1809-1812.

Wachira, T., McPherson, C.N.L., Gathuma, J.M. (1990) Hydatid disease in the Turkana District of Kenya VII. Analysis of the infection pressure on definitive and intermediate hosts of *E. granulosus*. Ann Trop Med Parasitol. 84: 361-368.

Zhang, W., Li, J., McManus, P. (2003) Concepts in immunology and diagnosis of hydatid disease. Clin Microbiol Rev. 16: 18-36.

21

Molecular detection of *Toxoplasma gondii* infection in aborted fetuses in sheep in Khorasan Razavi province, Iran

Danehchin, L.[1], Razmi, Gh.[2*], Naghibi, A.[3]

[1]*Department of Pathobiology, Faculty of Veterinary Medicine, Ferdowsi University of Mashhad, Mashhad, Iran*

[2]*Center of Excellence in Ruminant Abortion and Neonatal Mortality, Faculty of Veterinary Medicine, Ferdowsi University of Mashhad, Mashhad, Iran*

[3]*Department of Pathobiology, Faculty of Veterinary Medicine, Ferdowsi University of Mashhad, Mashhad, Iran*

Key words:

abortion, brain, nested-PCR, sheep, *Toxoplasma gondii*

Correspondence

Razmi, Gh.
Center of Excellence in Ruminant Abortion and Neonatal Mortality, Faculty of Veterinary Medicine, Ferdowsi University of Mashhad, Mashhad, Iran

Email: razmi@um.ac.ir

Abstract:

BACKGROUND: *Toxoplasma gondii* is a significant cause of abortion in sheep and goats in the world. Toxoplasmosis causes reproduction disorders such as fetal resorption, early embryonic death, mummification, abortion, stillbirth, neonatal and fetal death in sheep. **OBJECTIVES:** The aim of this study was to detect *T. gondii* infection in ovine aborted fetuses in Khorasan Razavi province. Methods: From June 2009 to July 2013, 112 brain samples of aborted ovine fetuses were collected and examined to detect *T.gondii* DNA by nested- PCR. The association of the frequency of *T.gondii* infection with age and geographical location of aborted fetuses was also studied. **RESULTS:** The results showed that 18 (16.07%) brain samples of aborted fetuses were Toxoplasm positive in PCR reaction. The frequency of *T.gondii* in the age group ≥120 days was more than other age groups of infected aborted fetuses (p<0.05). All the infected fetuses belonged to the sheep flocks in the northern part of the province. **CONCLUSIONS:** The results showed the moderate *T.gondii* infection among ovine aborted fetuses in the northern part of Khorasan Razavi province.

Introduction

Toxoplasma gondii was recognized for the first time as a significant cause of abortion in sheep in New Zealand and later in many countries (Buxton et al. 2007; Dubey, 2009). *T.gondii* infection during pregnancy can result in embryo/early fetal loss, fetal death and abortion/mummification and birth of weak lambs. (Buxton 1991; Scott 2007). This parasite is transmitted to sheep via ingesting food and water contaminated with oocysts which are excreted by cats or by other transmission rout from mother to fetus (Buxton et al. 2007). Furthermore, recent molecular studies showed that repeated transmission of *T. gondii* from dam to fetuses may be more common than previously observed in sheep (Duncanson et al. 2001; Morley et al. 2007; Hide et al. 2009).

The diagnosis of *T. gondii* infection is usually based on serological assay, histopathological examination and mouse bioassay. Many epidemiological studies have been carried out on ovine toxoplasmosis in different regions of Iran. The seroprevalence of ovine toxoplasmosis was reported between 13.8% -35% in different areas of Iran (Ghorbani et al. 1983; Rahbari&Razmi1992; Hashemi-Fesharki et al. 1996; Sharif et al. 2007). *T.gondii* infection was also detected in ovine fetuses using PCR and bioassay methods from Iran (Rassouli et al. 2011; Razmi et al. 2010; Zia-ali et al. 2007; Habibi et al. 2012). The aim of this study was to determine the frequency of Toxoplasma infection in aborted ovine fetuses in the province using molecular method.

Materials and Methods

The field of study: Khorasan Razavi province is located in northeastern Iran between 33°30'-37°41' N latitude and 56°19'-61°18' E longitude, with an area of more than 127,000 km2. The northern part of the province has a mountainous climate and suitable conditions for agricultural activity and animal husbandry. The southern part is mostly semi-desert and desert, with poor vegetation cover.

Sampling: From June 2009 to July 2013, one hundred-twelve aborted ovine fetuses were examined. The fetuses and fetal membranes were grossly examined for any macroscopic lesions and the age of the aborted fetuses was also determined by crown-rump length (Evans & Sack 1973).

The fetuses were necropsied and the brain samples were collected and stored at −20 °C for PCR analysis. The frozen fetal brain tissues were homogenized by mortar and pestle in Tris-HCl (pH 8•0) followed by treatment with proteinase K (Fermentas®, Lithuania) at a final concentration of 200 μgml. The phenol-chloroform and ethanol precipitation method was used for DNA extraction procedures. The purified DNA

samples were resuspended in 20 μl of TE (10mM Tris and 1mM EDTA, pH8•0) and stored at −20 °C. DNA extracted from 10^6 particles of the RH strain of *T. gondii* was used as a source of positive control sample. DNA samples were tested by nested-PCR based on the amplification of B1 gene (35 copies per parasite) using 2 sets of oligonucleotide primers as was described by Burg et al. (1989). Amplification was performed in 20 μl reaction volumes (Accupower PCR premix kit,Bioneer®, South Korea) with a final concentration of each dNTP of 250 μM in 10mM Tris-HCl pH 9•0, 30mM KCl and 2mM MgCl2, 1U Taq DNA polymerase and 10 pmol of each PCR primer(Denazist. Iran). Then 1 μl of DNA template (250-500 ng) was added to each reaction and the remaining 20 μl reaction volume was filled with sterile distilled water. The PCR conditions were slightly modified. The following cycling conditions using a Bio-Rad thermocycler were applied: The first step of amplification was 3min of denaturation at 94 °C, this step was followed by 38 cycles, with 1 cycle consisting of 1min at 94 °C, 1min of annealing at 50°Cfor each pair of primers, and1min at72 °C, an extension step of 7min at 72 °C was planned after the eventual cycle. The PCR primer pair was derived from the B1 gene sequence (Burgetal.1989) , B1F0:5'GGAACTGCATCCGTTCAT-GAG3' and BIR0:5'TCTTTAAAGCGTTC-GTGGTC-3' (position 694-714 and 887-868 nucleotide respectively).The PCR products were electrophoresed through a 1.8% agarose gel to assess the presence of a 193 bp band (if any) in the first round. All PCR products were included in the second round of PCR. The nested-PCR reaction condition was similar to the first round, except for the annealing temperature which was 52 °C, the number of cycles was 30. The resulted amplification products were diluted to 1:10 in water and then a second amplification was done with the internal primers (Burg et al 1989), B1F1:5'-TGCATAGGTTG-CAGTCACTG-3andB1R1:5'-GGCGAC-CAATCTGCGAATACACC-3' (position 757-776 and 853-831 nucleotide , respectively), using 1µl of the diluted product as the template nested PCR. The amplified products were detected in 1.8% gel stained by electrophoresis and viewed under ultraviolet light.

The presence of specific bands of 193 bp in primary PCR and 96 bp in nested -PCR on agarose gel was considered as positive sample.

Statistical analysis: The Chi-square test was used to analyze the association between the *T.gondii* infection with fetal age and geographic region.

All risk factors were analyzed in a multivariable logistic regression model and Odds-ratios (OR) with 95% confidence intervals are calculated. Statistical analyses were performed with the statistics package SPSS, version 16.0 for Windows (IBM, New York, USA).

Results

T.gondii DNA was detected in 18 out of 112 (16.07%) brain samples of ovine fetuses by nested- PCR (Table.1) Three positive samples demonstrated a detectable reaction in both rounds of PCR (Fig.2) and 15 positive samples were detected in second round (Fig. 3). Based on the geographical location, all Toxoplasma infection was detected in the aborted fetuses of sheep in the north areas (p<0.01, Table 2). In this study, significant differences were found between Toxoplasma infection in different age groups of fe-

Table 1. Frequency of *T.gondii* infection in aborted fetuses of sheep in different areas of Khorasan province.

Location	Number of positive	Total
Mashhad	10	47
Chenaran	1	17
Kalat	2	14
Fariman	0	7
Ghochan	0	2
Dargaz	2	4
Serakhas	0	6
Toos	1	2
Bojnord	1	2
Shirvan	1	3
Esfaryein	0	1
Torbat heidareih	0	2
Neishabour	0	1
Gonabad	0	1
Torbat Jaam	0	1
Khaf	0	2
Total	18	112

Table 2. Frequency of *T.gondii* infection in aborted fetuses of sheep from the Khorasan Razavi Province, Iran, in relation to possible risk factors.

Variable	PCR results		Total
	Negative No	Positive No (%)	
Age			
<120 day	15	0 (0)	15
≥120 day	69	18 (20.6%)	87
unknown	10	0 (0)	10
Region			
The North	72	18(20%)	90
The South	22	0 (0)	22
Year			
2009-2010	28	4(12.5%)	32
2010-2011	10	3(23%)	13
2011-2012	19	1(5%)	20
2012-2013	37	10 (21.28)	47

tuses (p<0.05, Table 2). No significant difference was shown between the frequency of Toxoplasma infection in different time periods (p>0.05, Table2).

Discussion

Several PCR methods have been devel-

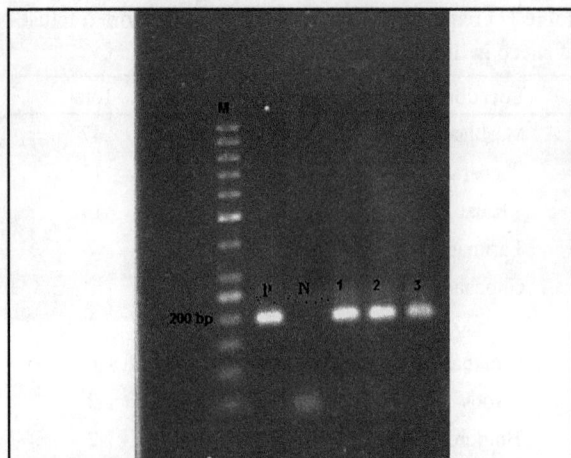

Figure 1. Electrophoretic analysis of PCR-amplified products stained with ethidium bromide in 1.8 % agarose gel. (M) Lane M, 50 bp DNA ladder marker; lane 1, negative control ; Lane2, positive control DNA sample of *T.gondii* (193 bp) ; lane 1-3 samples : DNA samples of blood.

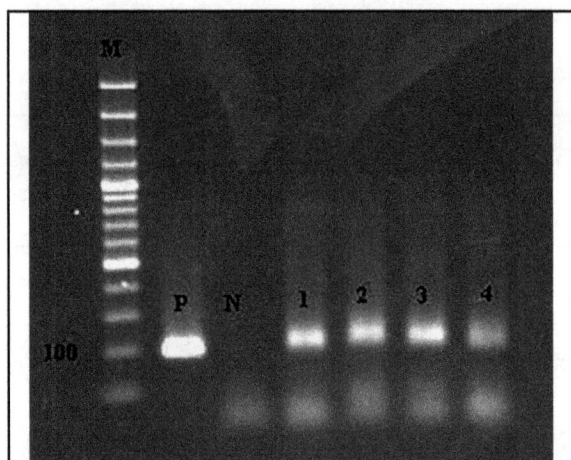

Figure 2. Electrophoretic analysis of PCR-amplified products stained with ethidium bromide in 1.8 % agarose gel . (M) Lane M, 50 bp DNA ladder marker; (P) lane P, positive control ; LaneN, negative control DNA sample of *T.gondii* (96 bp) ; lane 1-5 samples : DNA samples of blood.

oped for *T. gondii* detection in ovine abortion cases, (Hurtado and Aduriz 2007). Among these methods, the B1 gene is widely used as a target in many Toxoplasma PCR detection methods, mainly as a nested protocol based on that described by Burg et al (1989). In the present study, *T. gondii* infection was detected in 16.07% of aborted ovine fetuses by nested PCR.

Among the regions studied in Rio Grande do Norte, seroprevalence varied from 17.8%

in the Central Potiguar region to 26.3% in the Leste Potiguar region (24).

In Iran, *T.gondii* DNA has been detected in aborted fetuses to range between 13.5% to 69% in Khorasan, Qazvin and East Azarbeijan provinces by different PCR assays (Rassouli et al. 2009; Habibi et al. 2011; Mooazeni Jula et al. 2013). These results show that the moutainous climate of Qazvin and East Azarbeijan provinces are more favorable conditions to the development and maintenance of *T. gondii* oocysts in the environment. Oocysts can survive in the environment for months, depending on moisture and temperature. Thus, low humidity and high temperatures of the Khorasan Razavi province is deleterious to the viability of Toxoplasma oocysts in the pasture. In other countries, *T. gondii* PCR positivity was detected to range between 3.5 and11.1% in Italy (Masala et al. 2003; Pereira-Bueno et al. 2004; Chessa et al. 2014)., 5.4 to16.9% in Spain (Hurtado et al. 2001, Moreno et al. 2012), 14% in Ireland (Gutierrez et a l. 2012), 14.3% in Brazil (de Moraes, et al. 2011) and 29.8% in Jordan (Abu-Dalbouh et al. 2012). The differences of PCR results would be related to many factors such as different PCR methods, climatic condition in each country.

All infected fetuses in this study belonged to the areas that are located in the northern part of the province. The northern part of the province has mountainous climate and mean annual rainfall is more than the southern areas with semi desert climate. The mountainous climate confers favorable conditions for Toxoplasma oocysts survival, because the viability of *T. gondii* oocysts is dependent on the moisture and temperature of the soil (Lélu et al. 2012; Du et al. 2012 ;). The higher prevalence of ovine toxoplasmosis has been reported in the humid and temperate areas compared to dry areas (Kamani et al. 2010; Alvarado-Esquivel et al. 2013; Gebremedhin et al. 2013; Andrade et al. 2013; Hamidinejat et al. 2008).

In the present study, most of the infected fetuses had more than 120 days of age. The clinical signs of ovine toxoplasmosis in pregnant ewes depends on the age and immune status of fetus. Fetal death is more likely to occur from infection during the first trimester of pregnancy when the fetal immune system is relatively immature. Infection at mid-gestation can result in birth of a stillborn or weak lamb which may have an accompanying small mummified fetus, whereas infection in later gestation may result in birth of a live, clinically normal, but infected lamb (Buxton 1991; Scott 2007; Innes et al. 2009). Other studies have shown that the abortion associated ovine toxoplasmosis generally occurs during the mid pregnancy (Pereira-Bueno et al. 2004) when the *T. gondii* aborted fetuses have 110-130 days of age (Giadinis et al. 2011).

Based on our results, the moderate frequency of *T.gondii* infection was detected among ovine aborted fetuses in this area. However, a definite diagnosis of Toxoplasma infection in causing abortion in sheep needs to combine pathological and molecular examination

Conflict of interest: The authors declare that they have no conflict of interest

Acknowledgments

This study was supported by a grant VPRTFM-3.27748 from the Vice President of Research and Technology of Ferdowsi University of Mashhad, Iran. We would like to thank Dr Zahra Naseri for help sampling and Dr Fazaeli kindly provided the control positive PCR from the Institute of Public Health Research, Tehran University of Medical Sciences, Tehran, Iran.

References

Abu-Dalbouh, M.A., Ababneh, M.M., Giadinis, N.D., Lafi, S.Q. (2012) Ovine and caprine toxoplasmosis (*Toxoplasma gondii*) in aborted animals in Jordanian goat and sheep flocks. Trop Anim Health Prod. 44: 49-54.

Alvarado-Esquivel, C., Estrada-Malacón, M.A., Reyes-Hernández, S.O., Pérez-Ramírez, J.A., Trujillo-López, J.I.,Villena, I., Dubey, J.P. (2013) Seroprevalence of *Toxoplasma gondii* in domestic sheep in Oaxaca State, Mexico. J Parasitol. 99: 151-2 .

Andrade, M.M., Carneiro, M., Medeiros, A.D., Andrade Neto, V., Vitor, R.W. (2013) Seroprevalence and risk factors associated with ovine toxoplasmosis in Northeast Brazil. Parasite. doi: 10.1051/parasite/2013019.

Burg, J.L., Grover, C.M., Pouletty, P., Boothroyd, J.C. (1989) Direct and sensitive detection of a pathogenic protozoan, *Toxoplasma gondii*, by polymerase chain reaction. J Clin Microbiol. 27:1787-1792.

Buxton, D. (1991) Toxoplasmosis. In: Diseases of Sheep. Martin, W. B., Aitken, I.D. (eds.). (2nd ed.). CAB Wallingford, UK. p. 49-58.

Buxton, D., Maley, S.W., Wright, S. E., Rodger, S., Bartley, P., Innes, E. A. (2007) *Toxoplasma gondii* and ovine toxoplasmosis: new aspects of an old story. Vet Parasitol. 149: 25-28 .

Chessa, G., Chisu,V., Porcu, R., Masala, G. (2014) Molecular characterization of *Toxoplasma gondii* Type II in sheep abortion in sardinia, Italy. Parasite. Doi: 10.1051/parasite/2014007.

de Moraes, E.P., da Costa, M.M., Dantas, A.F., da Silva, J.C., Mota, R.A. (2011) *Toxoplasma gondii* diagnosis in ovine aborted fetuses and stillborns in the State of Pernambuco, Brazil. Vet Parasitol. 183: 152-5.

Dubey, J. P. (2009) Toxoplasmosis in sheep-The last 20 years.Vet Parasitol. 163: 1-14.

Duncanson, P., Terry, R.S., Smith, J.E., Hide, G. (2001) High levels of congenital transmission of *Toxoplasma gondii* in a commercial sheep flock. Int J Parasitol. 31: 1699-1703.

Du, F., Feng, H.L., Nie, H., Tu, P., Zhang, Q.L., Hu, M., Zhou, Y.Q., Zhao, J.L. (2012) Survey on the contamination of *Toxoplasma gondii* oocysts in the soil of public parks of Wuhan, China. Vet Parasitol. 184: 141-6.

Evans, H.E., Sack, W.O. (1973) Prenatal development of domesticand laboratory mammals: growth curves, external features and selected refrences. Anat Histol Embryol. 2: 11-45.

Gebremedhin, E.Z., Agonafir, A., Tessema, T.S., Tilahun, G., Medhin, G., Vitale, M., Di Marco, V. (2013) Some risk factors for reproductive failures and contribution of *Toxoplasma gondii* infection in sheep and goats of Central Ethiopia: a cross-sectional study. Res Vet Sci. 95: 894-900 .

Ghorbani, M., Hafizi, A., Shegerfcar, M.T., Rezaian, M., Nadim, A., Anwar, M., Afshar, A.(1983) Animal toxoplasmosis in Iran.J Trop Med Hyg. 86: 73-6.

Giadinis, N.D., Terpsidis, K., Diakou, A., Siarkou, V., Loukopolos, P., Osman, R., Karatzias, H., Papazahariadou, M. (2011) Massive Toxoplasma abortions in a dairy sheep flock and therapeutic approach with diff erent doses of sulfadimidine. Turk Vet Anim Sci. 35: 207-2011.

Gutierrez, J., O'Donovan, J., Williams, E., Proctor, A., Brady, C., Marques, P. X., Worrall, S., Nally, J. E., McElroy, M., Bassett, H., Sammin, D., Buxton, D., Maley, S., Markey, B.K. (2010) Detection and quantification of *Toxo-*

plasma gondii in ovine maternal and foetal tissues from experimentally infected pregnant ewes using real-time PCR.Vet Parasitol. 172: 8-15.

Hamidinejat, H., Goraninejad, S., Ghorbanpoor, M., Nabavi, L.,Akbarnejad, F. (2008) Role of *Toxoplasma gondii* in abortion of ewesin Ahvaz (South-West Iran). Bull Vet Inst Pulawy. 52: 369-371.

Hartley, W.J., Jebson, J.L., McFarlane, D. (1954) New Zealand type II abortion in ewes. Aust Vet J. 30: 216-218.

Habibi, G.R., Imani, A.R., Gholami, A.R., Hablolvarid, A.R., Behroozikhah, A.M., Lotfi, M., Kamalzade, M., Najjar, E., Esmaeil-Nia, K., Bozorgi, S. (2012) Detection and Identification of *Toxoplasma gondii* Type One Infection in Sheep Aborted Fetuses in Qazvin Province of Iran. Iran J Parasitol. 7: 64-72.

Hashemi-Fesharki, R. (1996) Seroprevalence of *Toxoplasma gondii* in cattle, sheep and goats in Iran. Vet Parasitol. 61: 1-3.

Hide, G., Morley, E.K., Hughes, J.M., Gerwash, O.M., Elmahaishi, S., Elmahaishi, K.H., Thomasson, D., Wright, E.A.,Williams, R.H., Murphy, R.G., Smith, J.E. (2009) Evidence for high levels of vertical transmission in *Toxoplasma gondii*. Parasitol. 136: 877-1885.

Hurtado, A., Aduriz, G., Moreno, B., Barandika, J., García-Pérez, A.L. (2001) Single tube nested PCR for the detection of *Toxoplasma gondii* in fetal tissues from naturally aborted ewes. Vet Parasitol. 102: 17-27 .

Hurtado, A., Aduriz, G. (2007) Polymerase Chain reaction. In: Protozoal Abortion in Farm Animal. Ortega, L.M., Gottstein, B., Conraths, F.J., Buxton, D. (eds.). Protozoal abortion in Farm animal. CAB International, Wallingford, UK. p. 136-141.

Innes, E.A., Barley, P.M., Buxton, D., Katzer, F. (2009) Ovine toxoplasmosis. Parasitol. 136:

1887-1894.

Kamani, J., Mani, A.U., Egwu, G.O. (2010) Seroprevalence of *Toxoplasma gondii* infection in domestic sheep and goats in Borno state, Nigeria. Trop Anim Health Prod. 42: 793-7.

Lélu, M., Villena, I., Dardé, M.L., Aubert, D., Geers, R., Dupuis, E., Marnef, F., Poulle, M.L., Gotteland, C., Dumètre, A., Gilot-Fromont, E. (2012) Quantitative estimation of the viability of *Toxoplasma gondii* oocysts in soil. Appl Environ Microbiol. 78: 5127-32.

Masala, G., Porch, R., Madau, L., Tanda, A., Ibba, B., Satta, G., Tola, S. (2003) Survey of ovine and caprine toxoplasmosis by IFAT and PCR assays in Sardinia, Italy. Vet Parasitol. 117: 15-21.

Morley, E.K., Williams, R.H., Hughes, J.M., Thomasson, D., Terry, R.S., Duncanson, P., Smith, J.E., Hide, G. (2007) Evidence that primary infection of Charollais sheep with *Toxoplasma gondii* may not prevent fetal infection and abortion in subsequent lambings. Parasitology. 135: 169-173.

Moreno, B., Collantes-Fernández, E., Villa, A., Navarro, A., Regidor-Cerrillo, J., Ortega-Mora, L.M. (2012) Occurrence of *Neospora caninum* and *Toxoplasma gondii* infections in ovine and caprine abortions. Vet Parasitol. 187: 312-318.

Moazeni Jula, F., Moazeni Jula1, G., Nowzari, N., Kavari1, H., Hashemzadeh Farhang, H. (2013) A Serological and Molecular study on *Toxoplasma gondii* infection in sheep and goat in Tabriz. Arch Razi Inst. 68: 29-35.

Pereira-Bueno, J., Quintanilla-Gozalo, A., Pérez-Pérez, V., Alvarez-García, G., Collantes-Fernández, E., Ortega-Mora, L.M. (2004) Evaluation of ovine abortion associated with *Toxoplasma gondii* in Spain by different diagnostic techniques. Vet Parasitol. 121: 33-43.

Rahbari, S., Razmi, G.R., Nurozian, E. (1991) A seroepidemiology survey for toxoplasmosis in sheep of Mazandran province. J Fac Vet Med Univ Tehran. 50: 39-49.

Rassouli, M., Razmi, G.R., Bassami, M., Movassaghi, A.R., Azizzadeh, M. (2011) Study on ovine abortion associated with *Toxoplasma gondii* in affected herds of Khorasan Razavi Province, Iran based on PCR detection of fetal brains and maternal serology. Parasitol. 138: 691-697.

Razmi, G.R., Ghezi, K., Mahooti, A., Naseri, Z. (2010) A Serological Study and Subsequent Isolation of *Toxoplasma gondii* From Aborted ovine Fetuses in Mashhad Area, Iran. J Parasitol. 96: 812-814.

Scott, P.R., Sargison, N.D., Wilson, D.J. (2007) The potential for improving welfare standards and productivity in U.K. sheep flocks using veterinary flock health plans. Vet J. 173: 522-531.

Sharifi, M., Gholami, Sh., Ziaei, H., Daryani, A., Laktarashi, B., Ziapour, S.P., Rafiei, A., Vahedi, M. (2007) Seroprevalence of *Toxoplasma gondii* in cattle, sheep and goats slaughtered for food in Mazandaran province, Iran, during 2005. Vet J. 174: 422-4.

Zia-Ali, N., Fazaeli, A., Khoramizadeh, M., Ajzenberg, D., Darde, M., Keshavarz-Valian, H. (2007) Isolation and molecular characterization of *Toxoplasma gondii* strains from different hosts in Iran. Parasitol Res. 101: 111-5.

22

A survey of pathogenic avian mycoplasma involvement in multicausal respiratory disease in broiler flocks

Rahmani, E.[1], Hosseini, H.[2*]

[1]Graduated from the Faculty of Veterinary Medicine, Karaj Branch, Islamic Azad University, Karaj, Iran

[2]Department of Clinical Sciences, Faculty of Veterinary Medicine, Karaj Branch, Islamic Azad University, Karaj, Iran

Key words:

broiler, molecular detection, multicausal respiratory disease, *Mycoplasma gallisepticum*, *Mycoplasma synoviae*

Correspondence

Hosseini, H.
Department of Clinical Sciences, Faculty of Veterinary Medicine, Karaj Branch, Islamic Azad University, Karaj, Iran

Email: hosseini.ho@gmail.com

Abstract:

BACKGROUND: *Mycoplasma gallisepticum* (MG) and *Mycoplasma synoviae* (MS) are the most important and pathogenic mycoplasma in chicken production. The tendency of avian mycoplasma for interaction with other pathogens is well-known. Interaction within several disease-producing factors in respiratory tract exacerbate the disease and is known as multicausal respiratory disease. **OBJECTIVES:** In recent years, high prevalence of multicausal respiratory disease in broiler flocks cause economic loss in Iran. The aim of the current study was to find the role of avian mycoplasma in recent outbreaks of respiratory diseases in broiler flocks. **METHODS:** Four hundred fifty tracheal or choanal cleft swabs were collected from 30 broiler farms with sever respiratory disease. The samples subjected to polymerase chain reaction (PCR) using specific primers for MG and MS. **RESULTS:** One flock (3.3%) and three flocks (10%) of broiler were found to be positive for MG and MS, respectively. **CONCLUSIONS:** The results show that mycoplasma (MG and MS) are not the major part of recent respiratory diseases and anti-mycoplasma drugs administration needs precise test to evaluated mycoplasma statues.

Introduction

Avian mycoplasma consist of more than 23 Mycoplasma species. *Mycoplasma gallisepticum* (MG) and *Mycoplasma synoviae* (MS) are the major avian pathogenic mycoplasmas and economically important pathogen in chicken flocks. *M. gallisepticum* known as chronic respiratory disease (CRD) and *M. synoviae* may cause respiratory disease or synovitis (Ferguson-Noel & Noormohammadi, 2013; Raviv & Ley, 2013). The tendency of avian mycoplasma for interaction with other pathogens is well-known. Interactions within several disease-producing factors in respiratory tract exacerbate the disease and are known as multicausal respiratory disease. Multicausal respiratory disease is a condition that multiple etiologies include a combination of infectious agents plus environmental factors may be involved. In this situation, harmless microbes which cause no disease in healthy bird imperil the bird's life (Glisson, 2013).

Recently, the high prevalence of multicausal respiratory disease in broiler flocks causes huge economic losses in Iran. While viral pathogens include Newcastle disease virus (NDV), infectious bronchitis virus (IBV) and avian influenza virus (AIV) are considered as the main cause of the mortality in broiler, it is believed that different agents may be involved in exacerbation of disease. The role of mycoplasma in recent outbreaks of respiratory disease in Iranian broiler flocks is ambiguous. Considering avian mycoplasma as the main part multicausal respiratory disease, it is important to find the possible role of MG and MS in the respiratory disease. The finding can be helpful in designing logical control, prevention and treatment.

Materials and Methods

Mycoplasma strains: Reference MG strains included S6 strain (University of Liverpool), MG SS strain (GD Animal Health Service Ltd., The Netherlands) and commercial vaccine ts-11 strain (Bioproperties, Australia) and MS-H (Bioproperties, Australia) were used as positive control.

Specimen: Samples were taken from thirty broiler flocks located in Qazvin province during the period from summer to autumn of 2015. Live or dead birds from these broiler flocks were submitted to a poultry clinic in Qazvin with acute respiratory signs and exponential increase in mortality rate. Before postmortem examination fifteen swabs from upper respiratory tract (tracheal or choanal cleft swabs) were carefully taken from each flocks with sterile swabs. Postmortem findings predominantly consist of conjunctivitis with watering eye, nasal discharge, congestion, catarrhal or caseous exudate in trachea, airsacculitis and in some advanced cases fibrinous pericarditis, perihepatitis and peritonitis. Samples which were collected from multicausal respirato-

ry disease-suspected flocks make up a total 450 swabs. Then, the tracheal or choanal cleft swabs submitted to PCR Veterinary Diagnostic Laboratory (Tehran, Iran).

DNA extraction: DNA was extracted from pooled swabs samples (three swabs) using CinnaPure-DNA (CinaClon, Iran) according to the manufacturer's procedure. Extracted DNA was stored at 4 °C for immediate or at -20 for later use.

Molecular detection: All samples were subjected to PCR using specific primers for MG and MS as described previously (Hosseini et al., 2006; Kleven & Bradbury 2008). Two pairs of oligonucleotide primers, (MG-14F: 5' GAG CTA ATC TGT AAA GTT GGT C 3' and MG-13R: 5' GCT TCC TTG CGG TTA GCA AC-3') and (MS-F: 5'-GAG AAG CAA AAT AGT GAT ATC A 3' and MS-R: 5' CAG TCG TCT CCG AAG TTA ACA A 3') were used for detection of MG and MS, respectively. The amplification was carried out in a total 20 μl reaction volume consisting of 2 μl 10 x PCR buffer, 1 μl of mixed primer (25 μM), 0.2 μl 10 mM dNTP, 1 μl 50 mM MgCl2, 0.25 μl Taq DNA polymerase (5U/μl) and 2 μl of template DNA. All amplification reactions were performed in a T100 Thermal Cycler (Bio-Rad, United States) as follows: 94 °C for 3 min, followed by 40 cycles of 94 °C for 10 sec, 55 °C for 10 sec, 72 °C for 10 sec, and a final extension at 72 °C for 5 min. The amplification products were electrophoresed on an agarose gel (2%) in TBE buffer. Gels were run for 1 hr. at 90 Volte, stained with ethidium bromide and visualized under UV light.

Results

A total of 30 broiler flocks with acute re-

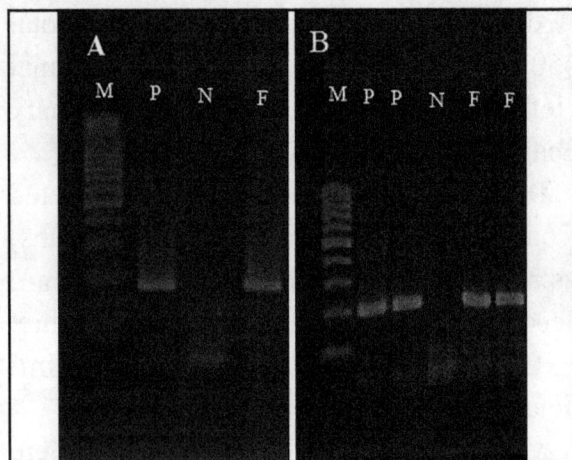

Figure 1. A: Amplification of 16S rRNA of *M. gallisepticum* B: Amplification of 16S rRNA of *M. synoviae*. M: GeneRuler 100 bp DNA Ladder (Thermo Fisher Scientific), P: positive N: negative F: field sample.

spiratory disease were investigated using specific PCR for MG and MS. In each flock 15 birds were swabbed. Swabs of each flock were pooled (three swabs) for examination. As a result, five pooled samples were tested for every affected flock.

The specific primers amplified a 185 bp and 207 bp of standard strains for MG and MS respectively (Fig. 1). Flock was considered positive if at least one sample gave positive result. Of all the flocks tested one flock (3/3%) only was positive in MG PCR and three flocks (10%) were positive in MS PCR. The majority of broiler flocks (26; 86.7%) were negative in MG and MS test.

Discussion

Poultry husbandry has changed since the 1950s. Keeping large numbers of birds in a small area with high density provides close contact between birds, in which infectious agent is easily transmitted. The respiratory tract of chicken harbors a variation of viruses and bacteria. In intensive poultry production infection with a single agent is an exception (Bradbury, 1984). In fact, in commercial condition multiple etiologies

that are involved in respiratory disease are known as multicausal respiratory disease. The outcome of multicausal disease depends on many factors including virulence of pathogens, age. Numerous studies showed that MG and MS are the best example of agent involved in multicausal respiratory disease (Glisson, 2013). Traditionally mycoplasma infection is considered as an important part of multicausal respiratory disease. Considering vertical transmission and the economic importance of mycoplasma, a great deal of effort has been targeted at producing mycoplasma free parent flocks. It seems reasonable that mycoplasma status of parent stocks reflects directly in their progenies.

A great upsurge in respiratory diseases along with high rate of morbidity and mortality in recent years in Iranian broiler flocks suggest more than an etiological contagious agent may be involved. Conventionally, MG and MS are considered as the main exacerbating factors in this situation and usually anti-mycoplasma medication is administered. While there is no pathognomonic gross lesion for mycoplasmosis in postmortem examination, airsacculitis is recognized as CRD in a routine investigation. However, there are few reports in terms of mycoplasma status in broiler flocks and in a study from 2004 to 2007 more than 30% of boiler breeder flocks were shown to be infected with MS (Bayatzadeh et al, 2011). In addition, an earlier survey revealed the high prevalence of MS in boiler flock and about 60% of flocks were found to be positive (Pourbakhsh et al, 2010).

However, status of mycoplasma in boiler breeder flocks has changed significantly in recent years. This may lead to change in mycoplasma status in broiler flocks. MG and MS transmit vertically and horizontally among poultry. As the mycoplasmas are susceptible outside of their host, transmission from hen to progeny through egg, i.e. vertical transmission is a very important route of spreading infection. So it is very important to acquire chicks from MG-free and MS-free parent stocks (Ferguson-Noel & Noormohammadi, 2013; Raviv & Ley, 2013; Kleven & Bradbury 2008). Strict biosecurity and sanitation along with depopulation of MG-positive flocks and repopulation with MG-free resulted in significant decrease in the MG-positive breeder broiler in Iran. While this approache was very effective for MG prevention and control, *M. synoviae* continued to circulate in broiler breeder. Vaccination of broiler breeder with MS-H was an alternative approach which was chosen in Iran from 2005. It is believed that vaccination can prevent the vertical transmission.

According to the results of this survey, the majority of broiler flocks were MG and MS-free and small number flocks were found to be positive. Low rate of mycoplasma infection in broiler can attribute to effectiveness of mycoplasma control applied in broiler breeder in recent years.

Anti-mycoplasma drugs including tylosin, tiamulin and tilmicosin are usually administered as part of the prevention or treatment program in broiler flocks. Medication is a short-term control method and has been of value in treating and controlling individual infected flocks (Ferguson-Noel & Noormohammadi, 2013; Raviv & Ley, 2013). However, the therapeutic and economic benefit of these expensive drugs in MG and MS-free flocks is a questionable decision and practice. It is not advisable to use anti-mycoplasma treatment based on

clinical signs and postmortem finding.

In conclusion, the finding of this survey reveals that the percentage of MG and MS infected flocks is less than expected and mycoplasma are not a dominate part of multicausal respiratory diseases like they used to be. As a result, any treatment of mycoplasma in broiler flocks should be based on laboratory diagnosis and confirmation.

Acknowledgments

The authors would like to thank the PCR Veterinary Diagnostic Laboratory experts for their technical support.

References

Bayatzadeh, M.A., Pourbakhsh, S.A., Homayounimehr, A.R., Ashtari, A. Abtin, A.R. (2011) Application of culture and polymerase chain reaction (PCR) methods for isolation and identification of *Mycoplasma synoviae* on broiler chicken farms. Arch Razi Inst. 66: 87-94.

Bradbury J. M. (1984) Avian mycoplasma infections: prototype of mixed infections with mycoplasmas, bacteria and viruses. Annales de l'Institut Pasteur / Microbiologie. 135: 83-89.

Ferguson-Noel, N., Noormohammadi, A. H. (2013) *Mycoplasma synoviae* Infection. In: Diseases of Poultry. David, E., Swayne, J. R., Glisson, L. R., McDougald, L. K., Nolan, D. L., Suarez, V. L. Nair (eds.). (13th ed.) Wiley-Blackwell Publishing, Ames, Iowa, USA. p. 900-906.

Glisson, J.R. (2103) Multicausal Respiratory Diseases In: Diseases of Poultry. David, E., Swayne, J. R., Glisson, L. R., McDougald, L. K., Nolan, D. L., Suarez, V. L. Nair (eds.). (13th ed.) Wiley-Blackwell Publishing, Ames,

Iowa, USA. p. 1320-1322.

Hosseini, H., Bozorgmehrifard, M.H., Peigham-
bari, S.M., Pourbakhsh, S.A., Razzazian,
M. (2006) Random amplified polymorphic
DNA (RAPD) fingerprinting of *Mycoplasma
gallisepticum* isolates from chickens. Arch
Razi Inst. 61: 67-71.

Pourbakhsh, S.A., Shokri, G.R., Banani, M., El-
hamnia, F., Ashtari, A. (2010) Detection of
Mycoplasma synoviae infection in broiler
breeder farms of Tehran province using PCR
and culture methods. Arch Razi Inst. 65: 75-
81.

Kleven, S.H., Bradbury, J.M. (2008) Avian mycoplasmosis (*Mycoplasma gallisepticum, M.
synoviae*). In: OIE Terrestrial Manual chapter 2. 3. 5: 482-496.

Raviv, Z., Ley, D. H. (2013) *Mycoplasma galli-
septicum* Infection. In: Diseases of Poultry.
David, E., Swayne, J. R., Glisson, L. R., Mc-
Dougald, L. K., Nolan, D. L., Suarez, V. L.
Nair (eds.). (13th ed.) Wiley-Blackwell Pub-
lishing, Ames, Iowa, USA. p. 877-893.

23

Toxoplasma gondii infection in slaughtered ewes in Khorramabad, western Iran

Olfaty-Harsini, S., Shokrani, H.*, Nayebzadeh, H.

Department of Pathobiology, Faculty of Veterinary Medicine, Lorestan University, Khorramabad, Iran

Key words:

frequency, PCR, protozoa, sheep, *Toxoplasma gondii*

Correspondence

Shokrani, H.
Department of Pathobiology,
Faculty of Veterinary Medicine,
Lorestan University, Khorramabad, Iran

Email: hamidreza_shokrani@
yahoo.com

Abstract:

BACKGROUND: The parasitic protozoa *Toxoplasma gondii* is widely prevalent in humans and warm-blooded animals. Humans are usually infected with *T. gondii* by ingesting oocysts shed by cats or by ingesting viable tissue cysts present in raw or undercooked meat. **OBJECTIVES:** This preliminary study was conducted to assess the frequency of *Toxoplasma gondii* infection in tissue samples of ewes slaughtered in Khorramabad, in the west of Iran. **METHODS:** We examined the brain tissue, diaphragm, tongue and masseter muscles of 30 ewes. A nested-PCR which targets the 25-50 copies of B1 sequence has been used for tissue samples. **RESULTS:** The parasite was identified in 21 brain samples (70%) and 8 muscle samples (26.6%). Twenty-three sheep (76.6%) were infected with *T. gondii*. **CONCLUSIONS:** *T. gondii* might be considered as one of the major causes of ovine abortion in this region. According to the result, edible parts of sheep may play a greater role as a source of infection for individuals living in this area.

Introduction

Toxoplasma gondii is a cosmopolitan zoonotic parasite, which is widely prevalent in humans and other warm-blooded animals. This parasite is an important cause of abortion in sheep and is a significant cause of economic loss to sheep industry. Furthermore, *T. gondii* infection is listed as the third-biggest cause of life threatening food-borne diseases (Kravetz and Federman, 2005). Up to one-third of the human world population is chronically infected with this obligate intracellular protozoan parasite (Tenter et al., 2000). The life cycle of *T. gondii* is facultatively heteroxenous and divides into an asexual cycle with little host specificity and a sexual cycle resulting

in the production of oocysts by cats (Tenter et al., 2000). Humans are usually infected with the parasite as a result of consuming raw or undercooked meat containing viable tissue cysts (Dubey, 2009).

Sheep meat is an important source of food for humans living in developing countries such as Iran. Numerous studies on prevalence of *T. gondii* in sheep have been carried out in different countries. Most of these studies have revealed a wide variation in the prevalence rates ranging between 3% and 95.7% within and across different countries (Dubey, 2009). In general, the variation in the prevalence rates among different regions is related to several factors such as the presence of oocysts (density of stray cats or wild felines), climatic conditions, farm management, age distribution as well as the different techniques employed for the sampling and diagnosis (Bayarri et al., 2012; Silva et al., 2013; Tenter et al., 2000).

To our knowledge, little is known about the prevalence and molecular detection of *T. gondii* in sheep in Khorramabad, in the west of Iran. Therefore, the present preliminary study was conducted to assess the frequency of infection in several tissue samples of ewes slaughtered for food in Khorramabad.

Materials and Methods

Sample collection: Samples were collected randomly from Khorramabad slaughterhouse, during a three month period, between April and June 2015. Totally 60 tissue samples were obtained from 30 slaughtered ewes, directly from skulls and diaphragms. Brain samples and meat samples (containing diaphragm, tongue and masseter muscles) were removed from each examined sheep. The tissue samples were immediately transported to the laboratory and kept at 4 °C until further processing. Firstly, 50 g each of meat and of brain were separately minced into small pieces. For each sample, freshly cleaned instruments were used to prevent crossover contamination of DNA. Subsequently, 1 g of each minced sample was thoroughly powdered under liquid nitrogen, transferred to a 1.5 ml sterile tube and stored at -20 °C until DNA extraction.

DNA extraction: DNA extraction was performed using a commercial DNA isolation kit (MBST, Iran) following the supplier's instructions. Briefly, 180 µl lysis buffer and 20 µl proteinase K were added per 50 mg powdered tissue sample, followed by incubation at 55 °C as long as no vis-

Table 1. Results of B1 gene detection in different tissue samples. *Mix of diaphragm, tongue and masseter muscles.

Tested samples	Nested-PCR positive samples		Nested-PCR negative samples		Total
	No.	(%)	No.	(%)	
Brain	21	(70)	9	(30)	30
Meat*	8	(26.7)	22	(73.3)	30
Total	29	(48.3)	31	(51.7)	60

Table 2. Percentage and number of infected tissues in examined ewes. *Mix of diaphragm, tongue and masseter muscles.

Infected tissues	No.	Percentage
Brain	15	50%
Meat*	2	6.6%
Mixed infection (brain & meat)	6	20%
Total	23	76.6%

ible indigested fibers were observed. After adding 360 µl binding buffer and incubation for 10 min at 70 °C, 270 µl ethanol was added to the solution and mixed by gentle vortexing. Subsequently, the complete volume was transferred to the MBST column. The MBST column was first centrifuged and then washed twice with 500 µl washing buffer. Finally, DNA was eluted from the carrier with 60 µl elution buffer and stored at -20 °C.

Nested PCR: A nested-PCR which targets the 25-50 copies of B1 sequence has been used for all DNA samples. PCR reaction was performed as previously described using specific primers P1 (5' GGAACTGCATCCGTTCATGAG 3') and P4 (5' TCTTTAAAGCGTTCGTGGTC 3') to amplify a 193 bp fragment of the B1 gene. The internal primer pairs used for secondary round were P2 (5' TGCATAGGTTGCAGTCACTG 3') and P3 (5' GGCGACCAATCTGCGAATACACC 3') to amplify a 94 bp DNA fragment (Wastling et al., 1993).

Nested-PCR was carried out on 2-5 µl of DNA solution as template for the initial PCR reaction and 1 µl of each PCR product as template for the second round in a total volume of 50 µl, including 5 µl PCR buffer (10X PCR buffer), 1.5 U Taq polymerase, 2 mM MgCl2, 0.2 µM each primer (SinaClon, Iran) and 100 µM of each dNTP (Fermentas, Germany), using a Primus thermal cycler (MWG-Biotech, Germany). The following program was performed for each PCR round: initial denaturation at 94 °C for 5 min; 35 cycles of 15 s at 94 °C, 30 s at 56 °C and 45 s at 72 °C; final extension at 72 °C for 5 min (Mason et al., 2010).

In each PCR experiment DNA isolated from *T. gondii* (RH strain, obtained from Pasteur Institute of Iran) was used as positive control template and also sterile distilled water was used as negative control template. PCR runs in which a negative control indicated contamination were discarded.

Results

From 60 tissue samples that were examined by two pairs of primers in two rounds of amplification, 29 samples (48.3%) were positive. Toxoplasma DNA was detected in 21 (70%) brain samples and 8 (26.7%) meat samples (Table 1). In the first round, the amplified DNA fragment (193 bp) was not always visible. Tissue samples were considered positive if the secondary round band (94bp) appeared (Fig. 1).

Results of B1-PCR revealed the presence of *T. gondii* in 76.6% (23 out of 30) of the examined ewes. In 15 ewes (50%), Toxoplasma DNA was detected only in brain. Mixed infection of meat and brain tissues was found in 6 animals (20%). In 2 ewes

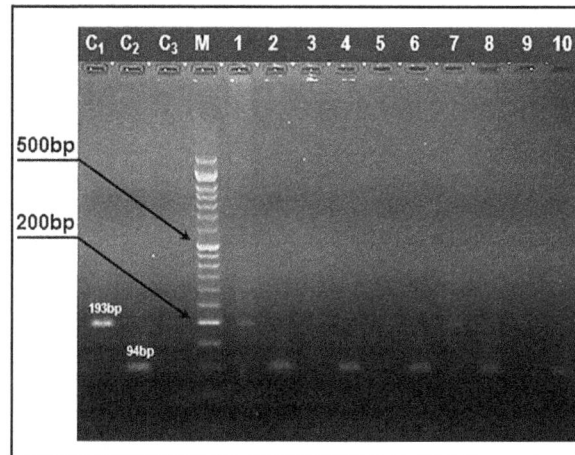

Figure 1. Electrophoretic separation of nested B1-PCR products. C1: positive control (RH strain, first round); C2: positive control (second round); C3: negative control (distilled water, second round); M: DNA ladder (50 bp); lanes 1, 3, 5, 7 and 9: tissue samples (first round, 193 bp which was not always visible); lanes 2, 4, 6, 8 and 10: positive tissue samples (second round, 94 bp).

(6.6%), Toxoplasma DNA was found only in muscles (Table 2). The results of present study showed that the nested-PCR is very sensitive to detection of parasite DNA, especially in samples harboring low amount of parasite.

Discussion

Ovine meat is the most common red meat type consumed in Iran as well as many other Muslim countries. Therefore, edible parts of sheep probably should be considered as the main sources of Toxoplasma infection in humans living in these countries. Results from the present study indicate that 76.6% of the examined sheep are infected with *T. gondii* which currently appears to be the highest infection rate reported in Iran.

These results may reflect some epidemiologic factors such as traditional sheep farming, wide distribution of stray cats and high relative humidity which can affect on the viability and sporulation of oocysts. In contrast, prior studies have shown that these factors are common in some other regions of the country with lower prevalence rates. In this regard, Asgari et al. (2011) analyzed several tissue samples taken from 56 sheep in Fars province (South Iran) and found that only 21 sheep (37.5%) were Toxoplasma DNA positive.

The majority of reports relating to the prevalence of the parasite are achieved from serological methods. High seroprevalence levels in mature sheep were found in the USA (65.5%) (Dubey and Kirkbride, 1989), France (65.6%) (Dumètre et al., 2006), Scotland (73.8%) (Katzer et al., 2011), Serbia (84.5%) (Klun et al., 2006) and Turkey (88%) (Yildiz et al., 2014). Similar seroprevalences were obtained in previous studies performed in Ahvaz, southwestern Iran (72.6%) (Hamidinejat et al., 2008) and Roudsar, northern Iran (62.2%) (Havakhah et al., 2014); while lower values (from 21.1% to 35%) were observed in some other regions of the country (Raeghi et al., 2011; Sharif et al., 2007). These differences can be attributed mainly to the age of the animals (Asgari et al., 2011; Dubey and Kirkbride, 1989; Dumètre et al., 2006; Halos et al., 2010; Katzer et al., 2011). Berger-Schoch et al. (2011) reported the seropositivity of animals slaughtered for meat production in Switzerland and found that increasing age of the sheep is a more important risk factor than housing conditions. In this study, all tissue samples were obtained from mature ewes that were older than two years. These results are expected because aged animals are exposed to oocysts for longer periods.

The difference in frequency among the present and previous studies may be partly due to the different sample preparation methods used for the PCR. In this study, each tissue sample (up to 50 mg) was taken from the homogenate of a large sample (50 g) containing brain or a pool of diaphragm, tongue and masseter muscles to increase the chance of detecting the parasite in each animal. In this respect, our findings seem more comprehensive than those of some previous studies in which samples were obtained by direct sampling and/or from only one sheep's tissue.

Another explanation for these differences is the employment of different techniques for *T. gondii* DNA detection. It is well known that DNA extracts from tissues contain a high ratio of host:parasite genome, which might lead to inhibition of the PCR. In the present study, a second PCR cycle using nested-PCR primers was performed to increase the probability of isolating parasite DNA. A number of PCR assays based on different target genes, including B1, ITS1, SAG1, 3´SAG2, 5´SAG2, SAG3 and 529 bp repeat element, have been used for the detection of *T. gondii* in different tissue samples (Aspinall et al., 2002; Burrells et al., 2013; Homan et al., 2000; Jalal et al., 2004). Some previous studies have shown that the B1-PCR is more sensitive than other PCR assays (Mason et al., 2010; Wastling et al., 1993).

The present study showed that the Toxoplasma infection was significantly high in the brain samples (70%) compared to the meat samples (26.6%). Sheep brain is occasionally consumed by Iranian consumers and it is often well cooked. Therefore, consumption of undercooked meat is a more potent risk factor than consumption of brain. It is now widely accepted that ingestion of inadequately cooked meat is a major source of infection for humans in the United States and Europe (Cook et al., 2000; Dubey et al., 2011). It has been estimated that up to 63%

of Toxoplasma infections in pregnant women in Europe could be attributed to meat consumption (Cook et al., 2000). However, the importance of ingestion of infected meat in the epidemiology of human toxoplasmosis in Iran is unknown.

In the period of 2006 to 2007, a serological study of 390 pregnant women was performed in Khorramabad. Anti-*T. gondii* IgG antibodies were identified in 31%, which was higher than the country's average level (Cheraghipour et al., 2010). These results are somewhat in line with our findings. However, the study does not contain any information to show that the infection was acquired by ingestion of undercooked meat.

Taken together, our findings suggest that the range of problems associated with toxoplasmosis in humans and sheep in Khorramabad is higher than what has been thought so far. The high frequency of infection among examined ewes indicates that edible parts of sheep may play a greater role as a source of infection for individuals living in this area. Furthermore, *T. gondii* is might be considered as one of the major causes of ovine abortion in this region.

Acknowledgments

This work was financially supported by Lorestan University. We are grateful to the meat inspectors of Khorramabad abattoir and the slaughterhouse workers for their co-operation during the present study.

References

Asgari, Q., Sarnevesht, J., Kalantari, M., Sadat, S.J.A., Motazedian, M.H., Sarkari, B. (2011) Molecular survey of Toxoplasma infection in sheep and goat from Fars province, Southern Iran. Trop Anim Health Prod. 43: 389-392.

Aspinall, T., Marlee, D., Hyde, J.E., Sims, P.F.G. (2002) Prevalence of Toxoplsama gondii in commercial meat products as monitored by polymerase chain reaction-food for thought?. Int J Parasitol. 32: 1193-1199.

Bayarri, S., Gracia, M.J., Lázaro, R., Perez-Arquillué, C., Herrera, A. (2012) *Toxoplasma gondii* in meat and food safety implications-a review. In: Zoonosis. Lorenzo-Morales J. (ed.). InTech. p. 229-254.

Berger-Schoch, A.E., Bernet, D., Doherr, M.G., Gottstein, B., Frey, C.F. (2011) *Toxoplasma gondii* in Switzerland: A serosurvey based on meat juice analysis of slaughtered pigs, wild boar, sheep and cattle. Zoonoses Public Health. 58: 472-478.

Burrells, A., Bartley, P.M., Zimmer, I.A., Roy, S., Kitchener, A.C., Meredith, A., Wright, S.E., Innes, E.A., Katzer, F. (2013) Evidence of the three main clonal *Toxoplasma gondii* lineages from wild mammalian carnivores in the UK. Parasitology. 140: 1768-1776.

Cheraghipour, K., Taherkhani, H.A., Falah, M., Sheykhian, A., Sardarian, K.H., Rostamnezhad, M., Maghsoudi, A.H. (2010) Seroprevalence of toxoplasmosis in pregnant women admitted to the health centers of Khorram-Abad city, Iran. Sci J Hamadan Univ Med Sci. 17: 46-51.

Cook, A.J.C., Holliman, R., Gilbert, R.E., Buffolano, W., Zufferey, J., Petersen, E., Jenum, P.A., Foulon, W., Semprini, A.E., Dunn, D.T. (2000) Sources of toxoplasma infection in pregnant women: European multicentre case-control study. BMJ. 321: 142-147.

Dubey, J.P., 2009. Toxoplasmosis in sheep-the last 20 years. Vet Parasitol. 163: 1-14.

Dubey, J.P., Kirkbride, C.A. (1989) Enzootic toxoplasmosis in sheep in north-central United States. J Parasitol. 39: 673-676.

Dubey, J.P., Rajendran, C., Ferreira, L.R., Martins, J., Kwok, O.C.H., Hill, D.E., Villena,

I., Zhou, H., Su, C., Jones, J.L. (2011) High prevalence and genotypes of *Toxoplasma gondii* isolated from goats, from a retail meat store, destined for human consumption in the USA. Int J Parasitol. 41: 827-833.

Dumètre, A., Ajzenberg, D., Rozette, L., Mercier, A., Dardé, M.L. (2006) *Toxoplasma gondii* infection in sheep from Haute-Vienne, France: seroprevalence and isolate genotyping by microsatellite analysis. Vet Parasitol. 142: 376-379.

Halos, L., Thébault, A., Aubert, D., Thomas, M., Perret, C., Geers, R., Alliot, A., Escotte-Binet, S., Ajzenberg, D., Dardé, M.L., Durand, B., Boireau, P., Villena, I. (2010) An innovative survey underlining the significant level of contamination by *Toxoplasma gondii* of ovine meat consumed in France. Int J Parasitol. 40: 193-200.

Hamidinejat, H., Goraninejad, S., Ghorbanpoor, M. (2008) Role of *Toxoplasma gondii* in abortion of ewes in Ahvaz (south-west Iran). Bull Vet Inst Puawy. 52: 369-371.

Havakhah, Y., Reza, A., Rastaghi, E., Amiri, S., Babaie, J., Aghighi, Z., Golkar, M. (2014) Prevalence of *Toxoplasma gondii* in sheep and goats in three counties of Gilan province, north of Iran; the more humid climate the higher prevalence. J Med Microbiol Infec Dis. 2: 80-283.

Homan, W.L., Vercammen, M., De Braekeleer, J., Verschueren, H. (2000) Identification of a 200- to 300-fold repetitive 529 bp DNA fragment in *Toxoplasma gondii*, and its use for diagnostic and quantitative PCR. Int J Parasitol. 30: 69-75.

Jalal, S., Nord, C.E., Lappalainen, M., Evengård, B. (2004) Rapid and sensitive diagnosis of *Toxoplasma gondii* infections by PCR. Clin Microbiol Infect. 10: 937-939.

Katzer, F., Brülisauer, F., Collantes-Fernández, E., Bartley, P.M., Burrells, A., Gunn, G., Maley, S.W., Cousens, C., Innes, E.A. (2011) Increased *Toxoplasma gondii* positivity relative to age in 125 Scottish sheep flocks; evidence of frequent acquired infection. Vet Res. 42: 121.

Klun, I., Djurković-Djaković, O., Katić-Radivojević, S., Nikolić, A. (2006) Cross-sectional survey on *Toxoplasma gondii* infection in cattle, sheep and pigs in Serbia: seroprevalence and risk factors. Vet Parasitol. 135: 121-131.

Kravetz, J.D., Federman, D.G. (2005) Prevention of toxoplasmosis in pregnancy: knowledge of risk factors. Infect Dis Obstet Gynecol. 13: 161-165.

Mason, S., Quinnell, R.J., Smith, J.E. (2010) Detection of *Toxoplasma gondii* in lambs via PCR screening and serological follow-up. Vet Parasitol. 169: 258-263.

Raeghi, S., Akaberi, A., Sedeghi, S. (2011) Seroprevalence of *Toxoplasma gondii* in sheep, cattle and horses in Urmia North-West of Iran. Iran J Parasitol. 6: 90-94.

Sharif, M., Gholami, S., Ziaei, H., Daryani, A., Laktarashi, B., Ziapour, S.P., Rafiei, A., Vahedi, M. (2007) Seroprevalence of *Toxoplasma gondii* in cattle, sheep and goats slaughtered for food in Mazandaran province, Iran, during 2005. Vet J. 174: 422-424.

Silva, A.F., Brandão, F.Z., Oliveira, F.C.R., Ferreira, A.M.R. (2013) *Toxoplasma gondii* in the sheep industry: a global overview and the situation in Brazil. R bras Ci Vet. 20: 179-188.

Tenter, A.M., Heckeroth, A.R., Weiss, L.M. (2000) *Toxoplasma gondii*: from animals to humans. Int J Parasitol. 30: 1217-1258.

Wastling, J.M., Nicoll, S., Buxton, D. (1993) Comparison of two gene amplification methods for the detection of *Toxoplasma gondii* in experimentally infected sheep. J Med Microbiol. 38: 360-365.

Yildiz, K., Kul, O., Gokpinar, S., Atmaca, H.T.,

Gencay, Y.E., Gazyagci, A.N., Babur, C., Gurcan, İ.S. (2014) The relationship between seropositivity and tissue cysts in sheep naturally infected with *Toxoplasma gondii*. Turk J Vet Anim Sci. 38: 169-175.

24

Comparing inhibitory potential of *Eugenia caryophyllus* and *Origanum compactum* against the growth and gene expression of enterotoxins in *Staphylococcus aureus* ATCC 29213

Azizkhani, M.[1]*, Akhondzadeh Basti, A.[2], Tooryan, F.[1]

[1]*Department of Food Hygiene, Faculty of Veterinary Medicine, Amol University of Special Modern Technologies, Amol, Iran*

[2]*Department of Food Hygiene, Faculty of Veterinary Medicine, University of Tehran, Tehran, Iran*

Key words:

enterotoxin, *Eugenia caryophyllus*, gene expression, *Origanum compactum*, *Staphylococcus aureus*

Correspondence

Azizkhani, M.
Department of Food Hygiene,
Faculty of Veterinary Medicine,
Amol University of Special
Modern Technologies, Amol,
Iran

Email: m.azizkhani@ausmt.ac.ir

Abstract:

BACKGROUND: Bacterial resistance to antibiotics is a crucial public health problem. Essential oils (EOs) possess antimicrobial effects and have been screened as potential natural antimicrobial compounds. **OBJECTIVES:** This study was conducted to compare the effects of *Eugenia caryophyllus* (clove) and *Origanum compactum* (oregano) EOs on the growth of *Staphylococcus aureus* and the expression of the SEA, SEC and SEE genes. **METHODS:** The minimum inhibitory concentrations (MIC) of EOs and growth of bacterium at subMIC levels of EOs were determined. Enterotoxin detection was done using a commercial SE visual immunoassay kit after 18, 24, 48 and 72 h. Gene expression of enterotoxins was evaluated through RNA extraction, DNA synthesis and performing real time-PCR using specific primers for each SE. **RESULTS:** MIC of clove and oregano were 2 µl/ml and 1µ l/ml, respectively. Colony counts at 48 and 72h of cultures grown at 75% MIC of clove oil showed the growth rate was reduced 1.67 and 1.83 log10 cfu/ml compared to the control, and in the case of oregano at 75% MIC the decreases in growth rate were 2.25 and 2.68 log10 cfu/ml, respectively. When the target bacterium is cultured in the presence 75% subMIC of EOs, the transcript levels of sea, sec, see and the regulatory gene (agrA) were decreased 8.81, 9.13, 9.08 and 8.32 fold in the case of clove, and 11.56, 9.96, 11.07 and 11.15 fold in the case of oregano, compared to the control. **CONCLUSIONS:** The growth, gene expression and as a result secretion of enterotoxins A, C and E by *S. aureus* were decreased significantly at subMIC levels of EOs, especially at 75% MIC.

Introduction

The importance of *Staphylococcus aureus* in diseases ranging from acute infections (localised or invasive) to acute toxaemia is well-known (Baird-Parker, 1990). Staphylococcal food-poisoning syndrome is an intoxication caused by ingestion of staphylococcal enterotoxins (SEs). These toxins are classified on the basis of their immunological reactivities and have been designated SEA, SEB, SEC1, SEC2, SEC3, SED, SEE and SEH (Omoe et al., 2002).

There is currently an impetus for the discovery of natural antimicrobial agents for use as alternatives to synthetic compounds in food preservation and human remedies. The excessive and inappropriate use of antibiotics in agriculture and in human health to treat infectious diseases is responsible for the emergence of resistant organisms (Farahnik and Murase, 2016; Zhao et al., 2017). Essential oils (EOs) obtained by steam distillation from aromatic plants have recently gained in popularity and scientific interest as natural preservative compounds. EOs are a potentially useful source of molecules of diverse biological activities, and numerous scientific reports have highlighted antimicrobial activities of them (Bajer et al., 2017; Oussalah et al., 2007). Some studies have evaluated the inhibitory effects of natural compounds and EOs on growth, toxin production and gene expression of enterotoxins in S.aureus (Azizkhani et al., 2013; Qiu et al., 2010).

Cloves are the aromatic dried flower buds of a tree (*Eugenia caryophyllus*) of the family Myrtaceae (Chaieb et al., 2007a). They exhibit anti-mutagenic (Miyazawa and Hisama, 2003), anti-inflammatory (Mektrirat et al., 2016), antioxidant (Chaieb et al., 2007b), anti-ulcerogenic (Li et al., 2005), anti-thrombotic (Srivastava and Malhotra, 1991) and anti-parasitic (Yang et al., 2003) properties.

Oregano, a plant belonging to the Laminaceae family, is mainly used as a culinary condiment and is largely employed in popular medicine for the treatment of ailments such as digestive and pulmonary disorders (Asadbeigi et al., 2014). In addition, it is used as a preservative in many kinds of food (Asensio et al., 2015; Bhargava et al., 2015). The EO of oregano also exhibits significant antimicrobial activity (De Falco et al., 2014) and various extracts of the oregano plant have been tested for their biological activities (Fratini et al., 2017; Dutra et al., 2016).

The present study is the first work that investigated the antimicrobial effect of clove and oregano EOs at molecular level. This work was conducted to determine the MICs value of clove and oregano EOs that would inhibit the growth of *S. aureus* ATCC 29213 on the one hand, and that required to kill this bacterium (minimum bactericidal concentration: MBC) on the other. In addition, the effect of subMIC levels of EOs on the growth of the microorganism and the gene expression of enterotoxins A, C and E has also been evaluated.

Materials and Methods

Essential oils: Commercially available oregano and clove essential oils supplied by Pranarôm International (Ghislenghien, Belgium) were used in this study. The EOs were analysed by gas chromatography, ThermoQuest Co. (Manchester, UK).

Bacterial strains and reagents: *S. aureus* ATCC 29213, which has the ability to secrete SEA, SEC and SEE, was obtained as a lyophilized culture from the Pasteur Research Institute, Tehran, Iran. All chemicals and culture media were purchased from Merck (Darmstadt, Germany).

Determination of MIC and MBC: In order to determine the lowest concentration (MIC) in which visible growth of the bacterium is inhibited, a broth microdilution assay was employed (NCCLS, 2000).

Table 1. Primers used for quantitative RT-PCR.

Primer	Sequence (5'à3')	Primer length (bp)	Tm (°C)
sea-F	ATGGTGCTTATTATGGTTATC	120	54
sea-R	CGTTTCCAAAGGTACTGTATT		
sea-F	TTTTTGGCACATGATTTAATTT	257	55
sec-R	CAACCGTTTTATTGTCGTTG		
see-F	CAGTACCTATAGATAAAGTTAAAACAAGC	178	55
see-R	TAACTTACCGTGGACCCTTC		
16S rRNA-F	GCTGCCCTTTGTATTGTC	278	54
16S rRNA-R	AGATGTTGGGGTTAAGTCCC		
agrA-F	TGATAATCCTTATGAGGTGCTT	274	56
agrA-R	CACTGTGACTCGTAACGAAAA		

The assay was carried out with Tryptic soy broth (TSB) culture medium. To obtain and maintain a stable oil-water emulsion in the broth substrate during the experiment, the method of Mann and Markham (1998) was used with some modifications. Briefly, 5 ml/100ml dimethylsulphoxide (DMSO) as an emulsifier and 0.05 g/100ml agar-agar as a stabilizer were added to the broth substrate. Dilutions of EOs were set up using a 96-well microtitre plate (180μl of TSB containing specified concentrations of EO and 20μl of inocula were transferred to each microwell). The final bacterial inoculation titre in each microwell was 10^5 cfu/ml. As a control, the same amount of DMSO and agar-agar were also added to broth lacking EOs to take into account any effects these additives might have on the growth and/or toxin production of the test organism. The plate was covered with a sterile plate sealer. The contents of each well were mixed on a plate shaker at 300 rpm for 20 s and then incubated at 35 °C for 24 h. Bacterial growth was determined by measuring absorbance at 600 nm. In order to determine the minimum bactericidal concentration (MBC) as the lowest concentration that reduces the bacterial population 99.9% after incubation at 35-37 °C for 24 h, 100 μl of those microtitre cultures with no visible growth in the MIC

determination assay were spread on Tryptic soy agar (TSA) and incubated at 35 °C for 24 h. The concentration of EOs in those wells that yielded plates with no visible colonies was considered to be the MBC.

Growth of bacterium: EOs were added at subMIC levels (25, 50 and 75%MIC; subMICs of clove: 0.5, 1 and 1.5 μl/ml; subMICs of oregano: 0.25, 0.5 and 0.75 μl/ml) to 10 ml liquid TSB culture media containing 5 ml/100ml DMSO and 0.05 g/100ml agar-agar. The inoculation dose of *S. aureus* was 10^5 cfu/ml. Bacteria were cultured at 35 °C with aeration. The control culture contained 5 ml/100ml DMSO and 0.05 g/100ml agar-agar only. For colony counting, serial dilutions were prepared from TSB cultures incubated for 0, 18, 24, 48 and 72 h and spread on TSA plates (Azizkhani et al., 2013).

Enterotoxin detection: The RIDAS-CREEN SET kit from R-Biopharm Co. (Darmstadt, Germany), a commercial SE visual immunoassay kit with a minimum detectable limit of 0.50 to 0.75 ng of SEs per ml or g of sample, was used for SE detection. Strain ATCC 29213 was cultured in TSB with subMIC levels of EOs at 35 °C for 72 h and enterotoxin detection was done according to the manufacturer's instructions after 18, 24, 48 and 72 h.

RNA extraction and purification: Strain ATCC 29213 was cultured in TSB in the presence of subMIC levels of EOs at 35 °C for 72 h. RNA was prepared after 18, 24, 48 and 72 h of culture using the Tripure isolation reagent (Roche Applied Science, Bavaria, Germany) according to the manufacturer's instructions. RNA was quantified by measuring the absorbance at 260 nm and purity was assessed measuring the A260nm/A280nm ratio using a NanoDrop Spectrophotometer 2000 (Thermo Scientific, Illinois, USA). RNA quality and integrity was visualized by ethidium bromide staining after electrophoresis of RNA on a 1 g/100ml agarose gel. DNA-free RNA was dissolved in DEPC-water (diethyl pyrocarbonate treated double-distilled water) and stored at -70 °C.

cDNA synthesis: RNA was reverse transcribed into cDNA using the Omniscript Reverse Transcription kit, Qiagen Co. (Hilden, Germany) according to the manufacturer's instructions. cDNA was stored at -20 °C until needed.

Real-time PCR: PCR reactions of 20µl total volume and containing Power SYBR Green (Applied Biosystems Co., Courtaboeuf, France) as recommended by the manufacturer were performed using the ABI PRISM 7500 Sequence Detection System from Applied Biosystems Co. (Courtaboeuf, France). The primer pairs used are listed in Table 1. Cycling conditions were as follows: one cycle at 95 °C for 10 min, 40 cycles at 95 °C for 15 s and 60 °C for 1 min. All samples were analyzed in triplicate and normalized against 16S rRNA expression (Azizkhani et al., 2013). Since sec and see are positively regulated by the agrA two-component system, the transcription of agrA was also investigated.

For SYBR Green based amplicon detection it is important to run a dissociation curve following the RT- PCR. This is due to the fact that SYBR Green will detect any double-stranded DNA including primer dimers, contaminating DNA, and PCR products from misannealed primers. The derivative plot of the melting curve of each gene in the reaction was therefore evaluated. Relative expression levels were determined by the $\Delta\Delta Ct$ method described in Applied Biosystems User Bulletin no. 2.

Statistical analysis: All experiments (MIC and MBC determination, growth experiments, enterotoxin detection and PCR experiments) were repeated three times. Data were expressed as the mean ± STD Dev. Statistical differences were calculated using the independent Student t-test. A p value less than 0.05 was considered to be statistically significant.

Results

Chemical composition of EOs: The main compounds present in oregano EO are carvacrol (46.88%), thymol (15.26%), p-cimene (13.10%) and g-terpinene (11.61%), and those in clove EO are eugenol (83.96%), eugenile acetate (10.75%) and b-caryophyllene (3.25%).

MIC and MBC results: The MIC and MBC values of clove EO against *S. aureus* ATCC 29213 were 2 ± 0.001 and 4 ± 0.05µ l/ml respectively. The MIC and MBC values obtained for oregano EO against *S. aureus* were 1 ± 0.004 and 1.2 ± 0.007µ l/ml respectively.

Growth of S. aureus: From the results given in Fig. 1A, after 24, 48 and 72 h of incubation at 35 °C, 75% MIC of clove EO decreased the final cell density of *S. aureus*

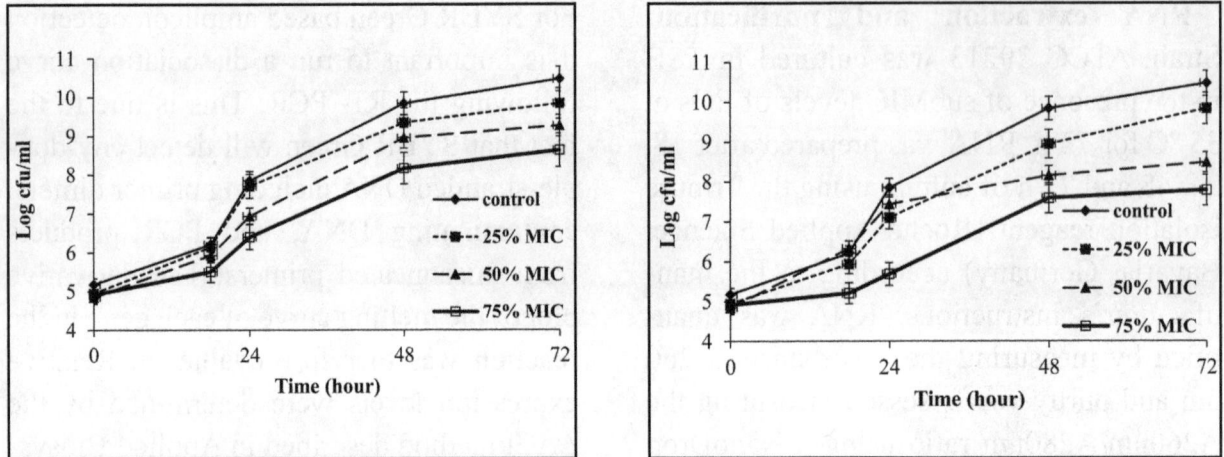

Figure 1. Colony counts of *S. aureus* cultured in the presence of subinhibitory levels of (1A) *Eugenia caryophyllus* and (1B) *Origanum compactum* EOs. The data are means and the associated error bars represent standard deviations. Deviation for three independent experiments (p<0.05).

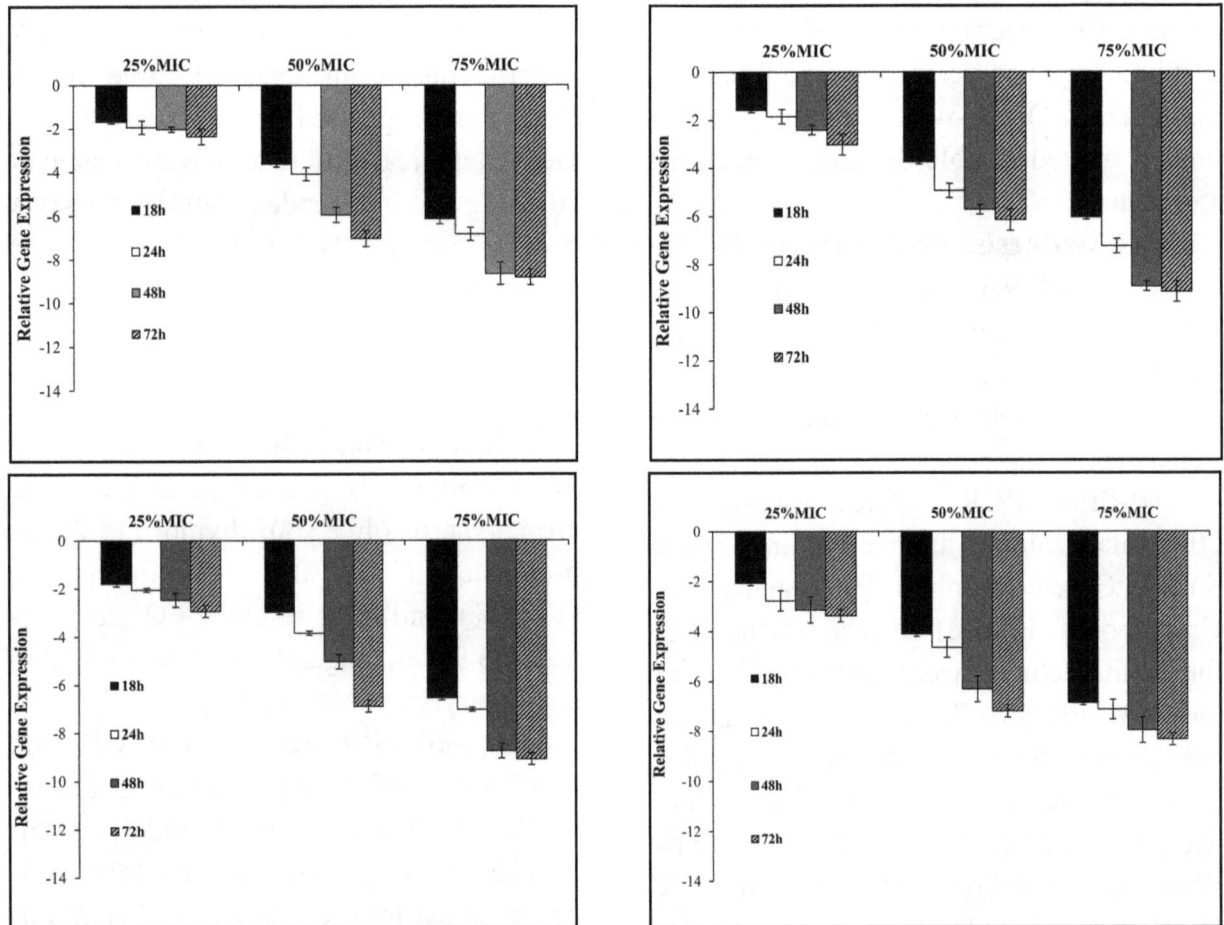

Figure 2. Relative expression of sea (2A), sec (2B), see (2C) and agrA (2D) in S. aureus. *S. aureus* ATCC 29213 was cultured with subinhibitory concentrations of *Eugenia caryophyllus* EO for 72 hours. Transcript levels were monitored by quantitative RT-PCR as described in the text. The fold reduction of gene expression in EO treatments is reported in comparison to the control culture lacking EO. The data are means and the associated error bars represent standard deviations. Deviation for three independent experiments (p<0.05).

by 1.45, 1.67 and 1.83 log10 (cfu/ml) respectively (p<0.05), compared to the control culture; colony counts of cultures grown in the presence of 75% MIC of oregano EO

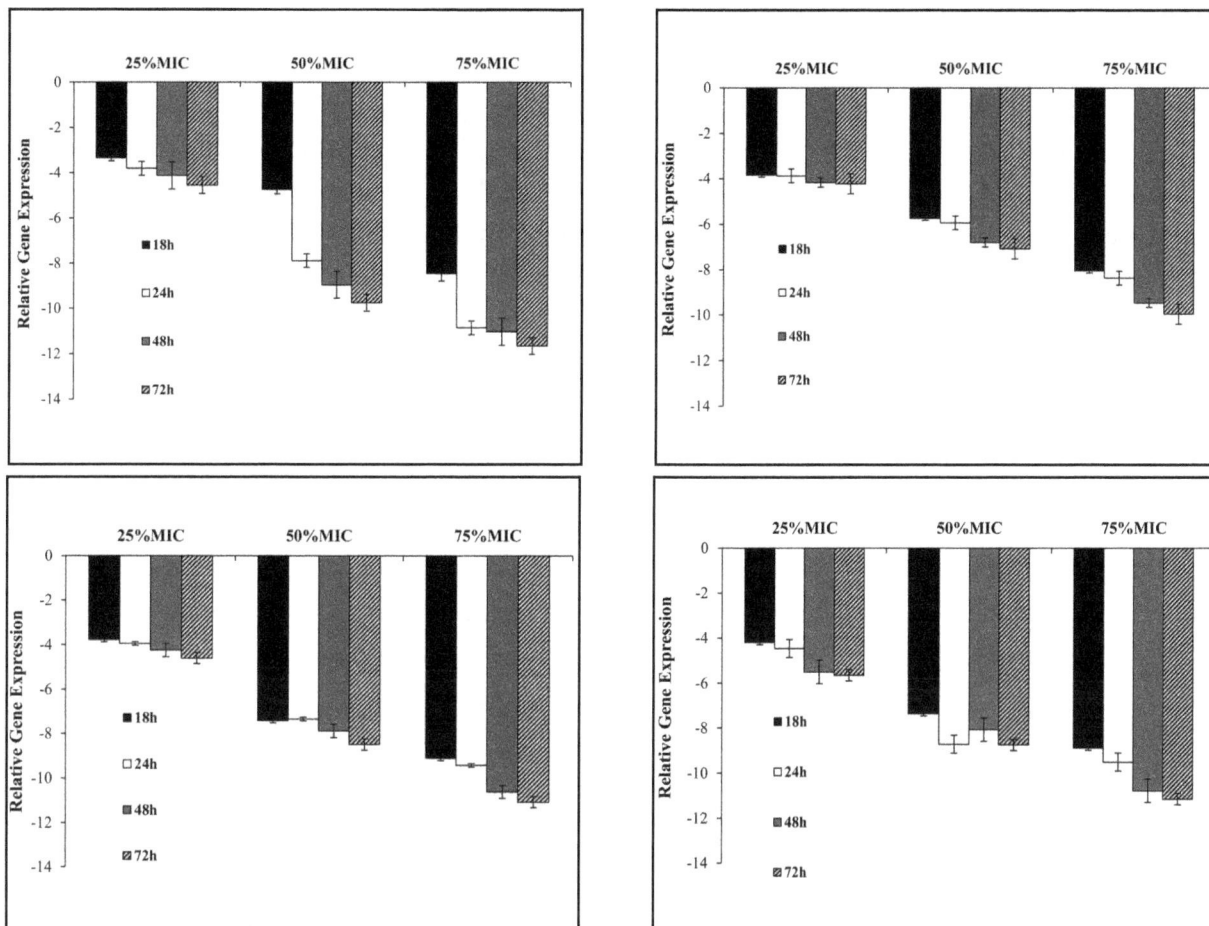

Figure 3. Relative expression of sea (3A), sec (3B), see (3C) and agrA (3D) in S. aureus. *S. aureus* ATCC 29213 was cultured with subinhibitory concentrations of *Origanum compactum* EO for 72 hours. Transcript levels were monitored by quantitative RT-PCR as described in the text. The fold reduction of gene expression in EO treatments is reported in comparison to the control culture lacking EO. The data are means and the associated error bars represent standard deviations. Deviation for three independent experiments ($p < 0.05$).

for the same incubation periods (Fig. 1B) showed growth to be reduced 2.16, 2.25 and 2.68 log10 cfu/ml respectively ($p < 0.05$). These reductions were found to be statistically significant compared to the controls for both EOs ($p < 0.05$). There was also a statistically significant difference between the results for the different incubation periods ($p < 0.001$).

ELISA results: In this study it can be seen that the EOs at 25% MIC had no inhibitory effect on enterotoxin production by *S. aureus* at any of the time periods analysed (18, 24, 48 and 72 h) compared to the control in the absence of EO. Increasing the concentration of EO to 50% and 75% MIC produced significant ($p < 0.05$) inhibitory effects on enterotoxin production.

Transcription of the sea, sec, see and argA genes: It was apparent from the melting curve data (not shown) that no contaminating products were present in the reactions since contaminating DNA or primer dimers would have shown up as additional peaks separate from the desired amplicon peak. The melting temperatures (Tm) of the genes are presented in Table 1. A dose-dependent reduction in sea, sec, see and agrA transcription was observed in *S. aureus* upon treatment with the EOs (Fig. 2 & 3). For example, when cultured with 75% MIC of clove EO, the transcriptional levels of sea, sec, see and agrA were decreased 6.13, 6.05, 6.54 and 6.85 fold after 18 h and 8.81, 9.13, 9.08 and 8.32 fold after 72 h in comparison to the control, respectively, (p<0.05). In the case of oregano EO, the expression of sea, sec, see and agrA was reduced 8.45, 8.06, 9.11 and 8.89 fold after 18 h and 11.65, 9.96, 11.07 and 11.15 fold after 72 h in comparison to control, respectively, (p<0.05).

Discussion

A number of reports have highlighted the potential that plant EOs (and their components) may, in food preservation, give the inhibitory effects they exert on microbial growth (Aumeeruddy-Elalfi et al., 2016; Kwon et al., 2017; Xiang et al., 2017). Several studies have focused specifically on the strongly antibacterial properties of clove EO (Cui et al., 2016; Fu et al., 2007; Khaleque et al., 2016; Li et al., 2005; Mulla et al., 2017), the high degree of its inhibitory activity probably derived from the antibacterial activities exhibited by a wide range of its constituent compounds: eugenol [2-methoxy-4- (2-propenyl) phenol], eugenyl acetate, beta-caryophyllene, 2-heptanone (Chaieb et al., 2007b), acetyl- eugenol, alpha-humulene, methyl salicylate, iso-eugenol, methyl-eugenol (Yang et al., 2003), phenyl propanoides, dehydrodieugenol, trans-coniferyl aldehyde, biflorin, kaempferol, rhamnocitrin, myricetin, gallic acid, ellagic acid and oleanolic acid (Khaleque et al., 2016).

It would appear that there are diverse mechanisms by which EOs - and their constituents - adversely affect microorganisms. It has been hypothesized that phenolic compounds are involved in microbial growth inhibition because these compounds sensitize the phospholipid bilayer of the microbial cytoplasmic membrane resulting in increased permeability, the absence of vital intracellular constituents and/or the impairment of bacterial enzyme systems (Juven et al., 1994). Phenolic components such as eugenol are highly active against microorganisms, and in the present study we found the principal constituent of clove oil to be eugenol (83.96%). It is known that the bactericidal or bacteriostatic activities of compounds of this type are determined by their concentration (Dorman and Deans, 2000).

The even stronger antibacterial activity of oregano EO compared to that of clove observed in this study correlates with the greater contents of carvacrol (46.88%) and thymol (15.26%) in *O. compactum* oil. These phenolics are among the most effective plant antibacterial agents known to date (Nazer et al., 2005), and several studies have demonstrated their ability to inactivate bacterial strains in synthetic media as well as in food systems (Knowles et al., 2005; Lambert et al., 2001; Valero and Frances, 2006). It has been proposed that the antibacterial activity of carvacrol derives from the physical distortion it induces in the membrane as a result of its accumulation in this hydrophobic environment, combined with the electron transporter activity conferred in part by its delocalised electron system resulting in further disruption of the transmembranal pH gradient. The consequent loss of the proton motive force results in ATP depletion and ultimately cell death (Ultee et al., 2002).

The MIC values obtained in the present study for clove and oregano EOs against *S. aureus* were 2µ l/Ml and 1µ l/ml, respectively, and are approximately in accordance with those of Fu et al. (2007) and Nostro et al. (2006). Both EOs reduce the growth of *S. aureus* and its production of SE in a dose-dependent manner. The data (Fig. 1A, 1B) also reveal a greater inhibitory effect of oregano EO compared to that of clove. In this regard, a number of previous observations reported significant inhibitory effects of carvacrol-containing EOs on *Bacillus cereus*, *Salmonella typhimurium* and *S. aureus* (Azizkhani et al., 2013; Basti et al., 2007; Misaghi and Basti, 2007; Moosavy et al., 2008). The greater the carvacrol content of the EO, the greater the inhibitory activity observed.

Our data highlight the potential of oregano EO for significantly reducing and inhibiting enterotoxin production. Similar findings were made by de Souza et al. (2010) and Palmer et al. (2004) who reported the strong effects of subMIC levels of bay, cinnamon, clove and oregano EOs in decreasing the production of enterotoxins by S. aureus, as well as the antimicrobial activity of Z. multiflora Boiss. EO on enterotoxin C production (Azizkhani et al., 2013; Parsaeimehr et al., 2010). In their study, de Souza et al. (2010) observed total suppression of enterotoxin production in the broth to which *Origanum vulgare* L. EO had been added at subMIC levels (0.3 and 0.15 µl/ml). Qiu et al. (2010) evaluated the effect of subMIC levels of thymol (a phenolic fraction of some EOs such as that of oregano in this study) on methicillin sensitive and resistant isolates of S. aureus, revealing dose-dependent decreases in the growth of the microorganism and the production of SEA, SEB and α-hemolysin. We have made similar observations in the present study.

Inhibitors of protein synthesis at subMIC levels significantly reduce the production of

virulence factors (including α-hemolysin, SEA, SEB and protein A) by *S. aureus* (Bernardo et al., 2004; Herbert et al., 2001) and many currently used synthetic preservatives affect the secretion of exotoxins, especially when used at suboptimal concentrations. Certain plant compounds (e.g. oleuropein and epicatechin gallate) and EOs (e.g. the oils of bay, cinnamon and cloves) can also influence the production of exotoxins when used at low concentrations (Palmer et al., 2004; Shah et al., 2008).

Previous reports have indicated that subMIC levels of antimicrobials may interfere with the translation of one or more regulatory gene products in *S. aureus* and by this means affect the transcription of exoprotein-encoding genes (Kuroda et al., 2007). Also, electron microscopy of EO-treated cells revealed the formation of holes in bacterial cell surfaces and the loss of cytoplasmic material (de Souza et al., 2010). In the current study, quantitative RT-PCR was used to investigate the influence of EOs on the expression of the agr locus of S. aureus. Our data show that the EOs tested significantly inhibit agrA transcription. However, the mechanisms by which *S. aureus* controls virulence gene expression are fairly intricate and involve an interactive, hierarchical regulatory cascade of the products of the agr gene along with other components (Chan and Foster, 1998). We therefore presume that the reduced production of virulence factors observed in our study may partially depend on EO-induced inhibition of the agr two-component system.

Oregano and clove EOs both show strong inhibitory effects against *S. aureus* in vitro, the most effective of the two being oregano. The ability of both EOs to inhibit the growth of this microorganism and its production of enterotoxin indicates a potential for these oils as natural food preservatives. The activity observed is attributable to the phenolic compounds present in the oils. The results presented here may explain the traditional culinary and medicinal uses of these plants. Further work is necessary to assess the effectiveness of these EOs in food systems and to extend the molecular analysis of gene expression to other enterotoxin encoding genes and enterotoxigenic microorganisms.

Acknowledgments

This work has been supported by a research grant (no. 8.2709) from the Amol University of Special Modern Technologies, Amol, Iran. We are also grateful to Dr. Andrew MacCabe of the Instituto de Agroquímica y Tecnología de Alimentos (IATA), Valencia, Spain, for critical reading of the manuscript.

References

Applied Biosystems, User bulletin no. 2. (1997) Relative quantification of gene expression. Applied Biosystems. Massachusetts, USA.

Asadbeigi, M., Mohammadi, T., Rafieian-Kopaei, M., Saki, K., Bahmani, M., Delfan, M. (2014) Traditional effects of medicinal plants in the treatment of respiratory diseases and disorders: an ethnobotanical study in the Urmia. Asian Pac J Trop Dis. 7: 364-368

Asensio, C.M., Grosso, N.R., Juliani, H.R. (2015) Quality preservation of organic cottage cheese using oregano essential oils. LWT - Food Sci Technol. 60: 664-671.

Aumeeruddy-Elalfi, Z., Gurib-Fakim, A., Fawzi Mahomoodally, M. (2016) Chemical composition, antimicrobial and antibiotic potentiating activity of essential oils from 10 tropical medicinal plants from Mauritius. J Herb Med. 6: 88-95.

Azizkhani, M., Misaghi, A., Basti, A.A., Gandomi, H., Hosseini, H. (2013) Effects of Zataria multiflora Boiss. essential oil on growth and gene expression of enterotoxins A, C and E in Staphylococcus aureus ATCC 29213. Int J Food Microbiol. 166: 249–255.

Bajer, T., Šilha, D., Ventura, K., Bajerová, P. (2017) Composition and antimicrobial activity of the essential oil, distilled aromatic water and herbal infusion from Epilobium parviflorum Schreb. Ind Crop Prod. 100: 95-105.

Basti, A.A., Misaghi, A., Khaschabi, D. (2007) Growth response and modeling of Zataria multiflora Boiss. essential oil, pH and temperature on Salmonella typhimurium and Staphylococcus aureus. LWT-Food Sci Technol. 40: 973-981.

Bernardo, K., Pakulat, N., Fleer, S., Schnaith, A., Utermohlen, O., Krut, O., Muller, S., Kronke, M. (2004) Subinhibitory concentrations of linezolid reduce Staphylococcus aureus virulence factor expression. Antimicrob Agents Chemother. 48: 546–555.

Betoni, J.E., Mantovani, R.P., Barbosa, L,N., De-Stasi, L,C., Junior, F.A. (2006) Synergism between plant extract and antimicrobial drugs used on Staphylococcus diseases. Memórias do Instituto Oswaldo Cruz. 101: 387-390.

Bhargava, K., Conti, D.S., da Rocha, SR.P., Zhang, Y. (2015) Application of an oregano oil nanoemulsion to the control of foodborne bacteria on fresh lettuce. Food Microbiol. 47: 69-73

Chaieb, K., Hajlaoui, H., Zmantar, T., Nakbi, K.A.B., Rouabhia, M., Mahdouani, K., Bakhrouf, A. (2007) The chemical composition and biological activity of essential oil, Eugenia cryophyllata (Syzygium aromaticum

L. Myrtaceae): a short review. Phytother Res. 21: 501-506.

Chaieb, K., Zmantar, T., Ksouri, R., Hajlaoui, H., Mahdouani, K., Abdelly, C., Bakhrouf, A. (2007) Antioxidant properties of essential oil of *Eugenia caryophyllata* and its antifungal activity against a large number of clinical *Candida* species. Mycosis. 50: 403-406.

Chan, P.F., Foster, S.J. (1998) Role of SarA in virulence determinant production and environmental signal transduction in *Staphylococcus aureus*. J Bacteriol. 180: 6232–6241.

Cui, H., Ma, C., Lin, L. (2016) Synergetic antibacterial efficacy of cold nitrogen plasma and clove oil against *Escherichia coli* O157:H7 biofilms on lettuce. Food Control. 66: 8-16.

De Falco, E., Roscigno, G., Landolfi, S., Scandolera, E., Senatore, F. (2014) Growth, essential oil characterization, and antimicrobial activity of three wild biotypes of oregano under cultivation condition in Southern Italy. Ind Crop Prod. 62: 242-249.

De Souza, E.L., de Barros, J.C., de Oliveira, C.E., da Conceição, M.L. (2010) Influence of *Origanum vulgare* L. essential oil on enterotoxin production, membrane permeability and surface characteristics of *Staphylococcus aureus*. Int J Food Microbiol. 137: 308-311.

Dorman, H. J.D., Deans, S.G. (2000) Antimicrobial agents from plants: antibacterial activity of plant volatile oils. J Appl Microbiol. 88: 308–316.

Dutra, R. C., Campos, M.M., Santos, A.R.S., Calixto J.B. (2016) Medicinal plants in Brazil: Pharmacological studies, drug discovery, challenges and perspectives. Pharmacol Res. 112: 4-29.

Farahnik, B., Murase, J.E. (2016) Antibiotic safety considerations in methicillin-resistant *Staphylococcus aureus* postpartum mastitis. J Am Acad Dermatol. 75: 140-149.

Fratini, F., Mancini, S., Turchi, B., Friscia, E.,

Pistelli, L., Giusti, G., Cerri, D. (2017) A novel interpretation of the Fractional Inhibitory Concentration Index: The case *Origanum vulgare* L. and *Leptospermum scoparium* J. R. et G. Forst essential oils against *Staphylococcus aureus* strains. Microbiol Res. 195: 11-17.

Fu, Y., Zu, Y., Chen, L., Shi, X., Wang, Z., Sun, S., Efferth, T. (2007) Antimicrobial activity of clove and rosemary essential oils alone and in combination. Phytother Res. 21: 989-994.

Herbert, S., Barry, P., Novick, R.P. (2001) Subinhibitory clindamycin differentially inhibits transcription of exoprotein genes in *Staphylococcus aureus*. Infect Immun. 69: 2996–3003.

Juven, B.J., Kanner, J., Sched, F., Weisslowicz, H. (1994) Factors that interact with the antibacterial of thyme essential oil and its active constituents. J Appl Microbiol. 76: 626-631.

Khaleque, M.A., Keya, C.A., Hasan, K.N., Hoque, M.M., Inatsu, Y., Bari, M.L. (2016) Use of cloves and cinnamon essential oil to inactivate *Listeria monocytogenes* in ground beef at freezing and refrigeration temperatures. LWT - Food Sci Technol. 74: 219-223.

Knowles, J.R., Roller, S., Murray, D.B., Naidu, A. (2005) Antimicrobial action of carvacrol at different stages of dual-species biofilm development by *Staphylococcus aureus* and *Salmonella* enteric serovar typhimurium. Appl Environ Microbiol. 7: 797-803.

Kuroda, H., Kuroda, M., Cui, L., Hiramatsu, K. (2007) Subinhibitory concentrations of beta-lactam induce haemolytic activity in *Staphylococcus aureus* through the SaeRS two-component system. FEMS Microbiol Lett. 268: 98–105.

Kwon, S.J., Chang, Y., Han, J. (2017) Oregano essential oil-based natural antimicrobial packaging film to inactivate *Salmonella enterica* and yeasts/molds in the atmosphere surrounding cherry tomatoes. Food Microbio. 65: 114-121.

Lambert, R.J.W., Skandamis, P.N., Coote. P.J., Nychas, G.J.E. (2001) A study of the minimum inhibitory concentration and mode of action of oregano essential oil, thymol and carvacrol. J Appl Microbiol. 91: 453–462.

Li, Y., Xu, C., Zhang, Q., Liu, J.Y., Tan, R.X. (2005) In vitro anti-Helicobacter pylori action of 30 Chinese herbal medicines used to treat ulcer diseases. J Ethnopharmacol. 98: 329-333.

Lopez, P., Sanchez, C., Batlle, R., Nerin, C. (2005) Solid- and Vapor-phase antimicrobial activities of six essential oils: susceptibility of selected food borne bacterial and fungal strains. J Agric Food Chem. 53: 6939-6946.

Mann, C.M., Markham, J.L. (1998) A new method for determining the minimum inhibitory concentration of essential oils. J Appl Microbiol. 84: 538–544.

Mektrirat, R., Janngeon, K., Pikulkaew, S., Okonogi, S. (2016) Evaluation of cytotoxic and inflammatory properties of clove oil microemulsion in mice. Asian J Pharm Sci. 11: 231-232

Misaghi, A., Basti, A.A. (2007) Effects of *Zataria multiflora* Boiss. essential oil and nisin on *Bacillus cereus* ATCC 11778. Food Control. 18: 1043–1049.

Miyazawa, M., Hisama, M. (2003) Antimutagenic activity of phenylpropanoides from clove (*Syzygium aromaticum*). J Agric Food Chem. 51: 6413-6422.

Moosavy, M.H., Basti, A.A., Misaghi, A., Salehi, T.Z., Abbasifar, R., Mousavi, H.A.E., Alipour, M., Razavi, N.E., Gandomi, H., Noori, N. (2008) Effect of *Zataria multiflora* Boiss. essential oil and nisin on *Salmonella typhimurium* and *Staphylococcus aureus* in a food model system and on the bacterial cell membranes. Food Res Int. 41: 1050–1057.

Mulla, M., Ahmed, J., Al-Attar, H., Castro-Aguirre, E., Arfat, Y.A., Auras, R. (2017) Antimicrobial efficacy of clove essential oil infused into chemically modified LLDPE film for chicken meat packaging. Food Control. 73: 663-671.

Nazer, A.I., Kobilinsky, A., Tholozan, J.L., Dubois-Brissonnet, F. (2005) Combinations of food antimicrobials at low levels to inhibit the growth of *Salmonella sv. typhimurium*: a synergistic effect. Food Microbiol. 22: 391-398.

NCCLS (National Committee for Clinical Laboratory Standards). (2000) Methods for Dilution Antimicrobial Susceptibility Tests for Bacteria that Grow Aerobically. Approved Standard, M7-A5.

Nostro, A., Sudano Roccaro, A., Bisignano, G., Marino, M., Cannatelli, M. A., Pizzimenti, F.C., Cioni, P.L., Procopio, F., Blanco, A.R. (2006) Effects of oregano, carvacrol and thymol on *Staphylococcus aureus* and Staphylococcus epidermidis biofilms. J Med Microbiol. 56: 519-523.

Omoe, K., Ishikawa, M., Shimoda, Y., Hu, D.L., Ueda, S., Shinagawa, K. (2002) Detection of seg, seh, and sei genes in *Staphylococcus aureus* isolates and determination of the enterotoxin productivities of *S. aureus* isolates Harboring seg, seh, or sei genes. J Clin Microbiol. 40: 857–62.

Oussalah, M., Caillet, S., Saucier, L., Lacroix, M. (2007) Inhibitory effects of selected plant essential oils on the growth of four pathogenic bacteria: *E. coli* O157:H7, *Salmonella typhimurium*, *Staphylococcus aureus* and *Listeria monocytogenes*. Food Control. 18: 414-420.

Palmer, A., Stewart, J., Fyfe, L. (2004) Influence of subinhibitory concentrations of plant essential oils on the production of enterotoxins A and B and alpha-toxin by *Staphylococcus aureus*. J Medi Microbiol. 53: 1023–1027.

Parsaeimehr, M., Akhondzadeh Basti, A., Rad-mehr, B., Misaghi, A., Abbasifar, A., Karim, G., Rokni, N., Sobhani Motlagh, M., Gandomi, H., Noori, N., Khanjari, A. (2010) Effect of Z. multiflora Boiss. essential oil, nisin, and their combination on the production of enterotoxin C and a-hemolysin by *Staphylococcus aureus*. Foodborne Pathog Dis. 7: 456-463.

Qiu, J., Wang, D., Xiang, H., Feng, H., Xia, L., Jiang, Y., Xia, L., Dong, J., Lu, J., Lu, Y., Deng, X. (2010) Subinhibitory concentrations of thymol reduce enterotoxins A and B and a-Hemolysin production in *Staphylococcus aureus* isolates. Plos ONE. 5: 9736-9742.

Shah, S., Stapleton, P.D., Taylor, P.W. (2008) The polyphenol (2)-epicatechin gallate disrupts the secretion of virulence-related proteins by *Staphylococcus aureus*. Lett Appl Microbiol. 46: 181–185.

Srivastava, K.C., Malhotra, N. (1991) Acetyl euginol, a component of oil of cloves (*Syzygium aromaticum* L.) inhibits aggregation and alters arachidonic acid metabolism in human blood platelets. Prostaglandins Leukot Essent Fatty Acids. 42: 73-81.

Ultee, A., Bennik, M. H., Moezelaar, R. (2002) The phenolic hydroxyl group of carvacrol is essential for action against the food-borne pathogen *Bacillus cereus*. Appl Environ Microbiol. 68: 1561–1568.

Valero, M., Frances, E. (2006) Synergistic bactericidal effect of carvacrol, cinnamaldehyde or thymol and refrigeration to inhibit *Bacillus cereus* in carrot broth. Food Microbiol. 23: 68-73.

Xiang, H., Zhang, L., Yang, Z., Chen, F., Zheng, X., Liu, X. (2017) Chemical compositions, antioxidative, antimicrobial, anti-inflammatory and antitumor activities of *Curcuma aromatica* Salisb. essential oils. Indl Crop Prod. 108: 6-16.

Yang, Y.C., Lee, S.H., Lee, W.J., Choi, D.H., Ahn, Y.J. (2003) Ovicidal and adulticidal effects of *Eugenia cryophyllata* bud and leaf oil compounds on Pediculus capitis. J Agri Food Chem. 51: 4884-4888.

Zhao, X., Wang, J., Zhu, L., Ge, W., Wang, J. (2017) Environmental analysis of typical antibiotic-resistant bacteria and ARGs in farmland soil chronically fertilized with chicken manure. Sci Total Environ. 593–594: 10-17.

25

Genetic variation among *Escherichia coli* isolates from human and calves by using RAPD PCR

Afshari, A.[1], Rad, M.[1*], Seifi, H.A.[2], Ghazvini, K.[3]

[1]*Department of Pathobiology, School of Veterinary Medicine, Ferdowsi University of Mashhad, Mashhad, Iran*

[2]*Center of Excellence in Ruminant Abortion and Neonatal Mortality and Department of Clinical Sciences, School of Veterinary Medicine, Ferdowsi Unversity of Mashhad, Mashhad, Iran*

[3]*Antimicrobial Resistance Research Center, Faculty of Medicine, Mashhad University of Medical Sciences, Mashhad, Iran*

Key words:

E. coli, genetic variation, RAPD-PCR

Correspondence

Rad, M.
Department of Pathobiology,
School of Veterinary Medicine,
Ferdowsi University of Mashhad, Mashhad, Iran

Email: rad@um.ac.ir

Abstract:

BACKGROUND: Various strains of *Escherichia coli* (*E. coli*) are known as major causes of intestinal and extraintestinal infections in humans and various animal species. Molecular methods are important for the identification of bacterial isolates and nucleotide sequence variations, as well as information on tracking bacterial agents related to the outbreaks, the frequency of the bacterial genetic structure, and the evolution of microbial populations. **OBJECTIVES:** The purpose of the present study was to evaluate the efficiency of the RAPD method to differentiate *E. coli* strains. **METHODS:** In this study, 110 isolates of *E. coli* were analyzed by the RAPD PCR method using two 10bp oligonucleotides. These strains were isolated from humans with urinary tract infections and neonatal calves affected by diarrhea or septicemia. **RESULTS:** Data analysis showed that 87.5% of human *E. coli* isolates were correctly classified in the human host group, while 94.3% of calf *E. coli* isolates were correctly placed in calf groups. It also demonstrated that 100% and 93.3% of isolates were accurately assigned to diarrheic and septicemic calf groups, respectively. **CONCLUSIONS:** Genetic variation analysis indicated that the percentage of polymorphism among *E. coli* isolates from humans with urinary tract infections, diarrheic calves, and septicemic neonatal calves were 54.71%, 61.22%, and 62.5%, respectively.

Introduction

Different strains of *Escherichia coli* (*E. coli*) are known as important agents in intestinal and extraintestinal infections in humans and various animal species. Clinical infections in young animals may be confined to the intestines (intestinal colibacillosis and diarrhea), or may occur as septicemia (colisepticemia and general colibacillosis) or as toxemia (toxemic colibacilli) (Rostamzad et al., 2010). This organism is also a major cause of community-acquired urinary tract infections (Zalewska'Piatek, 2011).

Many methods are used for the identification of *E. coli* isolates. Bacteriological and serological methods are not sensitive enough for distinguishing bacterial isolates (Anand, 2001). Molecular methods are important for the identification of bacterial strains and nucleotide sequence variations, as well as information on tracking the outbreaks, genetic structure, and evolution of microbial populations. However, these methods can help to differentiate strains that are specific to certain hosts. Moreover, they are useful guides for epidemiological studies in identifying the source of infection and the mode of disease transmission.

RAPD-PCR is one of the molecular techniques in which single oligonucleotides with arbitrary sequences are used for the synthesis of DNA. The strain-specific DNA fragments were amplified which require no prior knowledge of the nucleotide sequence of the target DNA. Since this method is PCR-based, small amounts of DNA (even at nanograms) are sufficient (Shehata, 2008). This method was successfully used for typing bacteria such as *Camphylobacte rjejuni* (Owen and Hernandez, 1993), *Listeria monocytogenes* (Mazurier and Wernars, 1992), and *Pseudomonas fragi* (Tanaka et al., 1993). Several studies were performed for typing *E. coli* strains by using RAPD PCR. In all of these studies, RAPD PCR was evaluated as an effective and important method in epidemiological surveys (Wang et al., 1993; Bando et al., 1998; Carvalho et al., 2007; Al-Darahi et al., 2008; Maityand Guru, 2008).

In the present study, the genetic diversity and clonal relationships of 110 isolates of *E. coli* from calves with septicemia and diarrhea along with humans with urinary tract infection were evaluated using the RAPD-PCR technique.

Materials and Methods

Bacteria: In this study, a total of 110 isolates of *E. coli*, including 40 human isolates from urinary tract infections, 40 isolates from diarrheic calves, and 30 isolates from septicemic calves, were used. Human isolates were collected from several medical diagnostic lab-

oratories in Mashhad, Iran, during the summer and autumn of 2010. Septicemic and diarrheic calf isolates were collected from commercial dairy farms around Mashhad, Iran, in the summer of 2010. The isolates were confirmed as *E. coli* by using standard biochemical methods, and they were kept in nutrient broth with 15 % glycerol at -20 °C.

RAPD PCR: The random amplified polymorphic DNA fingerprinting method was used to differentiate *E. coli* isolates. Two primers with the size of 10 bp, OPAC 7 (GTGGCCGATG), and OPAC 11 (CCTGGGTCAG) were used (Gomes et al., 2005).

Extraction of DNA: DNA was extracted from the isolates using a commercial DNA extraction kit (Bioneer, South Korea).

Amplification of DNA: Amplification of bacterial DNA was performed using premix PCR kit (20 µl volumes) (Bioneer, Southern Korea). Every reaction contained 1 µl of oligonucleotide primer, 6 µl of the DNA template, and 13 µl of deionized distilled water. The PCR condition was carried out as follows: 94°C for 3 minutes for initial denaturation, followed by 45 cycles of 94°C for 1 minute, 40°C for 1 minute, and 72°C for 2 minutes, plus a final extension of 72°C for 7 minutes.

Gel electrophoresis: The amplified products were visualized by standard gel electrophoresis on 1.5% agarose gel in TAE buffer (89 mMTris, 89 mM glacial Acetic acid, 0.5 M EDTA) containing 1 µg ml-1ethidium bromide for 45 min at 100 V.

A 100 bp DNA ladder molecular weight marker (Fermentas, UK) was included in each electrophoretic run to allow the identification of the amplified products. PCR products were visualized under UV illumination and catalogued with a gel documentation system.

Interpretation of PCR fingerprint images: Scanned images were analyzed using the Photocap software. Bands were assigned on a presence-absence basis. The software estimated band sizes for RAPD PCR data.

Statistical analysis: The data were analyzed using the SPSS software, version 16. Because the data were binary, the Jaccard distance matrix and Ward's hierarchical cluster technique were used. Isolates were clustered and displayed in the Dendrogram form. On the other hand, for differentiating isolates on the basis of host and the kind of infection, the discriminant method was applied, using the SPSS software, version16.

Results

A total of 28 bands were produced by primer OPAC7 among human isolates with sizes ranging from 350 to 3000 bp. Bands with the sizes of 900 and 650bp were repeated 16 and 15 times, respectively (Fig. 1). The electrophoresis of PCR products with primer OPAC11 among human strains revealed 26 bands with the sizes of 500 to 3000bp. Band 900bp was repeated 16 times.

The electrophoresis of PCR products with primer OPAC7 and OPAC11 for diarrheic calf isolates showed 22 and 24 bands, respectively. Band sizes ranged from 350 to 3000bp. A typical band with the size of 1000bp was repeated 19 times with primer OPAC7 (Fig. 2), and the typical bands with the sizes of 2000bp and 500bp were repeated 18 and 17 times, respectively. The electrophoresis of PCR products with primer OPAC7 for isolates from septicemic calves showed 28 bands with the sizes of 500 to 3000bp (Fig. 3). Band 900bp with 17 repeats was the typical band. A total of 20 bands by primer 2 with sizes ranging from 450 to 3000bp were produced among septicemic isolates. Typical bands with the sizes of 2300bp and 900bp were repeated 22 and 24 times, respectively. All *E. coli* isolates were grouped into 5 major groups, A, B, C, D, and E (Fig. 4). Group A included 50% of septicemic isolates from calves and 50% of isolates from urinary tract infections (UTI). Group B included 85 isolates from diarrheic calves and

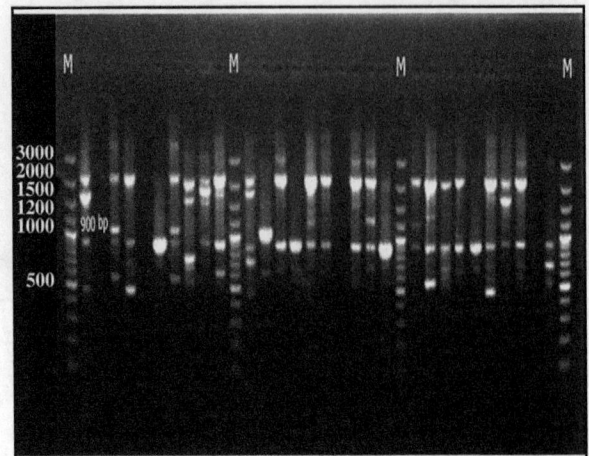

Figure 1. RAPD patterns of *E. coli* isolates from human using primer OPAC7. M: Marker 100 bp plus (Fermentas).

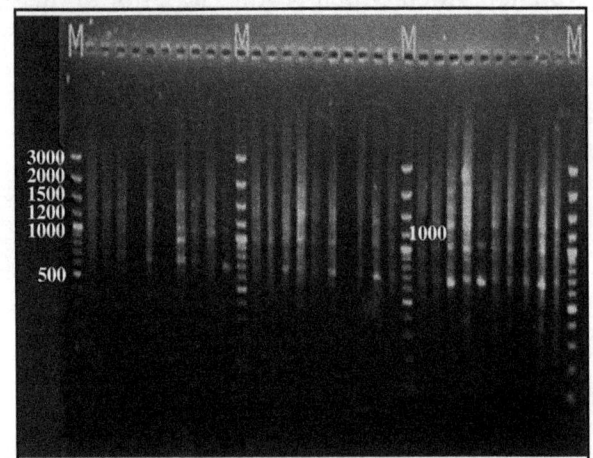

Figure 2. RAPD patterns of *E. coli* isolates from from diarrheic calves using primer OPAC7. M: Marker 100 bp plus (Fermentas).

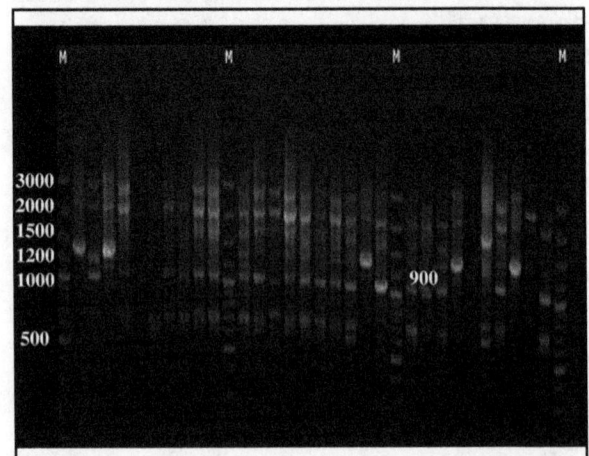

Figure 3. RAPD patterns of E. coli isolates from septicemic calves using primer OPAC11. M: Marker 100 bp plus (Fermentas).

15% of isolates from septicemic calves. Group C contained 5.5% of isolates of UTI samples and 4.44% of isolates from diarrheic calves.

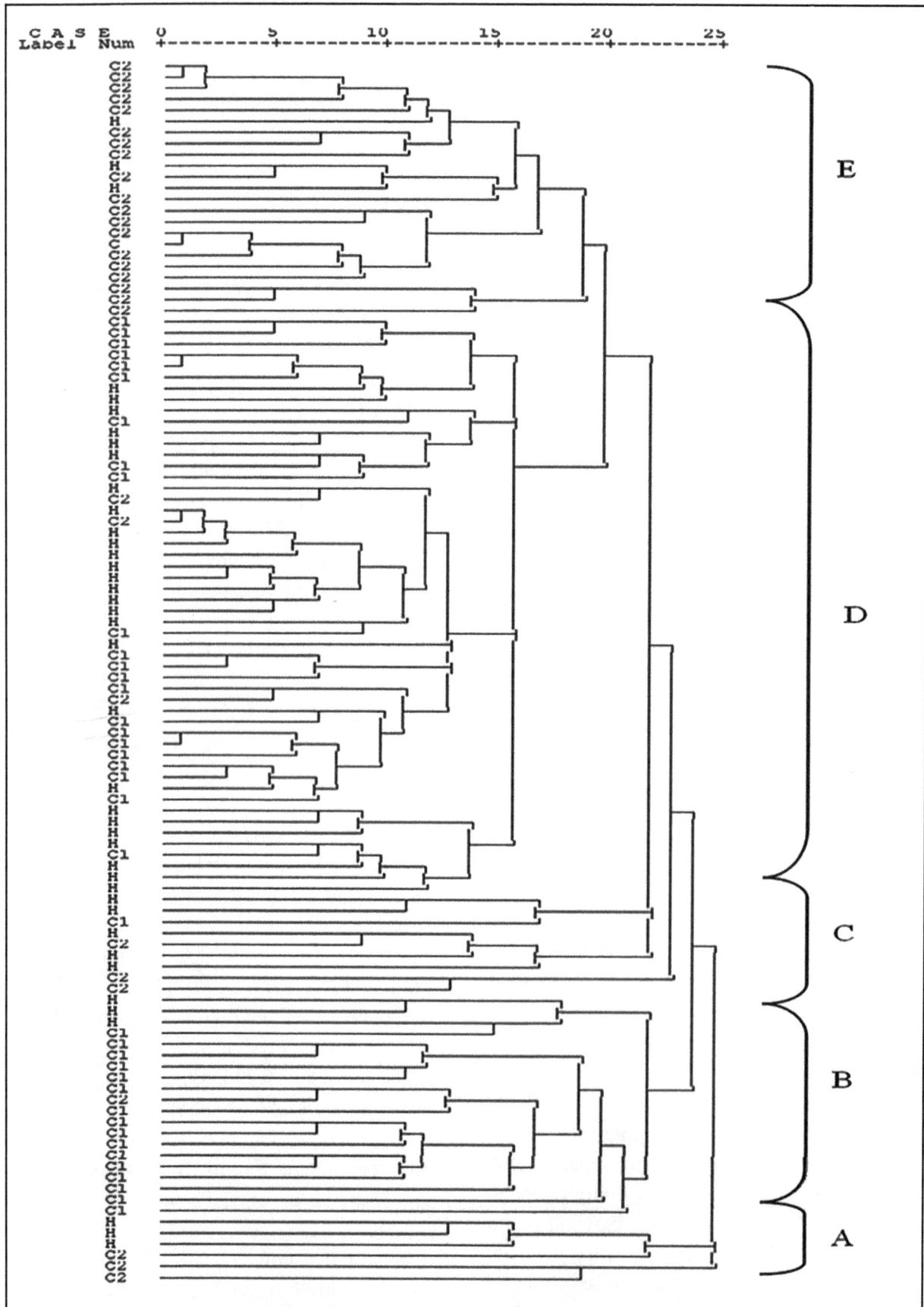

Figure 4. Dendrogram based on two RAPD primers (OPAC7 and OPAC11). H: human isolates, C1 : diarrheaic calves isolates, C2: septicaemic calves isolates.

Group D comprised of 50% of isolates from UTI, 3.42% of isolates from diarrheic calves, and 7.5% of isolates from septicemic calves. Group E contained 9.86% of isolates from septicemic calves, 6.8% of isolates from UTI, and 3.4% of isolates from diarrheic calves.

The results showed that there were clonal relationships among *E. coli* from different sources. On the other hand, genetic variation was clear among the isolates from each source.

Discriminant analysis of the results showed that *E. coli* isolates were significantly different based on the host. However, isolates from diarrheic and septicemic calves can correctly be differentiated. Isolates from diarrheic and septicemic calves were significantly placed with 100% and 93.3% accuracy in their own groups, respectively. Additionally, based on these results, human isolates were significantly classified with the accuracy of 87.5% in their own group. However, 94.3% of the isolates from calves were significantly assigned in their own group.

Discussion

E. coli is a normal flora in the digestive tract of animals. However, some pathogenic strains can cause severe disease in humans (Griffin and Tauxe, 1991). Cattle are the main reservoir of *E. coli*, with different prevalence ranges (Hancock et al., 1997). *E. coli* is an indicator organism for the fecal contamination of water. Some strains of *E. coli* known as O157: H7 can contaminate drinking water and can lead to disease outbreaks (Leung et al., 2004). Following the outbreak of the disease caused by this organism in 1982, in many countries, including America, Britain, and Japan, E coli infections were considered as a public health threat (Lih-Ching et al., 2001). Several major diseases, including urinary tract infection, septicemia, meningitis, and diarrhea were caused by E coli. Therefore, methods of microbial source tracking have drawn attention to themselves. Several methods are designed to classify the strains of E.coli. The evaluation of classification systems in epidemiological studies were based on important criteria, including the differential ability of the technique, typeability, and repeatability. Several methods based on phenotype and genotype are designed to differentiate *E. coli* strains (Tenover, 1997). Phenotypic methods like serotyping and phage typing have little discriminating power. Thus, genotypic methods with high discriminating power, low cost, and quick and easy usage had to be utilized for the classification of *E. coli* isolates (Rostamzad et al., 2010).

Recently, many methods have been applied for microbial source tracking. Methods such as ribotyping (Rodtong and Tannock, 1993), ERIC PCR (Parabhu et al., 2010), RAPD PCR (Gomes et al., 2005; Nowrouzian et al., 2001), and RFLP (Kamerbeek et al., 1997) were successfully applied for the differentiation of different bacterial strains. One of the most widely used methods, especially for the differentiation of *E. coli*, is RAPD-PCR. In this study, RAPD PCR was used to differentiate strains of *E. coli* based on the host and also the kind of infection.

A study on the differentiation of E.coli strains isolated from humans and animals was carried out using RAPD-PCR by Tseng et al. (2001). They reported the RAPD-PCR technique as a sensitive method for the fingerprinting of E.coli strains (Tseng et al., 2001). The genetic and molecular characterizations of pathogenic *E. coli* in laboratory rodent species were analyzed effectively using RAPD PCR (MaityandGuru, 2007). In the study of Carvalho et al. (2007), a clonal relationship was shown between the enteropathogenic *E. coli* isolates from human and primates using RAPD-PCR (Carvalho et al., 2007).

This study showed that this method has a relatively high power for differentiating *E. coli* strains. The isolates were divided into five groups. Most of the isolates in each group had

a common source. In many epidemiological studies, RAPD PCR was used to trace the origin. RAPD-PCR was also used for the molecular typing of other bacteria such as Shigella, *Staphylococcus aureus*, and *Pasteurella multocida* (RostamZad et al., 2010; Shehata, 2008; Ozbey et al., 2004). In our study, *E. coli* isolates were divided into 5 major groups based on 35 pleomorphic bands, using two different primers.

In a similar study, RAPD PCR was effectively used for the differentiation of *E. coli* strains from human and animal origin (Tseng et al., 2001). The results of the present study showed that *E. coli* isolates from humans and calves with the correct rates of 87.5% and 94.3% were classified in their own groups, respectively. On the other hand, our results showed that RAPD PCR was able to differentiate *E. coli* isolates from diarrheic and septicemic calves with the correct rates of 100% and 93.3%. The selection of suitable primers for RAPD PCR is an important aspect. In this study, we used two primers which were already used in other studies. However, using several primers for typing by RAPD PCR can increase the typeability of the method. The results of several other studies have proved the greater effectiveness of RAPD PCR in comparison to other molecular typing methods (Wang et al., 1993; Leung et al., 2004; ZahraeiSalehi et al., 2008; Saxena et al., 2014).

In this study, there were genetic variations among *E. coli* isolates from each source. This may be due to different origins, occurrence of mutations, and horizontal gene transmission. On the other hand, because of the difference of intestinal tract conditions among different species, the clonal relationship of *E. coli* isolates in specific hosts can be considered.

Conclusion: RAPD PCR was used to differentiate the isolates of *E. coli* based on the host and kind of infection. *E. coli* isolates from humans and calves with the correct rates of 87.5% and 94.3% were classified in their own

groups, respectively. In addition, our results showed that RAPD PCR was able to differentiate *E. coli* isolates from diarrheic and septicemic calves with the correct rates of 100% and 93.3%, respectively.

Acknowledgments

This project was supported by the research grant (grant no. 1170) of the Ferdowsi University of Mashhad. The authors wish to thank Dr. Abbas Bahari and Mrs. Gholamhosseini Moghadam for their technical assistance.

References

1. Al-Darahi, K.F., KhalidMahdi, L., Al-Naib, K.T., Jubreal, J. (2008) Molecular characterization of *E. coli* O157:H7 strains using Random Amplified Polymorphic DNA (RAPD). J Doh Uni. 11: 198-204.

2. Anand, N.N., Bukanov, T.U., Westblum, S. Kresovich., Berg, D.E. (2001) DNA diversity among clinical isolates of *Helicobacter pylori* detected by PCR based RAPD fingerprinting. Nucleic Acids Res. 20: 5137-5142.

3. Bando, S.Y., do Valle, G.R., Martinez, M.B., Trabulsi, L.R., Moreira-Filho, C.A. (1998) Characterization of entero invasive *Escherichia coli* and Shigella strains by RAPD analysis. FEMS Microbiol Lett. 165: 159-65.

4. Carvalho, V.M., Irino, K., Onuma, D., Pestana de Castro, A.F. (2007) Random amplification of polymorphic DNA reveals clonal relationships among enteropathogenic *Escherichia coli* isolated from non-human primates and humans. Braz J Med Res. 40: 237-24.

5. Gomes, A.R., Muniyappa, L., Krishnappa, G., Suryanarayana, V.V.S., Isioor, S., Prakash, B., and Hugar, P.G. (2005) Genotypic characterization of avian *Escherichia coli* by random amplification of polymorphic DNA. Int J Poult Sci. 4: 378-381.

6. Griffin, P.M., Tauxe, R.V. (1991) The epide-

miology of infections caused by *Escherichia coli* O157:H7, other enterohemorrhagic *E. coli*, and the associated hemolytic uremic syndrome. Epidemiol Rev. 13: 60-98.

7. Hancock, D.D., Rice, D.H., Thomas, L.A., Dargatz, D.A., Besser, T.E. (1997) Epidemiology of *Escherichia coli* O157 in feedlot cattle. J Food Prot. 4: 462-604.

8. Kamerbeek, J., Schouls, L., Kolk, A., van Agterveld, M., van Soolingen, D., Kuijper, S., Bunschoten, A., Molhuizen, H., Shaw, R., Goyal, M., van Embden, J. (1997) Simultaneous detection and strain differentiation of *Mycobacterium tuberculosis* for diagnosis and epidemiology. J Clin Microbiol. 35: 907-914.

9. Leung, K.T., Mackereth, R., Tien, Y.C., Topp, E. (2004) A comparison of AFLP and ERIC-PCR analyses for discriminating *Escherichia coli* from cattle, pig, and human sources. FEMS Microbiol Ecol. 47: 111-119.

10. Lih-Ching, CH., Wey-Huey, SH., Chih, D. (2001) Characterization of *Escherichia coli* serotype O157 strains isolated in taiwan by PCR and multilocus enzyme analysis. J Food Drug Anal. 9: 12-19.

11. Maity, B., Guru, P.Y. (2007) Genetic diversity and molecular characterization of pathogenic *Escherichia coli* from different species of laboratory rodents. Indian J Biotechnol. 6: 210-215.

12. Mazurier, J., Wernars, T. (1992) Molecular epidemiological study of a mass outbreak caused by enteropathogenic *Escherichia coli* O157:H45. J Microbiol Immunol. 43: 381-4

13. Nowrouzian, F., Wold, A.E., Adlerberth, I. (2001) Computer-based analysis of RAPD (Random Amplified Polymorhic DNA finger-prints for typing of intestinal *Eschericia coli*. Mol Biol Today. 2: 5-10.

14. Ozbey, G., Kilic, A., Ertas, H.B., Muz, A. (2004) Random amplified polymorphic DNA (RAPD) analysis of *Pasteurella multocida* and Manheimia haemolytica strains isolated from cattle, sheep and goats. Vet Med Czech. 49: 65-69.

15. Owen, R.J., Hernandez, T.H. (1993) Chromosomal DNA fingerprinting- a new method ofspecies and identification applicable to microbial pathogens. J Med Microbiol. 30: 89-90.

16. Parabhu, V., Isloor, S., Balu, M., Suryanarayana, V.V., Rathnamma, D. (2010) Genotyping by Eric PCR of *Escherichia coli* isolated from bovine mastitis cases. Indian J Biotechnol. 9: 298-301.

17. Rodtong, S.,Tannock, G.W. (1993) Differentiation of Lactobacillus strains by ribotyping. Appl Environ Microbiol. 59: 3480-3484.

18. RostamZad, A., Zarkesh Esfahani, H., Enteshari, J. (2010) The investigation of molecular epidemiology of *Shigella soneii* isolated from clinical cases in Tehran using RAPD-PCR method. Sci Med J. 9: 279-289.

19. Saxena, S., Verma, J., Shikha., Mod, D.R. (2014) RAPD-PCR and 16S rDNA phylogenetic analysis of alkaline protease producing bacteria isolated from soil of India: Identification and detection of genetic variability. J Genet Engineer Biotechnol. 12: 27-35.

20. Shehata, A.I. (2008) Phylogenetic diversity of *Staphylococcus aureus* by random amplification of polymorphic DNA. Aust J Basic Appl Sci. 2: 858-863.

21. Tanaka, N.F., MacRae, M., Johnston, M., Mooney, J., Ogden, I.D. (1993) Optimizing enrichment conditions for the isolation of *Escherichia coli* O157 in soils by immunomagnetic separation. Lett Appl Microbiol. 34: 365-369.

22. Tenover, F., Arbeit, R., Goering, R. (1997) How to select and interpret molecular strain typing methods for epidemiological studies of bacterial infections: A review for healthcare epidemiologists. Infect Control Hosp Epidemiol. 18: 426-439.

23. Tseng, C., Ting, E., Johnson, D., Saluta, M., Dunst, R. (2001) RAPD fingerprinting as a potential means for differentiating human and animal *E. coli*. Life Sci News. 7: 10-11.

24. Wang G., Whittam, T.S., Berg, C.M., Berg, D.E. (1993) Rapd (arbitarary primer) PCR is more sensitive than multilocus enzyme elec-

trophoresis for distinguishing related bacterial strains. Nucleic Acid Res. 21: 5930-5933.

25. Zahraei Salehi, T., Madani, S.A., Karimi, V., Arab Khazaeli, F. (2008) Molecular genetic differentiation of avian *Escherichia coli* by RAPD-PCR. Brac J Microbiol. 39: 494-497.

26. Zalewska 'Piatek, B.M. (2011) Urinary tract infections of *Escherichia coli* strains of chaperone-usher system. Pol J Microbiol. 60: 279-285.

Permissions

List of Contributors

Jabbari, A. R. and Azizian, Kh.
Department of Anaerobic Bacterial Vaccines Research and Production, Razi vaccine and Serum Research Institute, Agricultural Research Education and Extension Organization (AREEO), Karaj, Iran

Esmaelizad, M.
Department of Biotechnology, Razi Vaccine and Serum Research Institute, Agricultural Research Education and Extension Organization (AREEO), Karaj, Iran

Mahboubi, M.
Department of Microbiology, Biology Center, Medicinal Plant Center of Barij, Kashan, Iran

Falsafi, T.
Department of Biology, Faculty of Basic Sciences, Alzahra University, Vanak, Tehran, Iran

Torabi Goodarzi, M.
Razi Vaccine & Serum Research Institute (Central Area branch), Arak, Iran

Eftekharian, S., Ghorbanpoor, M. and Seyfi Abad Shapouri, M. R.
Department of Pathobiology, Faculty of Veterinary Medicine, Shahid Chamran University of Ahvaz, Ahvaz, Iran

Ghanbarpour, R.
Molecular Microbiology Research Group, Faculty of Veterinary Medicine, Shahid Bahonar University, Kerman, Iran

Jafari, R.
Department of Clinical Sciences, Faculty of Veterinary Medicine, Shahid Chamran University of Ahvaz, Ahvaz, Iran

Amani, A.
DVSc (Poultry Diseases) Graduate, Faculty of Veterinary Medicine, Shahid Chamran University of Ahvaz, Ahvaz, Iran

Sharifzadeh, A., Khosravi, A. R. and Balal, A.
Mycology Research Center, Faculty of Veterinary Medicine, University of Tehran, Tehran, Iran

Shokri, H.
Department of Pathobiology, Faculty of Veterinary Medicine, Amol University of Special Modern Technologies, Amol, Iran

Arabkhazaeli, F.
Department of Parasitology, Faculty of Veterinary Medicine, University of Tehran, Tehran, Iran

Soltani, M., Moghimi, S. M. and Ebrahimzade Mousavi, H.
Department of Aquatic Animal Health, Faculty of Veterinary Medicine, University of Tehran, Tehran, Iran

Abdi, K.
Aquatic Animal Health Expert, Office of Health and Control of Aquatic Animal Diseases, Iranian Veterinary Organization, Tehran, Iran

Soltani, E.
Department of Microbiology, Faculty of Science, University of Tehran, Tehran, Iran

Ghasemi B.
Gratuated from the Faculty of Veterinary Medicine, University of Zabol, Zabol, Iran

Najimi, M.
Department of Pathobiology, Faculty of Veterinary Medicine, University of Zabol, Zabol, Iran

Dastmalchi Saei, H.
Department of Microbiology, Faculty of Veterinary Medicine, Urmia University, Urmia, Iran

Javadi, S.
Department of Clinical Sciences, Faculty of Veterinary Medicine, Urmia University, Urmia, Iran

Akbari, S., Hadian, N. and Zarza, E.
Graduated from the Faculty of Veterinary Medicine, Urmia University, Urmia, Iran

Shokri, H.
Department of Pathobiology, Faculty of Veterinary Medicine, Amol University of Special Modern Technologies, Amol, Iran

Sharifzadeh, A. and Khosravi, A. R.
Mycology Research Center, Faculty of Veterinary Medicine, University of Tehran, Tehran, Iran

Jahani, Z., Meshgi, B. and Amininia, N.
Department of Parasitology, Faculty of Veterinary Medicine, University of Tehran, Tehran-Iran (Center of Excellent of Ecosystem and Ultrastructural Changes of Helminthes)

Jamshidi, A. and Fallah, N.
Department of Food Hygiene, Faculty of Veterinary Medicine, Ferdowsi University of Mashhad, Mashhad, Iran

Razmyar, J.
Department of Clinical Sciences, Faculty of Veterinary Medicine, Ferdowsi University of Mashhad, Mashhad, Iran

Pouramini, A.
Department of Internal Medicine, Faculty of Veterinary Medicine, University of Tehran, Tehran, Iran

Jamshidi, Sh.
Department of Internal Medicine, Faculty of Veterinary Medicine, University of Tehran, Tehran, Iran
Department of Pathology, School of Veterinary Medicine, Shahrekord University, Shahrkord, Iran

Shayan, P. and Ebrahimzadeh, E.
Department of Parasitology, Faculty of Veterinary Medicine, University of Tehran, Tehran, Iran

Namavari, M.
Razi Vaccine and Serum Research Institute, Agricultural Research, Educationanl Extention Organization (AREEO),Shiraz, Iran

Shirian, S.
Shefa Neuroscience Research Center, Khatam-Al-Anbia Hospital, Tehran, Iran

Rezaei, S., Haji Hajikolaei, M. R. and Ghadrdan Mashhadi, A. R.
Department of Clinical Sciences, Faculty of Veterinary Medicine, Shahid Chamran University of Ahvaz, Ahvaz, Iran

Ghorbanpour, M.
Department of Pathobiology, Faculty of Veterinary Medicine, Shahid Chamran University of Ahvaz, Ahvaz, Iran

Abdollahpour, G.
Department of Internal Medicine, Faculty of Veterinary Medicine, University of Tehran, Tehran, Iran

Mokhtari A. and Mahzounieh M.
Department of Pathobiology, Faculty of Veterinary Medicine, University of Shahrekord, Shahrekord, Iran

Frossard J. P.
Department of Virology, Veterinary Laboratories Agency, Addlestone, United Kingdom

Nazemi, K., Ghalyanchi Langeroudi, A. and Ehsan, M.R.
Department of Microbiology and Immunology, Faculty of Veterinary Medicine, University of Tehran, Tehran, Iran

Seger, W.
Department of Microbiology and Immunology, Faculty of Veterinary Medicine, University of Tehran, Tehran, Iran
Department of Pathology and Poultry Diseases, Faculty of Veterinary Medicine, University of Basra, Basra, Iraq

Hashemzadeh, M.
Department of Research and Production of Poultry Viral Vaccine, Razi Vaccine and Serum Research Institute, Karaj, Iran

Karimi, V.
Department of Avian Medicine, Faculty of Veterinary Medicine, University of Tehran, Tehran, Iran

Tatari, Z., Peighamabri, S. M. and Madani, S. A.
Department of Avian Diseases, Faculty of Veterinary Medicine, University of Tehran, Tehran, Iran

Namroodi, S., Rezaie, H. and Milanlou, D.
Department of Environmental Sciences, Faculty of Fisheries and Environmental Sciences, Gorgan University of Agricultural Sciences & Natural Resources, Gorgan, Iran

Rostami, A. and Shahabi, M.
Department of Internal Medicine, Faculty of Veterinary Medicine, University of Tehran, Tehran, Iran

Madani, A.
Department of Poultry Diseases, Faculty of Veterinary Medicine, University of Tehran, Tehran, Iran

Borhani Zarandi, M., Hoseini, S. H., Jalousion, F. and Etebar, F.
Department of Parasitology, Faculty of Veterinary Medicine, Tehran University, Tehran, Iran

Vojgani, M.
Department of Immunology and Biology, School of Medicine, Tehran University of Medical Sciences, Tehran, Iran

Mohebbi, M. R., Lotfollahzadeh, S. and Mokhber Dezfouli, M.
Department of Internal Medicine, Faculty of Veterinary Medicine, University of Tehran, Tehran, Iran

Madadgar, O.
Department of Microbiology, Faculty of Veterinary Medicine, University of Tehran, Tehran, Iran

Jalousian, F., Hosseini, S. H., Fathi, S., Aghaei, S. and Kordafshari, S.
Department of Parasitology, Faculty of Veterinary Medicine, University of Tehran, Tehran, Iran

Shirani, D.
Department of Internal Medicine, Faculty of Veterinary Medicine, University of Tehran, Tehran, Iran

Danehchin, L.
Department of Pathobiology, Faculty of Veterinary Medicine, Ferdowsi University of Mashhad, Mashhad, Iran

Razmi, Gh.
Center of Excellence in Ruminant Abortion and Neonatal Mortality, Faculty of Veterinary Medicine, Ferdowsi University of Mashhad, Mashhad, Iran

Naghibi, A.
Department of Pathobiology, Faculty of Veterinary Medicine, Ferdowsi University of Mashhad, Mashhad, Iran

Rahmani, E.
Graduated from the Faculty of Veterinary Medicine, Karaj Branch, Islamic Azad University, Karaj, Iran

Hosseini, H.
Department of Clinical Sciences, Faculty of Veterinary Medicine, Karaj Branch, Islamic Azad University, Karaj, Iran

Olfaty-Harsini, S., Shokrani, H. and Nayebzadeh, H.
Department of Pathobiology, Faculty of Veterinary Medicine, Lorestan University, Khorramabad, Iran

Azizkhani, M. and Tooryan, F.
Department of Food Hygiene, Faculty of Veterinary Medicine, Amol University of Special Modern Technologies, Amol, Iran

Akhondzadeh Basti, A.
Department of Food Hygiene, Faculty of Veterinary Medicine, University of Tehran, Tehran, Iran

Afshari, A. and Rad, M.
Department of Pathobiology, School of Veterinary Medicine, Ferdowsi University of Mashhad, Mashhad, Iran

Seifi, H. A.
Center of Excellence in Ruminant Abortion and Neonatal Mortality and Department of Clinical Sciences, School of Veterinary Medicine, Ferdowsi Unversity of Mashhad, Mashhad, Iran

Ghazvini, K.
Antimicrobial Resistance Research Center, Faculty of Medicine, Mashhad University of Medical Sciences, Mashhad, Iran

Index